Eosinophilic Gastrointestinal Diseases

Editors

GLENN T. FURUTA
DAN ATKINS

IMMUNOLOGY AND ALLERGY CLINICS OF NORTH AMERICA

www.immunology.theclinics.com

Consulting Editor
ROHIT KATIAL

May 2024 • Volume 44 • Number 2

ELSEVIER

1600 John F. Kennedy Boulevard • Suite 1800 • Philadelphia, Pennsylvania, 19103-2899

http://www.theclinics.com

IMMUNOLOGY AND ALLERGY CLINICS OF NORTH AMERICA Volume 44, Number 2

May 2024 ISSN 0889-8561, ISBN-13: 978-0-443-12903-2

Editor: Taylor Hayes

Developmental Editor: Nitesh Barthwal

Immunology and Allergy Clinics of North America (ISSN 0889–8561) is published quarterly by Elsevier Inc., 360 Park Avenue South, New York, NY 10010-1710. Months of issue are February, May, August, and November. Periodicals postage paid at New York, NY and additional mailing offices. Subscription prices are $375.00 per year for US individuals, $100.00 per year for US students and residents, $458.00 per year for Canadian individuals, $100.00 per year for Canadian students, $484.00 per year for international individuals, $220.00 per year for international students. For institutional access pricing please contact Customer Service via the contact information below. To receive student/resident rate, orders must be accompanied by name of affiliated institution, date of term, and the *signature* of program/residency coordinator on institution letterhead. Orders will be billed at individual rate until proof of status is received. Foreign air speed delivery is included in all *Clinics* subscription prices. All prices are subject to change without notice. **POSTMASTER:** Send address changes to Immunology and Allergy Clinics of North America, Elsevier Health Sciences Division, Subscription Customer Service, 3251 Riverport Lane, Maryland Heights, MO 63043. **Customer Service: 1-800-654-2452 (U.S. and Canada); 314-447-8871 (outside U.S. and Canada). Fax: 314-447-8029. E-mail:journalscustomerservice-usa@elsevier.com (for print support); journalsonlinesupport-usa@elsevier.com (for online support).**

Reprints. For copies of 100 or more, of articles in this publication, please contact the Commercial Reprints Department, Elsevier Inc., 360 Park Avenue South, New York, New York 10010-1710. Tel. 212-633-3874, Fax: 212-633-3820, E-mail: reprints@elsevier.com.

Immunology and Allergy Clinics of North America is covered in MEDLINE/PubMed (Index Medicus), Current Contents/Life Sciences, Science Citation Index, ISI/BIOMED, Chemical Abstracts, and EMBASE/Excerpta Medica.

Contributors

CONSULTING EDITOR

ROHIT KATIAL, MD, FAAAAI, FACAAI, FACP
Professor of Medicine, Associate Vice President of Education, Director, Center for Clinical Immunology, Irene J. & Dr. Abraham E. Goldminz, Chair in Immunology and Respiratory Medicine, Division of Allergy and Clinical Immunology, Department of Medicine, National Jewish Health and University of Colorado, Denver, Colorado, USA

EDITORS

GLENN T. FURUTA, MD
Professor, Department of Pediatrics, Gastroenterology, Hepatology and Nutrition, University of Colorado School of Medicine, Section Head, Pediatric Gastroenterology, Hepatology and Nutrition, Digestive Health Institute; Director, Gastrointestinal Eosinophilic Diseases Program, Children's Hospital Colorado, Aurora, Colorado, USA

DAN ATKINS, MD
Associate Professor, Department of Pediatrics, University of Colorado School of Medicine; Pediatric Allergy and Immunology; Co-Director, Gastrointestinal Eosinophilic Diseases Program, Children's Hospital Colorado, Aurora, Colorado, USA

AUTHORS

SEEMA ACEVES, MD, PhD
Professor, Division of Pediatric Gastroenterology, Department of Pediatrics, University of California, La Jolla, California, USA

NICOLETA C. ARVA, MD, PhD
Pathologist, Department of Pathology, Nationwide Children's Hospital, Columbus, Ohio, USA

DAN ATKINS, MD
Associate Professor, Department of Pediatrics, University of Colorado School of Medicine; Pediatric Allergy and Immunology; Co-Director, Gastrointestinal Eosinophilic Diseases Program, Children's Hospital Colorado, Aurora, Colorado, USA

DOMINIQUE D. BAILEY, MD
Assistant Professor, Division of Pediatric Gastroenterology, Hepatology, and Nutrition, Department of Pediatrics, Columbia University Vagelos College of Physicians and Surgeons/New York-Presbyterian Morgan Stanley Children's Hospital, New York, New York, USA

MAUREEN BAUER, MD
Associate Professor, Department of Pediatric Allergy and Immunology, Gastrointestinal Eosinophilic Diseases Program, Children's Hospital Colorado, University of Colorado School of Medicine, Aurora, Colorado, USA

ANAS BERNIEH, MD
Assistant Professor, Division of Pathology and Laboratory Medicine, Cincinnati Children's Hospital Medical Center, University of Cincinnati College of Medicine, Cincinnati, Ohio, USA

LUC BIEDERMANN, MD
Gastroenterology and Hepatology Specialist, Department of Gastroenterology and Hepatology, University Hospital Zurich, Zurich, Switzerland

ALBERT J. BREDENOORD, MD, PhD
Gastroenterologist, Department of Gastroenterology and Hepatology, Amsterdam UMC, Amsterdam Gastroenterology Endocrinology Metabolism, Amsterdam, the Netherlands

JOY W. CHANG, MD, MS
Assistant Professor, Division of Gastroenterology, Department of Internal Medicine, Ann Arbor, Michigan, USA

MIRNA CHEHADE, MD, MPH
Professor of Pediatrics and Medicine, Founding Director, Mount Sinai Center for Eosinophilic Disorders, Icahn School of Medicine at Mount Sinai, New York, New York, USA

MARGARET H. COLLINS, MD
Professor, Division of Pathology and Laboratory Medicine, ML1035, Cincinnati Children's Hospital Medical Center, Cincinnati, Ohio, USA

EVAN S. DELLON, MD, MPH
Professor, Division of Gastroenterology and Hepatology, Department of Medicine, Center for Esophageal Diseases and Swallowing, University of North Carolina School of Medicine, Chapel Hill, North Carolina, USA

BETHANY DOERFLER, MS, RDN
Clinical Research Dietitian, Department of Gastroenterology and Hepatology, Northwestern Feinberg School of Medicine, Chicago, Illinois, USA

REBECCA J. DOIDGE, MS, CCC-SLP
Speech-Language Pathologist II, Department of Speech Pathology, Children's Hospital Colorado, Aurora, Colorado, USA

JULIA L.M. DUNN, PhD
Assistant Professor, Department of Pediatrics, Section of GI, Hepatology, and Nutrition, University of Colorado School of Medicine, and Digestive Health Institute, Children's Hospital Colorado, Aurora, Colorado, USA

GARY W. FALK, MD, MS
Professor, Division of Gastroenterology and Hepatology, Department of Medicine, Hospital of the University of Pennsylvania, University of Pennsylvania Perelman School of Medicine, Philadelphia, Pennsylvania, USA

NIRMALA GONSALVES, MD, AGAF, FACG
Professor of Medicine, Division of Gastroenterology and Hepatology, Northwestern University-Feinberg School of Medicine, Chicago, Illinois, USA

THOMAS GREUTER, MD
Consultant, Division of Gastroenterology and Hepatology, University Hospital Lausanne - CHUV, Lausanne, Switzerland; Department of Gastroenterology and Hepatology, University Hospital Zurich, Zürich, Switzerland; Department of Internal Medicine, GZO – Zurich Regional Health Center, Wetzikon, Switzerland

MARION GROETCH, MS, RDN
Associate Professor, Department of Pediatric Allergy and Immunology, Icahn School of Medicine at Mount Sinai, New York, New York, USA

SANDEEP K. GUPTA, MD
Professor, Division of Pediatric Gastroenterology, Hepatology and Nutrition, University of Alabama at Birmingham/Children's of Alabama, Birmingham, Alabama, USA

ANGELA M. HAAS, MA, CCC-SLP
Clinical Program Specialist, Department of Speech Pathology, Children's Hospital Colorado, Aurora, Colorado, USA

GIRISH HIREMATH, MD, MPH
Associate Professor, Department of Pediatrics, Monroe Carell Jr. Children's Hospital at Vanderbilt, Vanderbilt University, Nashville, Tennessee, USA

ELIZABETH T. JENSEN, MPH, PhD
Associate Professor, Department of Epidemiology and Prevention, Wake Forest University School of Medicine, Winston-Salem, North Carolina, USA

DAVID KATZKA, MD
Professor, Department of Gastroenterology and Hepatology, Columbia University Medical Center, New York, New York, USA

KANAK V. KENNEDY, MD
Pediatric Gastroenterologist, Division of Pediatric Gastroenterology, Hepatology, and Nutrition, Department of Pediatrics, The Children's Hospital of Philadelphia, Philadelphia, Pennsylvania, USA

PANEEZ KHOURY, MD, MHSc
Senior Clinician, Human Eosinophil Section, National Institute of Allergy and Infectious Diseases, National Institutes of Health, Bethesda, Maryland, USA

CHRIS A. LIACOURAS, MD
Professor, Department of Gastroenterology, Hepatology and Nutrition, Perelman School of Medicine, University of Pennsylvania, Attending Gastroenterologist, The Children's Hospital of Philadelphia, Philadelphia, Pennsylvania, USA

OSCAR LOPEZ-NUNEZ, MD
Staff Pathologist, Division of Pathology and Laboratory Medicine, Cincinnati Children's Hospital Medical Center, University of Cincinnati College of Medicine, Cincinnati, Ohio, USA

ALFREDO LUCENDO, MD, PhD
Head of the Department, Department of Gastroenterology, Hospital General de Tomelloso, Tomelloso, Spain; Centro de Investigación Biomédica en Red de Enfermedades Hepáticas y Digestivas (CIBERehd), Instituto de Investigación Sanitaria de Castilla-La Mancha (IDISCAM), Tomelloso, Ciudad Real, Spain

EMILY CLARKE McGOWAN, MD, PhD
Associate Professor, Division of Allergy and Immunology, Departments of Internal Medicine and Pediatrics, University of Virginia School of Medicine, Charlottesville, Virginia, USA

POOJA MEHTA, MD, MSCS
Assistant Professor, Department of Pediatrics, Children's Hospital Colorado, University of Colorado School of Medicine, Aurora, Colorado, USA

CALIES MENARD-KATCHER, MD
Associate Professor, Departments of Pediatrics, Section of Pediatric Gastroenterology, Hepatology and Nutrition, University of Colorado School of Medicine, Digestive Health Institute, Childrens Hospital Colorado, Anschutz Medical Campus, Aurora, Colorado, USA

AMANDA B. MUIR, MD, MSTR
Assistant Professor, Division of Gastroenterology, Hepatology, and Nutrition, Department of Pediatrics, Children's Hospital of Philadelphia, Perelman School of Medicine, University of Pennsylvania, Abramson Research Center, Philadelphia, Pennsylvania, USA

NATHALIE NGUYEN, MD
Associate Professor, Department of Pediatric Gastroenterology, Hepatology and Nutrition, Gastrointestinal Eosinophilic Diseases Program, Digestive Health Institute, Children's Hospital Colorado, University of Colorado School of Medicine, Aurora, Colorado, USA

SALVATORE OLIVA, MD, PhD
Associate Professor, Department of Maternal and Child Health, Pediatric Gastroenterology and Liver Unit, Sapienza University of Rome, Rome, Italy

ALEXANDRA PAPADOPOULOU, MD
Chief, Division of Gastroenterology and Hepatology, First Department of Pediatrics, University of Athens, Children's Hospital Agia Sophia, Athens, Greece

ROBBIE PESEK, MD
Associate Professor, Division of Allergy and Immunology, Department of Pediatrics, Arkansas Children's Hospital, University of Arkansas for Medical Sciences, Little Rock, Arkansas, USA

KATHRYN PETERSON, MD
Professor of Medicine, Division of Gastroenterology and Hepatology, Department of Internal Medicine, University of Utah, Salt Lake City, Utah, USA

MARIA PLETNEVA, MD, PhD
Associate Professor, Director, Department of Pathology, University of Utah School of Medicine, University of Utah, Salt Lake City, Utah, USA

MELANIE A. RUFFNER, MD, PhD
Assistant Professor, Division of Pediatric Allergy and Immunology, Department of Pediatrics, The Children's Hospital of Philadelphia, Philadelphia, Pennsylvania, USA; Perelman School of Medicine, University of Pennsylvania, Rutledge, Pennsylvania, USA

MARIA A. SACTA, MD, PhD
Allergist/Immunologist, Division of Allergy and Immunology, Children's Hospital of Philadelphia, Philadelphia, Pennsylvania, USA

EKATERINA SAFRONEEVA, PhD
Adjunct Professor, Institute of Social and Preventive Medicine, University of Bern, Bern, Switzerland

ALAIN M. SCHOEPFER, MD, AGAF
Professor of Medicine, Department of Gastroenterology and Hepatology, Centre Hospitalier Universitaire Vaudois and University of Lausanne, Lausanne, Switzerland

LISA A. SPENCER, PhD
Associate Professor, Department of Pediatrics, Section of GI, Hepatology, and Nutrition, University of Colorado School of Medicine, and Digestive Health Institute, Children's Hospital Colorado, Aurora, Colorado, USA

JONATHAN SPERGEL, MD, PhD
Professor and Chief, Division of Allergy and Immunology, Children's Hospital of Philadelphia, Philadelphia, Pennsylvania, USA

ALEX STRAUMANN, MD
Department of Gastroenterology and Hepatology, University Hospital Zurich, Zurich, Switzerland

MARIA L. VAN KLINK, MD
Standard PhD Candidate, Department of Gastroenterology and Hepatology, Amsterdam UMC, Amsterdam Gastroenterology Endocrinology Metabolism, Amsterdam, the Netherlands

JOSHUA B. WECHSLER, MD, MSci
Assistant Professor, Division of Gastroenterology, Hepatology and Nutrition, Simpson-Querrey 10-518, Stanley Manne Children's Research Institute, Ann & Robert H. Lurie Children's Hospital of Chicago, Northwestern University Feinberg School of Medicine Chicago, Chicago, Illinois, USA

BRIDGET E. WILSON, MD
Allergist/Immunologist, Division of Allergy, Asthma and Clinical Immunology, Department of Medicine, Mayo Clinic Arizona, Scottsdale, Arizona, USA; Division of Allergy and Immunology, Phoenix Children's, Phoenix, Arizona, USA

NICOLE WOLFSET, MD
Allergist/Immunologist, Division of Allergy and Immunology, Children's Hospital of Philadelphia, Philadelphia, Pennsylvania, USA

BENJAMIN L. WRIGHT, MD
Associate Professor, Division of Allergy, Asthma and Clinical Immunology, Department of Medicine, Mayo Clinic Arizona, Scottsdale, Arizona, USA; Division of Allergy and Immunology, Phoenix Children's, Phoenix, Arizona, USA

GUANG-YU YANG, MD, PhD
Professor, Department of Pathology, Northwestern University Feinberg School of Medicine, Chicago, Illinois, USA

NOAM ZEVIT, MD
Director, Eosinophilic Gastrointestinal Disease Service Institute of Gastroenterology, Hepatology, and Nutrition Schneider Children's Medical Center of Israel, Tel-Aviv University, Petach Tikvah, Israel

Contents

Eosinophilic esophagitis (EoE) is a chronic, progressive immune-mediated disease associated with antigen-driven type 2 inflammation and symptoms of esophageal dysfunction. Research over the last 2 decades has dramatically furthered our understanding of the complex interplay between genetics, environmental exposures, and cellular and molecular interactions involved in EoE. This review provides an overview of our current understanding of EoE pathogenesis.

Most of the major clinical signs and consequences of eosinophilic esophagitis seem to be related to tissue remodeling. Important data on remodeling activity in patients with eosinophilic esophagitis are provided by a range of current and new biologic markers and diagnostics. To completely clarify the possible advantages and restrictions of therapeutic approaches, clinical studies should take into consideration the existence and reversibility of esophageal remodeling. The degree of mucosal or submucosal disease activity may not be reflected by epithelial eosinophilic inflammation, which is used to define one criterion of disease activity".

Despite the rising prevalence and incidence of eosinophilic esophagitis (EoE), the etiology and pathophysiology remain unknown. Studies to date suggest that complex interactions between genetic and environmental risk factors result in the development and presentation of disease. Examining environmental factors both in the early life and later life exposures offers potential clues for the development of EoE, although challenges exist in making causal inferences due to diagnostic delay and access, ascertainment biases, and misclassification of cases. The authors review studies supporting early life factors as etiologic factors in the development of EoE.

from the area of greatest involvement of the esophagus should be reported. The EREFS grading system was formally validated as an endoscopy score and several randomized placebo-controlled trials have shown responsiveness of the EREFS score to therapeutic interventions.

Microscopic examination of esophageal biopsies is essential to diagnose eosinophilic esophagitis (EoE). Eosinophil inflammation is the basis for the diagnosis, but additional abnormalities may contribute to persistent symptoms and epithelial barrier dysfunction. Both peak eosinophil count and assessments of additional features should be included in pre-therapy and post-therapy pathology reports. Pathologic abnormalities identified in esophageal biopsies of EoE are reversible in contrast to esophageal strictures.

Eosinophilic esophagitis (EoE) is a chronic immune-mediated food allergy–driven disease characterized by eosinophilic inflammation of the esophagus leading to symptoms of esophageal dysfunction. Prior studies have supported the key role of food allergen exposure as the main driver behind the etiopathogenesis showing that removal of food antigens can result in disease remission in both children and adults. These landmark studies serve as the basis for the rising interest and evolution of dietary therapy in EoE. This article will focus on the rationale for dietary therapy in EoE and provide helpful tools for the implementation of dietary therapy in practice.

Proton pump inhibitors (PPIs), swallowed topical corticosteroids (STSs), and dupilumab are highly effective therapies for the treatment of eosinophilic esophagitis. Shared decision-making informs the choice of therapy and factors such as ease of use, safety, cost, and efficacy should be addressed. PPIs are the most common medication utilized early in the disease course; however, for nonresponders, STSs are an excellent alternative. Dupilumab is unlikely to replace PPIs or STSs as first-line therapy, except in highly specific circumstances. Identification of novel biologic pathways and the development of small molecules may lead to a wider range of treatment options in the future.

Measuring health-related quality of life (HRQOL) gained relevance in research and clinical practice in patients with eosinophilic esophagitis. The physical discomfort and social and psychological consequences of this food-related disease substantially affect HRQOL. Determinant of an impaired HRQOL include symptom severity, disease duration, biological disease activity, and psychological factors. Patients prioritize symptom relief and improved HRQOL as treatment objectives. Available treatment options can address these goals; however, there is a suboptimal adherence to treatment. There is a need for enhanced patient guidance and education. The assessment of HRQOL will help to prioritize patient's needs in management.

Immunotherapy is a treatment approach based on the principle of incremental allergen exposure to achieve desensitization. Recently, oral immunotherapy has been introduced as a treatment of IgE-mediated food allergy. Some patients receiving oral immunotherapy for food allergy may develop eosinophilic esophagitis. Here, we summarize the literature examining this association, its treatment, and outcomes and discuss possible explanations for this clinical phenomenon. We further identify potential associations with aeroallergen sensitivity and other forms of immunotherapy including subcutaneous immunotherapy and sublingual immunotherapy. Finally, we discuss management of immunotherapy-induced eosinophilic esophagitis. Epicutaneous immunotherapy is highlighted as an area of therapeutic investigation.

Eosinophilic gastrointestinal diseases (EGIDs) including eosinophilic esophagitis (EoE) are rare diseases in which eosinophils abnormally infiltrate the gastrointestinal tract. Because these are rare diseases, there is limited information regarding race and ethnicity in EGIDs and even less is known about the impact of socioeconomic factors. There is some evidence that access to care in rural settings may be affecting epidemiologic understanding of EGIDs in the pediatric populations. Future work should try to evaluate bias in research and strive for representation in clinical trials and medicine.

Eosinophilic gastrointestinal disorder (EGID) is an umbrella term encompassing a group of chronic, immune-mediated disorders characterized by eosinophil-rich inflammation affecting one or more segments of the gastrointestinal tract. A recent consensus in nomenclature and emerging data made possible through multi-center consortia are beginning to unravel the molecular and cellular underpinnings of EGIDs below the esophagus. These emerging findings are revealing both overarching commonalities related to a food allergen-driven, chronic, Th2-mediated immune response as well as location-specific nuances in the pathophysiology of the collective EGIDs. Altogether, these advances offer promise for improved diagnoses and more efficacious interventional strategies.

Mast cells play a central role in the pathogenesis of eosinophilic gastrointestinal disorders (EGIDs), including eosinophilic esophagitis. Their interactions with immune and structural cells, involvement in tissue remodeling, and contribution to symptoms make them attractive targets for therapeutic intervention. More is being discovered regarding the intricate interplay of mast cells and eosinophils. Recent studies demonstrating that depletion of eosinophils is insufficient to improve symptoms of EGIDs have raised the question of whether other cells may play a role in symptomatology and pathogenesis of EGIDs.

Eosinophilic gastrointestinal disorders (EGIDs) are becoming more common causing significant suffering and reduced quality of life. These conditions can affect different parts of the digestive system, either individually or in combination. Recognition of their link to allergic disorders or other gastrointestinal (GI) diseases has raised questions about their shared underlying mechanisms, which has had implications for diagnosis and management. The authors critically examine the current understanding of the connection between EGIDs and allergic conditions (ie, atopic dermatitis, allergic rhinitis, asthma, and food allergy) and GI diseases (ie, inflammatory bowel disease, celiac disease, gastroesophageal reflux disease, and motility disorders).

The clinical presentation of eosinophilic gastrointestinal diseases beyond eosinophilic esophagitis (non-EoE EGIDs) varies depending on the gastrointestinal segments affected by the eosinophilic inflammation, the extent of eosinophilic inflammation within the gastrointestinal tract and its depth through the bowel wall. Non-EoE EGIDs with mucosal involvement tend to present with diarrhea, malabsorption, and sometimes bleeding, those with muscular involvement may present with symptoms of obstruction or pseudo-obstruction, intussusception, and even perforation, whereas those with serosal involvement may present with eosinophilic ascites. Here we describe the differences in symptoms experienced by children with non-EoE EGIDs with varying degrees of eosinophilic inflammation through the bowel wall.

Endoscopic evaluation with biopsies is a mainstay of the diagnosis of eosinophilic esophagitis (EoE) and non-EoE eosinophilic gastrointestinal diseases (EGIDs). Increasing knowledge has resulted in the development of 2 standardized scoring systems: the Endoscopic REFerence Score (EREFS) for EoE and the EG-REFS for eosinophilic gastritis, although the latter has not been validated. In EGIDs, diagnosis and follow-up focus on eosinophil infiltration in biopsies. In this article, we will discuss the most commonly used endoscopic scores in EoE and non-EoE EGIDs, their validity for the diagnosis and follow-up of disease activity, as well as endoscopic interventions and areas of uncertainty.

Eosinophilic gastrointestinal diseases (EGID), such as eosinophilic gastritis (EoG), eosinophilic enteritis, and eosinophilic colitis (EoC), are chronic inflammatory conditions characterized by persistent gastrointestinal symptoms and elevated levels of activated eosinophils in the gastrointestinal tract. EoG and eosinophilic duodenitis (EoD) are strongly associated with food allergen triggers and T_H2 inflammation, whereas EoC shows minimal transcriptomic overlap with other EGIDs. The level of expression of certain genes associated with T_H2 immune response is associated with certain histopathologic findings of EoG, EoD, and EoC. Current immune therapy for EoG depletes tissue eosinophilia with persistence of other histopathologic features of disease.

Patients with non–eosinophilic esophagitis eosinophilic gastrointestinal diseases (non-EoE EGIDs) are prone to nutritional deficiencies due to food-avoidant behaviors, malabsorption, and high nutrition impact symptoms. Nutrient deficiencies correspond to the segment, depth, and extent of the gastrointestinal tract involved and can impact organs distant from the gut. Patients with non-EoE EGIDs are often atopic, and some appear to respond to dietary avoidance of specific food allergens. Tests to identify food triggers other than response to elimination diets are lacking. Dietary restriction therapy should be considered in such patients and is best implemented through a multidisciplinary approach to avoid nutritional complications.

Data for pharmacologic treatments for non–eosinophilic esophagitis (EoE) eosinophilic gastrointestinal diseases (EGIDs) are limited. Nevertheless, because of the increasing understanding of EGID pathogenesis, a number of medications are used to treat EGIDs, though all are currently off-label. Initial therapy generally starts with corticosteroids, and "topical" delivery is preferred over systemic due to long-term side effects. A number of other small molecules could potentially be used, ranging from allergy medications to immunosuppressants. Biologics are also being used and investigated for EGIDs and represent promising targeted therapies. Multiple therapeutic targets have also been identified, many of which overlap with EoE targets.

IMMUNOLOGY AND ALLERGY CLINICS OF NORTH AMERICA

SERIES OF RELATED INTEREST

Medical Clinics
https://www.medical.theclinics.com/

THE CLINICS ARE AVAILABLE ONLINE!
Access your subscription at:
www.theclinics.com

IMMUNOLOGY AND ALLERGY
CLINICS OF NORTH AMERICA

Foreword

Eosinophilic Gastrointestinal Diseases

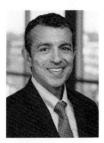

Rohit Katial, MD, FAAAAI, FACAAI, FACP
Consulting Editor

It is with great pleasure that I introduce this comprehensive issue, edited by eminent leaders in the field, Drs Furuta and Atkins. This issue is a significant contribution to the understanding and management of Eosinophilic Gastrointestinal Diseases (EGIDs) as well as a testament to the dedication and expertise of luminaries in the field, who have meticulously compiled and analyzed the latest research and clinical practices related to EGIDs.

The issue begins by delving into the pathophysiology of Eosinophilic Esophagitis (EoE), providing a solid foundation for understanding the disease's progression and impact, transitioning into exploring the clinical implications of esophageal remodeling and fibrosis in EoE.

The articles on the epidemiologic and clinical clues to the cause of EoE, and the clinical evaluation of children and adults with EoE, provide a reference to the evaluation of such patients. The recognition and management of feeding dysfunction in pediatric patients with EoE are also addressed, highlighting the unique challenges faced by this demographic. The issue further explores the endoscopic features and histopathology of EoE. The articles on dietary and pharmacologic management of EoE offer practical guidance for clinicians, while the section on health-related quality of life underscores the disease's impact beyond the physical symptoms. The article on embracing diversity, equity, inclusion, and accessibility in EGIDs is particularly noteworthy, emphasizing the importance of a patient-centered approach in managing these diseases.

The latter part of the issue expands the scope to non-EoE EGIDs, discussing their pathophysiology, the role of mast cells, and their associations with other gastrointestinal and allergic diseases. The final articles on the dietary and pharmacologic management of non-EoE EGIDs offer practical strategies for clinicians managing these complex conditions.

Immunol Allergy Clin N Am 44 (2024) xvii–xviii
https://doi.org/10.1016/j.iac.2024.01.012
immunology.theclinics.com
0889-8561/24/© 2024 Elsevier Inc. All rights reserved.

I highly recommend this issue to anyone wishing to learn about such diseases or those who provide care to such patients, as this issue is a valuable resource for clinicians, researchers, and anyone interested in EGIDs. It is my hope that it will inspire further research and innovation in the field, ultimately improving the lives of patients affected by these diseases. Enjoy the read!

Rohit Katial, MD, FAAAAI, FACAAI, FACP
Division of Allergy & Clinical Immunology
Department of Medicine
National Jewish Health
Denver, CO 80206, USA

E-mail address:
KatialR@NJHealth.org

Preface

Gastrointestinal Eosinophilic Diseases: Updates on Eosinophilic Esophagitis and Eosinophilic Gastrointestinal Diseases

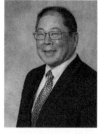 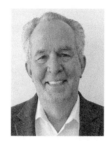

Glenn T. Furuta, MD   Dan Atkins, MD
Editors

Fifteen years after the last issue of *Immunology and Allergy Clinics of North America* on this topic, eosinophilic gastrointestinal diseases (EGIDs) continue to capture the attention of allergists/immunologists, gastroenterologists, pathologists, dietitians, speech therapists, and psychologists. Our understanding of the pathogenesis and clinical aspects of eosinophilic esophagitis (EoE) has advanced rapidly, whereas knowledge regarding the lower-tract EGIDs (eosinophilic gastritis [EoG], eosinophilic enteritis [EoN], eosinophilic colitis [EoC]) has accumulated at a slower, albeit increasing, pace. For instance, over the last 5 years, nomenclature has been clarified; genetic profiles have been developed for each; COM development is underway, and therapeutic trials have been completed. Thus, the collective awareness and accumulated knowledge of lower-tract EGIDs are also increasing, providing abundant hope for accelerated diagnosis and care. Due to the rapid and numerous advances in the understanding of and approach to diagnosis and treatment of EoE and other EGIDs in addition to the identification of their significant impact on each patient's quality of life, the intended goal of this issue is to provide a multidisciplinary comprehensive update for reference to improve clinical care and research focused on EGIDs.

Consequently, this issue of *Immunology and Allergy Clinics of North America* is divided into two sections, with the first thirteen articles focusing on EoE and the next eight articles addressing EoG, EoN, and EoC. Each section begins with reviews of pathophysiology followed by articles discussing clinical presentation, endoscopic features, histopathology, and dietary and pharmacologic management. Other key articles complement the overview of EoE by discussing epidemiologic and clinical

Immunol Allergy Clin N Am 44 (2024) xix–xx
https://doi.org/10.1016/j.iac.2024.01.011
0889-8561/24/© 2024 Published by Elsevier Inc.

immunology.theclinics.com

clues to the cause, recognition, and management of feeding dysfunction, quality-of-life issues, and diversity, equity, and inclusion. In addition, Drs Khoury and Wechsler review the roles of mast cells in EGIDs, and Drs Oliva and McGowan address the associations of EGIDs with other gastrointestinal and allergic diseases. As a pediatric gastroenterologist and an allergist, we appreciate the opportunity to coedit another issue of *Immunology and Allergy Clinics of North America* on EGIDs and are fortunate to have such an incredible group of valued colleagues rise to the occasion by authoring such thorough, informative reviews that we hope will serve as a valuable resource for those interested in research and/or caring for patients with these disorders.

Glenn T. Furuta, MD
Department of Pediatrics–Gastroenterology
Hepatology and Nutrition
University of Colorado School of Medicine
Digestive Health Institute
Children's Hospital Colorado
13123 East 16th Avenue
Aurora, CO 80045, USA

Dan Atkins, MD
Department of Pediatrics - Allergy and Immunology
University of Colorado School of Medicine
Children's Hospital Colorado
13123 East 16th Avenue
Aurora, CO 80045, USA

E-mail addresses:
Glenn.Furuta@childrenscolorado.org (G.T. Furuta)
Dan.Atkins@childrenscolorado.org (D. Atkins)

Pathophysiology of Eosinophilic Esophagitis

Kanak V. Kennedy, MD[a], Amanda B. Muir, MD, MSTR[b],*,
Melanie A. Ruffner, MD, PhD[b,c]

KEYWORDS

- Eosinophil • Esophagitis • Etiology • Pathogenesis • Food allergy • Genetics
- Epithelium

KEY POINTS

- Eosinophilic esophagitis (EoE) is a chronic, progressive immune-mediated disease associated with antigen-driven type 2 inflammation and symptoms of esophageal dysfunction.
- EoE affects patients of all ages, with typical clinical manifestations varying based on age at presentation.
- Infants and younger children are more likely to present with nonspecific symptoms or signs such as vomiting, feeding difficulties, and failure to thrive, whereas adolescents and adults more often present dysphagia and food impaction secondary to progressive fibrosis.

INTRODUCTION

Eosinophilic esophagitis (EoE) is a chronic, progressive immune-mediated disease associated with antigen-driven type 2 inflammation and symptoms of esophageal dysfunction.[1] EoE affects patients of all ages, with typical clinical manifestations varying based on age at presentation. Infants and younger children are more likely to present with nonspecific symptoms or signs such as vomiting, feeding difficulties, and failure to thrive, whereas adolescents and adults more often present dysphagia and food impaction secondary to progressive fibrosis.[2]

The etiology of EoE specifically is influenced by a complex interplay between genetic risk factors, environmental exposures, and baseline atopy (**Fig. 1**). Exposure to

[a] Division of Pediatric Gastroenterology, Hepatology, and Nutrition, Department of Pediatrics, The Children's Hospital of Philadelphia, 3400 Civic Center Boulevard, Philadelphia, PA 19104, USA; [b] Department of Pediatrics, Perelman School of Medicine, University of Pennsylvania, Abramson Research Center 902E, 3615 Civic Center Boulevard, Philadelphia, PA 19104, USA; [c] Division of Pediatric Allergy and Immunology, Department of Pediatrics, The Children's Hospital of Philadelphia
* Corresponding author. Abransom Research Center 902, 3615 Civic Center Boulevard, Philadelphia, PA 19104.
E-mail address: MUIRA@chop.edu

Immunol Allergy Clin N Am 44 (2024) 119–128
https://doi.org/10.1016/j.iac.2023.12.001
0889-8561/24/© 2024 Elsevier Inc. All rights reserved.

immunology.theclinics.com

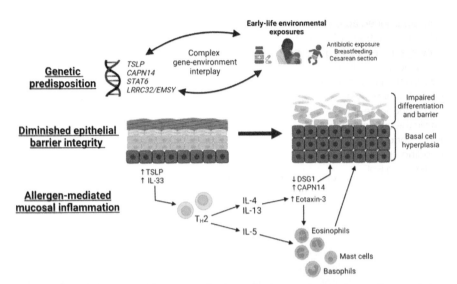

Fig. 1. EoE pathogenesis involves a complex interplay between genetics, environmental exposures, and cellular and molecular interactions. Multiple genetic risk loci (*TSLP, CAPN14, STAT6,* and *LRRC32/EMSY*) have been associated with EoE, many of which act through gene–gene and gene–environment interactions. The impaired epithelial barrier integrity and subsequent allergen-mediated T_H2 inflammation seen in EoE is influenced by these genetic polymorphisms and mediates chronic eosinophilic inflammation. (Created with BioRender.com.)

common food antigens through the diet drives esophageal inflammation by triggering the epithelial release of alarmins, including interleukin (IL)-33 and thymic stromal lymphopoietin (TSLP), which further stimulate T_H2 cell release of IL-4, IL-5, and IL-13, as well as downstream release of chemotaxis, including eotaxin-3. This mixed cytokine milieu stimulates epithelial structural changes, recruits granulocytes, and activates fibroblasts leading to collagen deposition and increased tissue stiffness.[3] Here, the authors review the genetic contributions, environmental factors, and cellular interactions currently known to contribute to EoE pathogenesis.

GENETIC CONTRIBUTIONS

EoE is more common among first-degree relatives of patients with EoE with a higher risk of developing EoE than the general population.[4,5] EoE has also been observed at higher rates in association with some monogenic disorders, but in general, EoE is not associated with a Mendelian inheritance pattern. The monogenic disorders associated with EoE have recently been comprehensively reviewed elsewhere,[6] but notably EoE has been observed in connective tissue disorders (Loeys–Dietz syndrome, Ehlers Danlos syndrome), as well as several inborn errors of immunity associated with atopy (Netherton syndrome, autosomal dominant [AD] signal transducer and activator of transcription 6 [*STAT6*] gain of function, AD-*STAT3* deficiency, *DOCK8* deficiency, and *ERBIN* deficiency).

Genetic studies aimed at identifying common genetic risk variants for EoE have been limited to small sample sizes owing to its relatively low prevalence (approximately 0.5–1 case per 1000 individuals).[6,7] Genome-wide association studies (GWASs) identified numerous genetic susceptibility loci shown to contribute to EoE. Several genetic loci, including 2p23 (*CAPN14*), 5q22 (*TSLP*), 11q13 (*LRRC32/EMSY*), and *STAT6*, have been reproduced across multiple GWASs.[6,8–12] Many of these genes influence epithelial barrier function or T_H2-mediated immune responses, supporting the role of these pathways in EoE pathogenesis. Interestingly, many of the above EoE genetic risk variants are located outside of gene-coding regions, frequently between genes (intergenic) or within the introns of genes (intronic), suggesting genotype-dependent gene regulation as the underlying mechanism for increased genetic risk.[6] Namjou and colleagues used a phenome-wide association study approach and further identified EoE risk variants in the cytokine cluster IL5–IL13 region, which is known to be associated with other atopic conditions.[13] Whole exome sequencing also identified variants in the genes encoding desmosomal-associated proteins desmoplakin and periplakin among 61 families with EoE.[14]

Calpain 14

Calpain 14 (*CAPN14*) is an intracellular calcium-activated regulatory protease highly expressed in the squamous epithelium of the esophagus, with increased expression in active EoE and upregulation in response to IL-13.[11,15–17] Overexpression of *CAPN14* in cultured esophageal cells has a disruptive effect on epithelial barrier function,[11,15,16] attributed at least in part to reduction of desmoglein-1 expression.[16] Lyles and colleagues demonstrated an association between specific *CAPN14* genetic variants and very early-onset EoE (diagnosed at age 12 months or less), making *CAPN14* the first identified EoE genetic susceptibility variant associated with early age of onset of EoE.[18]

Thymic Stromal Lymphopoietin

TSLP is a cytokine released by activated gastrointestinal, skin, and lung epithelial cells that promotes the maturation and activation of dendritic cells, which then secrete factors involved in T_H2 cell differentiation and migration. Elevated *TSLP* levels[8,19] are seen in esophageal biopsies from individuals with EoE compared with healthy controls. *TSLP* is the most dominant genetic variant associated with EoE risk.[20] Sherrill and colleagues identified a single single nucleotide polymorphism (SNP) in the TSLP receptor gene on the Y chromosome associated with EoE in male patients, which may play a role in the male predominance of EoE.[20] Transcriptional factor EMSY is upregulated in active EoE and has been shown to activate TSLP expression in vitro.[21] In addition to increasing the risk of acquiring EoE, the presence of an SNP at the 5q22 locus was found to be associated with an increased number of EoE food allergen triggers.[22] Martin and colleagues further found that the strength of the association between the *TSLP* genetic variation and EoE was highly dependent on genetic variation at the IL4 locus, suggesting that an underlying atopic phenotype may magnify the effects of *TSLP*.[23]

Signal Transducer and Activator of Transcription 6

STAT6 is a DNA-binding transcription factor that is phosphorylated in response to IL-4 and IL-13 and has an important role in the development of T_H2 cells. *STAT6* SNPs have previously been associated with serum immunoglobulin E (IgE) levels and allergic sensitization through GWAS.[11,24] Sleiman and colleagues identified two EoE-specific *STAT6* loci, one of which may induce *CAPN14* expression.[11] Specific *STAT6* variants have been tied to poor initial response to proton pump inhibitor (PPI) therapy,[25] as well as loss of PPI long-term response after 1 year in pediatric patients with EoE.[25,26]

EARLY-LIFE ENVIRONMENTAL EXPOSURES

The rapid increase in EoE prevalence in western countries suggests that environmental factors play a critical role in EoE pathogenesis; however, these factors have not been definitively identified. This is supported by multiple lines of evidence beyond the sharp increase in the few decades because EoE was first described. Dizygotic twins have a 10fold increase in disease concordance compared with non-twin siblings,[4] suggesting that there may be shared early-life exposures which impact disease risk. Increased risk was also observed among spouses of EoE patients, further supporting the role of a shared environment in EoE pathogenesis.[5]

Jensen and colleagues further examined early life exposures associated with the development of EoE, identifying antibiotic use in infancy, Cesarean delivery, preterm birth, and formula use as risk factors associated with later diagnosis of EoE.[27] Further, interplay between specific EoE-predisposing polymorphisms (notably at *CAPN14* and *LOX283710/KLF13*) and early-life environmental factors such as breastfeeding and neonatal intesive care unit (NICU) admission may contribute to increased EoE susceptibility.[28] Together, these data suggest a complex genetic etiology that acts in the context of environmental exposures.

Allergen-Mediated Mucosal Inflammation

There are several important lines of evidence that support an allergic etiology for EoE. The first line of evidence is that risk for development of EoE has been linked to a history of IgE-mediated food allergy, and individuals with EoE have been shown to be at increased risk for airway hyperresponsiveness.[29,30] This is believed to be due to a combination of shared genetic risk factors and environmental exposures leading to development of atopic disorders. Second, the success of dietary therapy in EoE has established a causal link between food allergen exposure and EoE. Kelly and colleagues described the first use of elemental diet therapy in EoE, demonstrating that patients significantly improved with removal of food antigens from the diet.[31] This has been redemonstrated in numerous studies using elimination diets,[32–35] and this body of work has shown that cow's milk is the most common food associated with EoE, followed by wheat and gluten-containing grains. Last, there is growing evidence that patients with type-I, IgE-mediated food allergy are at risk for development of EoE. In a pediatric cohort study, EoE prevalence was higher in the IgE food allergy patient cohort when compared with the general population (4.7% vs 0.04%).[36] EoE has been reported as a complication of food allergy oral immunotherapy in 3% to 5% of patients,[37,38] suggesting that this may be a population at unique risk for development of EoE.

Despite the evidence that EoE is an allergic disorder, data suggest that it is not dependent on IgE. The development of EoE in murine models does not require the presence of B cells.[39] Although there were initial promising clinical results using skin-prick testing, ultimately the efficacy of IgE-mediated food allergen testing in EoE is not superior to empirical elimination diets.[40] In addition, a randomized placebo-controlled trial of 14 adults with EoE demonstrated that omalizumab did not alter symptoms of EoE or eosinophil counts in biopsy samples compared with placebo.[41] However, there is evidence for local mucosal B-cell infiltration and IgE and IgG4 production, suggesting that these immunoglobulins may play a role within the context of a mixed, delayed hypersensitivity.

EoE was named for the eosinophil-rich inflammatory infiltrate present in the mucosa; however, during disease, a diverse population of inflammatory cells can be found. Eosinophils are recruited to the epithelium by alarmins (ie, TSLP, IL-33) and chemokines (ie, eotaxin-3) from the esophageal epithelium.[19,42,43] This local environment similarly promotes recruitment of T cells, group 2 innate lymphoid cells, mast cells, and an additional mixed inflammatory milieu into the esophageal mucosa.[44–46] However, the role of eosinophils as the cause of the inflammation or just a participant in the cascade caused by T2-cytokines has not been fully elucidated; the recent failure of anti-eosinophil targeted therapies in clinical trials have called into question their role as major effectors.

The important role of T2-cytokine production in EoE has been illustrated by trials demonstrating the clinical efficacy of anti-IL-4 receptor antagonists and anti-IL13 monoclonal antibody therapies for the treatment of EoE.[47,48] T2 cytokine production from pathogenic effector T2 (peT$_H$2) cells is thought to play an important role in the pathogenesis of EoE. Experimental models of EoE depend on CD3+ T cells, and T cells have been noted to be enriched in the mucosa of EoE patients.[39,46,49] peT$_H$2 cells are chemoattractant receptor-homologous molecule-positive, hematopoietic prostaglandin D synthase-positive, and CD161^{high} CD4 T cells capable of high levels of IL-5 production.[49–51] Recent single-cell sequencing studies of EoE biopsy tissue have identified the enrichment of esophageal homing receptor, GPR15, on peTH2 cells.[45] Additional data suggest that antigen-specific T cells can be found in the circulation of EoE patients and are increased in the setting of active disease.[45,52,53]

ROLE OF THE EPITHELIUM IN EOSINOPHILIC ESOPHAGITIS PATHOGENESIS

Although antigen stimulation leads to an inflammatory cascade of T cells, eosinophils, mast cells, and basophils that ultimately culminates in mucosal remodeling, the role of the epithelium in initiating this cascade and acting as an effector cell contributing to inflammation and symptomatology is only partially understood. One key question that remains unanswered is the role of the epithelium in allowing transmigration of particles and whether the barrier defects noted in the EoE epithelium are a cause of inflammation, a result of the inflammation, or both.

Barrier and Differentiation

As food is transported from the mouth to the stomach, a nonkeratinized epithelium lines the esophagus and acts as a barrier preventing damage from food particles, microbes, and acid. The esophageal epithelium is composed of a basal proliferative epithelium that undergoes differentiation and eventually de-nucleates and sloughs off into the lumen. Differentiation is a requisite for maintenance of an intact epithelial barrier in the esophagus with junctional protein expression in the later stages of differentiation.[54] The balance of proliferation and differentiation is altered in the inflammatory milieu of EoE, and as a result, there is expansion of the basal epithelium with decreased terminally differentiated cells and a depleted barrier.

Ultrastructural evaluation of the esophagus with active EoE using electron microscopy demonstrates that there are decreased desmosomes[55] compared with those with inactive EoE, patients with reflux, and healthy controls. Furthermore, there was a notable increase in the intercellular spaces between cells of the epithelia compared with healthy controls. Mucosal impedance performed at the time of endoscopy has shown that there is decreased impedance (and therefore decreased barrier integrity) in patients with EoE compared with healthy controls and reflux patients.[56] Of note, the degree of eosinophilia did not correlate with the mucosal impedance,[57] suggesting that factors beyond eosinophils and their granular proteins may be responsible for depletion of the barrier.

In vitro analysis has evaluated the role of various cytokines, microbial factors, and effector inflammatory cells in barrier dysfunction. These studies use three dimensional (3D) esophageal models such as air–liquid interface (ALI) culture, in which esophageal epithelial cells are stratified on a permeable membrane and electrical resistance and permeability are measured.[58] ALI coculture with mast cells[59] and EoE-relevant cytokines such as IL-13[54] or transforming growth factor-beta (TGF-β)[60] all demonstrated decreased electrical resistance and increased barrier permeability. Of note, stimulation with TLR2 agonists zymosan and peptidoglycan increased resistance in the cultures with enhanced expression of the tight junction proteins, tight junction protein 1, and claudin.[61] Taken together, these results suggest that the allergic milieu promotes disruption of the epithelial barrier, whereas microbial byproducts may increase resistance through effects on cellular tight junctions.

In conjunction with dilated intercellular spaces and diminished barrier function, differentiation of the epithelium is stalled.[62] Differentiation of the esophageal epithelium is canonically regulated in part by Notch and Bone Morphogenic Protein (BMP) signaling and both of these pathways are dysregulated in EoE. In the case of Notch signaling, Notch 1 and Notch 3 coordinate the transcription of differentiation markers including *HES5* and involucrin.[63] Patients with active EoE had decreased expression of intracellular Notch1 with decreased *NOTCH3* RNA, suggesting decreased Notch signaling. Similarly, esophageal epithelial cells stimulated with EoE-relevant cytokines (IL-4, IL-13, IL-5, and tumor necrosis factor-alpha [TNFα]) all demonstrated decreased Notch signaling in vitro[64] with resultant basal cell hyperplasia demonstrated in 3D organoid cultures. In addition to disruption of Notch signaling, IL-13 has been shown to decrease BMP-driven epithelial differentiation in a murine model of EoE. Specifically, mice that ectopically express IL-13 in the esophageal epithelium demonstrate decreased BMP signaling and accompanying basal cell hyperplasia.

Recent data demonstrate that in the EoE esophagus, depletion of protease inhibitor SPINK7 (serine peptidase inhibitor, kazal type 7) disrupts epithelial differentiation.[65] In fact, the loss of SPINK7 in in vitro culture decreased terminal differentiation marker filaggrin and increased alarmin TSLP expression. Further, treatment of murine models of EoE with a protease inhibitor resulted in improved epithelial thickness.

Clinically, basal cell hyperplasia was noted in 97% of EoE biopsies with active inflammation and 29% of biopsies with inactive disease; the presence of ongoing basal cell hyperplasia despite resolution of eosinophilia was associated with ongoing esophageal dysfunction.[66] Recent single-cell RNA sequencing suggested that the inactive esophageal epithelium was in an intermediate state, not completely healed with a unique transcriptome from both active EoE patients and healthy controls.[67] Taken together, these demonstrate that even in the inactive state, the EoE epithelium has ongoing structural abnormalities that may be driving symptomatology independent of inflammatory infiltrate.

SUMMARY

Research over the last 2 decades has dramatically furthered our understanding of EoE pathogenesis, revealing a complex interplay between genetics, environmental exposures, and cellular and molecular interactions. Studies linking specific genetic risk loci and environmental exposures, with subsequent barrier dysfunction and allergic hypersensitivity, provide a unifying mechanism for EoE development. Future advances elucidating the underlying allergic inflammatory pathways involved in EoE and the interactions between different elements of pathogenesis may help reveal potential noninvasive biomarkers of disease activity as well as new therapeutic targets.

CLINICS CARE POINTS

- Current literature has identified multiple genetic risk loci associated with EoE, many of which act through gene–gene and gene–environment interactions.
- Epithelial disruption and allergen-mediated T2 inflammation contribute to disease pathogenesis and may provide novel therapeutic targets.

> • Factors beyond eosinophils may be responsible for EoE-associated inflammation and barrier dysfunction.

ACKNOWLEDGMENTS

Thanks to Dr Tatiana Karakasheva for making the schematic using BioRender.

DISCLOSURE

The authors have declared that no conflict of interest exists for this article.

FUNDING

ABM: Recieves consulting fees from Nexstone Immunology, Regeneron/Sanofi, Bristol Meyers; SquibbABM: R01DK124266.

REFERENCES

1. Dellon ES, Liacouras CA, Molina-Infante J, et al. Updated International consensus diagnostic criteria for eosinophilic esophagitis: proceedings of the AGREE conference, 155. W.B. Saunders; 2018. p. 1022–33, e10.
2. Noel RJ, Putnam PE, Rothenberg ME. Eosinophilic esophagitis. N Engl J Med 2004;351:940–1.
3. Muir A, Falk GW. Eosinophilic esophagitis: a review. JAMA 2021;326:1310–8.
4. Alexander ES, Martin LJ, Collins MH, et al. Twin and family studies reveal strong environmental and weaker genetic cues explaining heritability of eosinophilic esophagitis. J Allergy Clin Immunol 2014;134:1084–92.e1.
5. Allen-Brady K, Firszt R, Fang JC, et al. Population-based familial aggregation of eosinophilic esophagitis suggests a genetic contribution. J Allergy Clin Immunol 2017;140:1138–43. Available at: https://pubmed.ncbi.nlm.nih.gov/28192145/.
6. Kottyan LC, Parameswaran S, Weirauch MT, et al. The genetic etiology of eosinophilic esophagitis. J Allergy Clin Immunol 2020;145:9–15.
7. Dellon ES, Hirano I. Epidemiology and Natural History of Eosinophilic Esophagitis. Gastroenterology 2018;154:319–32.e3.
8. Rothenberg ME, Spergel JM, Sherrill JD, et al. Common variants at 5q22 associate with pediatric eosinophilic esophagitis. Nat Genet 2010;42:289–91.
9. Kottyan LC, Maddox A, Braxton JR, et al. Genetic variants at the 16p13 locus confer risk for eosinophilic esophagitis. Gene Immun 2019;20:281–92.
10. Kottyan LC, Trimarchi MP, Lu X, et al. Replication and meta-analyses nominate numerous eosinophilic esophagitis risk genes. J Allergy Clin Immunol 2021;147:255–66.
11. Sleiman PMA, Wang M-L, Cianferoni A, et al. GWAS identifies four novel eosinophilic esophagitis loci. Nat Commun 2014;5:5593.
12. Chang X, March M, Mentch F, et al. A genome-wide association meta-analysis identifies new eosinophilic esophagitis loci. J Allergy Clin Immunol 2022;149:988 98.
13. Namjou B, Marsolo K, Caroll RJ, et al. Phenome-wide association study (PheWAS) in EMR-linked pediatric cohorts, genetically links PLCL1 to speech language development and IL5-IL13 to Eosinophilic Esophagitis. Front Genet 2014;5:401.
14. Shoda T, Kaufman KM, Wen T, et al. Desmoplakin and periplakin genetically and functionally contribute to eosinophilic esophagitis. Nat Commun 2021;12:6795.

15. Kottyan LC, Davis BP, Sherrill JD, et al. Genome-wide association analysis of eosinophilic esophagitis provides insight into the tissue specificity of this allergic disease. Nat Genet 2014;46:895–900.

16. Davis BP, Stucke EM, Khorki ME, et al. Eosinophilic esophagitis-linked calpain 14 is an IL-13-induced protease that mediates esophageal epithelial barrier impairment. JCI Insight 2016;1:e86355.

17. Litosh VA, Rochman M, Rymer JK, et al. Calpain-14 and its association with eosinophilic esophagitis. J Allergy Clin Immunol 2017;139:1762–71.e7.

18. Lyles JL, Martin LJ, Shoda T, et al. Very early onset eosinophilic esophagitis is common, responds to standard therapy, and demonstrates enrichment for CAPN14 genetic variants. J Allergy Clin Immunol 2021;147:244–54.e6.

19. Noti M, Wojno EDT, Kim BS, et al. Thymic stromal lymphopoietin-elicited basophil responses promote eosinophilic esophagitis. Nat Med 2013;19:1005–13.

20. Sherrill JD, Gao P-S, Stucke EM, et al. Variants of thymic stromal lymphopoietin and its receptor associate with eosinophilic esophagitis. J Allergy Clin Immunol 2010;126:160–5.e3.

21. Fahey LM, Guzek R, Ruffner MA, et al. EMSY is increased and activates TSLP & CCL5 expression in eosinophilic esophagitis. Pediatr Allergy Immunol 2018;29:565–8.

22. Fahey LM, Chandramouleeswaran PM, Guan S, et al. Food allergen triggers are increased in children with the TSLP risk allele and eosinophilic esophagitis. Clin Transl Gastroenterol 2018;9:139.

23. Martin LJ, He H, Collins MH, et al. Eosinophilic esophagitis (EoE) genetic susceptibility is mediated by synergistic interactions between EoE-specific and general atopic disease loci. J Allergy Clin Immunol 2018;141:1690–8.

24. Bønnelykke K, Matheson MC, Pers TH, et al. Meta-analysis of genome-wide association studies identifies ten loci influencing allergic sensitization. Nat Genet 2013;45:902–6.

25. Mougey EB, Williams A, Coyne AJK, et al. CYP2C19 and STAT6 variants influence the outcome of proton pump inhibitor therapy in pediatric eosinophilic esophagitis. J Pediatr Gastroenterol Nutr 2019;69:581–7.

26. Mougey EB, Nguyen V, Gutiérrez-Junquera C, et al. STAT6 variants associate with relapse of eosinophilic esophagitis in patients receiving long-term proton pump inhibitor therapy. Clin Gastroenterol Hepatol 2021;19:2046–53.e2.

27. Jensen ET, Kappelman MD, Kim HP, et al. Early life exposures as risk factors for pediatric eosinophilic esophagitis. J Pediatr Gastroenterol Nutr 2013;57:67–71.

28. Jensen ET, Kuhl JT, Martin LJ, et al. Early-life environmental exposures interact with genetic susceptibility variants in pediatric patients with eosinophilic esophagitis. J Allergy Clin Immunol 2018;141:632–7.e5.

29. Hill DA, Grundmeier RW, Ramos M, et al. Eosinophilic esophagitis is a late manifestation of the allergic march. J Allergy Clin Immunol Pract 2018;6:1528–33.

30. Krupp NL, Sehra S, Slaven JE, et al. Increased prevalence of airway reactivity in children with eosinophilic esophagitis. Pediatr Pulmonol 2016;51:478–83.

31. Kelly KJ, Lazenby AJ, Rowe PC, et al. Eosinophilic esophagitis attributed to gastroesophageal reflux: Improvement with an amino acid-based formula. Gastroenterology 1995;109:1503–12.

32. Kagalwalla AF, Sentongo TA, Ritz S, et al. Effect of six-food elimination diet on clinical and histologic outcomes in eosinophilic esophagitis. Clin Gastroenterol Hepatol 2006;4:1097–102.

33. Kliewer KL, Gonsalves N, Dellon ES, et al. One-food versus six-food elimination diet therapy for the treatment of eosinophilic oesophagitis: a multicentre, randomised, open-label trial. Lancet Gastroenterol Hepatol 2023;8:408–21.

34. Molina-Infante J, Arias Á, Alcedo J, et al. Step-up empiric elimination diet for pediatric and adult eosinophilic esophagitis: The 2-4-6 study. J Allergy Clin Immunol 2018;141:1365–72.

35. Gonsalves N, Yang G-Y, Doerfler B, et al. Elimination diet effectively treats eosinophilic esophagitis in adults; food reintroduction identifies causative factors. Gastroenterology 2012;142:1451–5.

36. Hill DA, Dudley JW, Spergel JM. The prevalence of eosinophilic esophagitis in pediatric patients with IgE-mediated food allergy. J Allergy Clin Immunol Pract 2017; 5:369–75.

37. Lucendo AJ, Arias A, Tenias JM. Relation between eosinophilic esophagitis and oral immunotherapy for food allergy: a systematic review with meta-analysis. Ann Allergy Asthma Immunol 2014;113:624–9.

38. Chu DK, Spergel JM, Vickery BP. Management of eosinophilic esophagitis during oral immunotherapy. J Allergy Clin Immunol Pract 2021;9:3282–7.

39. Mishra A, Schlotman J, Wang M, et al. Critical role for adaptive T cell immunity in experimental eosinophilic esophagitis in mice. J Leukoc Biol 2007;81:916–24.

40. Pitsios C, Vassilopoulou E, Pantavou K, et al. Allergy-test-based elimination diets for the treatment of eosinophilic esophagitis: a systematic review of their efficacy. J Clin Med Res 2022;11. https://doi.org/10.3390/jcm11195631.

41. Clayton F, Fang JC, Gleich GJ, et al. Eosinophilic esophagitis in adults is associated with IgG4 and not mediated by IgE. Gastroenterology 2014;147:602–9.

42. Blanchard C, Stucke EM, Rodriguez-Jimenez B, et al. A striking local esophageal cytokine expression profile in eosinophilic esophagitis. J Allergy Clin Immunol 2011;127:208–17, e1–7.

43. Spergel J, Aceves SS. Allergic components of eosinophilic esophagitis. J Allergy Clin Immunol 2018;142:1–8.

44. Doherty TA, Baum R, Newbury RO, et al. Group 2 innate lymphocytes (ILC2) are enriched in active eosinophilic esophagitis. J Allergy Clin Immunol 2015;136: 792–4.e3.

45. Morgan DM, Ruiter B, Smith NP, et al. Clonally expanded, GPR15-expressing pathogenic effector TH2 cells are associated with eosinophilic esophagitis. Sci Immunol 2021;6. https://doi.org/10.1126/sciimmunol.abi5586.

46. Greuter T, Straumann A, Fernandez-Marrero Y, et al. Characterization of eosinophilic esophagitis variants by clinical, histological, and molecular analyses: A cross-sectional multi-center study. Allergy 2022;77:2520–33.

47. Dellon ES, Rothenberg ME, Collins MH, et al. Dupilumab in adults and adolescents with eosinophilic esophagitis. N Engl J Med 2022;387:2317–30.

48. Hirano I, Collins MH, Assouline-Dayan Y, et al. RPC4046, a monoclonal antibody against IL13, reduces histologic and endoscopic activity in patients with eosinophilic esophagitis. Gastroenterology 2019;156:592–603.e10.

49. Mitson-Salazar A, Yin Y, Wansley DL, et al. Hematopoietic prostaglandin D synthase defines a proeosinophilic pathogenic effector human T(H)2 cell subpopulation with enhanced function. J Allergy Clin Immunol 2016;137:907–18.e9.

50. Islam SA, Chang DS, Colvin RA, et al. Mouse CCL8, a CCR8 agonist, promotes atopic dermatitis by recruiting IL-5+ T(H)2 cells. Nat Immunol 2011;12:167–77.

51. Wambre E, Bajzik V, DeLong JH, et al. A phenotypically and functionally distinct human TH2 cell subpopulation is associated with allergic disorders. Sci Transl Med 2017;9. https://doi.org/10.1126/scitranslmed.aam9171.

52. Cianferoni A, Ruffner MA, Guzek R, et al. Elevated expression of activated TH2 cells and milk-specific TH2 cells in milk-induced eosinophilic esophagitis. Ann Allergy Asthma Immunol 2018;120:177–83.e2.

53. Dilollo J, Rodríguez-López EM, Wilkey L, et al. Peripheral markers of allergen-specific immune activation predict clinical allergy in eosinophilic esophagitis. Allergy 2021;76:3470–8.

54. Wu L, Oshima T, Li M, et al. Filaggrin and tight junction proteins are crucial for IL-13-mediated esophageal barrier dysfunction. Am J Physiol Gastrointest Liver Physiol 2018;315:G341–50.

55. Capocelli KE, Fernando SD, Menard-Katcher C, et al. Ultrastructural features of eosinophilic oesophagitis: impact of treatment on desmosomes. J Clin Pathol 2015;68:51–6.

56. Patel DA, Higginbotham T, Slaughter JC, et al. Development and validation of a mucosal impedance contour analysis system to distinguish esophageal disorders. Gastroenterology 2019;156:1617–26.e1.

57. Alexander JA, Ravi K, Geno DM, et al. Comparison of mucosal impedance measurements throughout the esophagus and mucosal eosinophil counts in endoscopic biopsy specimens in eosinophilic esophagitis. Gastrointest Endosc 2019;89:693–700.e1.

58. Nakagawa H, Kasagi Y, Karakasheva TA, et al. Modeling epithelial homeostasis and reactive epithelial changes in human and murine three-dimensional esophageal organoids. Curr Protoc Stem Cell Biol 2020;3:52.

59. Kleuskens MTA, Bek MK, Al Halabi Y, et al. Mast cells disrupt the function of the esophageal epithelial barrier. Mucosal Immunol 2023. https://doi.org/10.1016/j.mucimm.2023.06.001.

60. Nguyen N, Fernando SD, Biette KA, et al. TGF-β1 alters esophageal epithelial barrier function by attenuation of claudin-7 in eosinophilic esophagitis. Mucosal Immunol 2018;11:415–26.

61. Ruffner MA, Song L, Maurer K, et al. Toll-like receptor 2 stimulation augments esophageal barrier integrity. Allergy: European Journal of Allergy and Clinical Immunology 2019;74:2449–60.

62. Rochman M, Travers J, Miracle CE, et al. Profound loss of esophageal tissue differentiation in patients with eosinophilic esophagitis. J Allergy Clin Immunol 2017; 140:738–49.e3.

63. Ohashi S, Natsuizaka M, Yashiro-Ohtani Y, et al. NOTCH1 and NOTCH3 coordinate esophageal squamous differentiation through a CSL-dependent transcriptional network. Gastroenterology 2010;139:2113–23.

64. Kasagi Y, Chandramouleeswaran PM, Whelan KA, et al. The esophageal organoid system reveals functional interplay between notch and cytokines in reactive epithelial changes. CMGH 2018;5:333–52.

65. Azouz NP, Ynga-Durand MA, Caldwell JM, et al. The antiprotease SPINK7 serves as an inhibitory checkpoint for esophageal epithelial inflammatory responses. Sci Transl Med 2018;10. https://doi.org/10.1126/scitranslmed.aap9736.

66. Whelan KA, Godwin BC, Wilkins B, et al. Persistent basal cell hyperplasia is associated with clinical and endoscopic findings in patients with histologically inactive eosinophilic esophagitis. Clin Gastroenterol Hepatol 2020;18:1475–82.e1.

67. Rochman M, Wen T, Kotliar M, et al. Single-cell RNA-Seq of human esophageal epithelium in homeostasis and allergic inflammation. JCI Insight 2022. https://doi.org/10.1172/jci.insight.159093.

Pathophysiology and Clinical Impact of Esophageal Remodeling and Fibrosis in Eosinophilic Esophagitis

Calies Menard-Katcher, MD[a],*, Seema Aceves, MD, PhD[b]

KEYWORDS

- Eosinophilic esophagitis • Remodeling • Fibrosis • Dysphagia • Stricture • Stenosis

KEY POINTS

- Eosinophilic esophagitis (EoE) is a chronic Th2-mediated inflammatory disease of the esophagus characterized by signs and symptoms related to esophageal dysfunction and histologically characterized by an eosinophil predominant inflammation. EoE has emerged as an important clinical entity with steadily rising prevalence.
- Difficulty swallowing in the esophageal phase is common. In children, this can manifest as feeding disorders, regurgitation, vomiting, abdominal pain, and poor weight gain. In adolescents and adult patients, EoE is one of the most common causes of solid food dysphagia.
- An increasing number of studies support that the primary symptoms in children and adults as well as clinical complications of EoE including food impaction and lumen narrowing are consequences of esophageal tissue remodeling. Tissue remodeling can lead to fibrosis, muscle hypertrophy, and esophageal stenosis.

INTRODUCTION

Eosinophilic esophagitis (EoE) is a chronic Th2-mediated inflammatory disease of the esophagus characterized by signs and symptoms related to esophageal dysfunction and histologically characterized by an eosinophil predominant inflammation. EoE has emerged as an important clinical entity with steadily rising prevalence.[1,2] Difficulty

[a] Departments of Pediatrics, Section of Pediatric Gastroenterology, Hepatology and Nutrition, University of Colorado School of Medicine, Digestive Health Institute, Childrens Hospital Colorado, Anschutz Medical Campus, 13123 East 16th Avenue, Aurora, CO 80045, USA; [b] Division of Pediatric Gastroenterology, Department of Pediatrics, University of California, Biomedical Research Facility 2, 4A17, 3147 Biomedical Sciences Way, La Jolla, CA, USA
* Corresponding author. 13123 East 16th Avenue, B-290, Aurora, CO 80045.
E-mail address: calies.menard-katcher@childrenscolorado.org

Immunol Allergy Clin N Am 44 (2024) 129–143
https://doi.org/10.1016/j.iac.2023.12.002
0889-8561/24/© 2024 Elsevier Inc. All rights reserved.

swallowing in the esophageal phase is common. In children, this can manifest as feeding disorders, regurgitation, vomiting, abdominal pain, and poor weight gain. In adolescents and adult patients, EoE is one of the most common causes of solid food dysphagia. An increasing number of studies support that the primary symptoms in children and adults as well as clinical complications of EoE including food impaction and lumen narrowing are consequences of esophageal tissue remodeling with resultant fibrosis, muscle hypertrophy, and esophageal stenosis. This article focuses on the current understanding of the pathogenesis, clinical detection, and therapeutic implications of esophageal remodeling in EoE.

DEFINING ESOPHAGEAL REMODELING IN EOSINOPHILIC ESOPHAGITIS

Remodeling can be defined as tissue changes in target organs that result in end-organ dysfunction. Remodeling can be physiologic, such as in wound healing, but when it continues beyond the need for tissue repair, it can be pathologic. Triggers for pathologic remodeling include unbridled inflammation and mechano-chemical changes in the extracellular environment, which alter cellular phenotypes. Together, these create negative consequences for organ function. Indeed, the usual natural history of untreated EoE is progression to stricture formation, at least in a majority of adolescents and adults.[3,4] Our studies show that pre-stricture changes of remodeling such as esophageal rigidity can occur even in young children.[5,6]

For the purpose of this review, tissue remodeling refers to both histologic and macroscopic changes. Epithelial remodeling changes include basal zone hyperplasia, dilated intercellular spaces, and increased invagination of the lamina propria vascular papillae into the epithelial space. Subepithelial changes include lamina propria fibrosis with increased collagen deposition and thickness and increased vascularity with vascular activation. Muscular remodeling changes include smooth muscle hypertrophy and hyperplasia. In turn, these histologic alterations result in the macroscopic findings of esophageal rings and diffuse or focal stenosis. Diffuse stenosis results in a narrow caliber esophagus, whereas focal stenosis is defined traditionally as an esophageal stricture.

Together these tissue remodeling events characterize likely mechanisms for the esophageal dysfunction that underlies EoE-related clinical symptoms and complications of dysphagia, food impactions, strictures, esophageal rigidity, and dysmotility. Therefore, by extension, a goal of treatment is to prevent, limit, and/or reverse tissue remodeling. Treating inflammation can impact histologic remodeling and even macroscopic remodeling in some patients. The degree of the remodeling response to anti-inflammatory therapies likely depends on multiple yet to be determined factors. Given the recommendation for and clinical practice of repeated endoscopic assessment and biopsies for EoE management, there is a unique opportunity to study the clinical complications, natural history, and reversibility of remodeling in the context of human tissue.

Pathogenesis of Remodeling in Eosinophilic Esophagitis

Inflammatory cells and mediators

Inflammatory mediators and cells, particularly eosinophils, clearly play a role in driving esophageal remodeling and have both epithelial and transmural impact. Animal models demonstrate that mice with decreased esophageal eosinophils have decreased basal zone hyperplasia.[7] In addition, mice lacking eosinophils or the eosinophilopoetic cytokine interleukin (IL)-5 have significantly less collagen deposition and fibronectin expression than their wild type littermates.[7,8] Transgenic mice that overexpress IL-5 have stricture formation and increased longitudinal and circular smooth muscle contraction force.[9] In this model, a lack of eosinophils, even in the presence of IL-5 overexpression, results in decreased stricture formation suggesting other eosinophilopoetic cytokines are at play.[9] In contrast, anti-IL-5 treatment in human EoE reduced esophageal eosinophilia but did not result in clear decreases in remodeling or clinical symptoms.[10–13]

In animal models, IL-13 overexpression causes esophageal strictures that are not reversed by subsequent IL-13 depletion.[9] Primary human epithelial cells and fibroblasts cultured with IL-13 express pro-remodeling proteins such as periostin.[14] In alignment with these findings, blockade of the common α chain of the IL-13 and IL-4 receptor with dupilumab improved markers of epithelial–mesenchymal transitions and esophageal compliance in a phase II study.[15,16]

Other inflammatory cells also contributed to EoE inflammation and likely to esophageal remodeling. For example, mast cells are expanded within each tissue layer in the esophagus during active EoE and can exceed the numbers of eosinophils.[17] Distinct mast cell transcript signatures demonstrate a pathogenic proliferative mast cell phenotype which could be supported by the production of mast cell chemotactic and survival factors such as IL-9.[17–19] Indeed, eosinophil-derived IL-9 is found within eosinophil-mast cell couplets, suggesting that there is an intricate balance between eosinophilia and mastocytosis in EoE.[20] Mast cell-deficient mice have decreased smooth muscle hypertrophy and proliferation.[21] As such, mast cells likely promote remodeling by stimulating fibrotic pathways and/or altering smooth muscle function.

Mice deficient in TSLP or basophils are protected from food impactions in an experimental EoE model, demonstrating that TSLP and basophils may play significant roles in esophageal dysfunction.[22]

Multiple infiltrating and resident inflammatory cells produce the profibrotic factor transforming growth factor beta (TGFβ) in EoE. Eosinophils, mast cells, and T cells have all been shown to produce TGFβ1. TGFβ1 increases extracellular matrix proteins such as collagen, fibronectin, and extracellular matrix (ECM) remodeling proteins such as matrix metalloproteinases (MMPs).[23–26] TGFβ1 messenger RNA (mRNA) and protein levels are elevated in the epithelium and subepithelium of pediatric and adult EoE subjects when compared with control subjects.[23] A TGFβ1 promoter functional single nucleotide polymorphism that increases its gene transcription associates with histologic remodeling.[27] Primary esophageal fibroblasts from EoE patients with the TT genotype at −509, the functional promoter single nucleotide polymorphism (SNP), have higher baseline levels of collagen I and MMP transcripts, poorer epithelial barrier protein expression, and altered wound healing.[28] Increased numbers of cells expressing the canonical TGFβ1 signaling molecules phosphorylated Smad 2 and 3 are found in active EoE patients.[23] Smad3-deficient mice are protected from esophageal remodeling, supporting the requirement for TGFβ signals in driving esophageal remodeling.[29]

Functionally, TGFβ1 affects multiple cell types beyond fibroblasts. Eosinophil or mast cell-derived TGFβ1 can cause direct contraction of primary esophageal smooth muscle cells in culture.[17,30] Esophageal smooth muscle hypertrophy is induced by TGFβ1, in part via a pathway involving the calcium channel regulator, phospholamban.[31] In the epithelium, TGFβ1 causes epithelial–mesenchymal transformation, decreases the expression of E-cadherin, and diminishes epithelial barrier function.[32,33] Fibroblast–epithelial crosstalk via tumor necrosis factor alpha (TNFα) and TGFβ1 induce collagen cross-linking in in vitro models via epithelial lysyl oxidase (LOX) expression.[34] This pathway occurs via the activation of nuclear factor κB and TGFβ-mediated signaling and suggests a positive feedback mechanism between fibroblasts and epithelial cells to promote remodeling.[34] In addition, TGFβ1 can interact with the TNF superfamily member, TNFSF14/LIGHT to create an inflammatory myofibroblasts.[35–37]

Epithelial mediators of remodeling

Epithelial cells also contribute to remodeling because they also produce TGFβ, respond to TNF, and make CCL26 recruiting inflammatory cells that drive remodeling. Periostin, a secreted extracellular matrix protein, is largely expressed by esophageal epithelial cells along with fibroblasts, is overexpressed in EoE, and associates with markers of esophageal remodeling.[26] Periostin captured in esophageal lumen eluate correlated with histologic markers of remodeling including basal zone hyperplasia and markers of epithelial–-mesenchymal transition.[38]

Fibroblasts in promoting remodeling in eosinophilic esophagitis

Fibroblasts are the main cells that produce ECM and thereby provide structural support for all organs. Perturbations in their function lead to altered transcriptional and functional phenotypes which can be organ-specific and drive disease exacerbations in disorders such as rheumatoid arthritis.[39,40] As noted above, fibroblasts secrete multiple pro-inflammatory and pro-fibrotic factors including TGFβ1 and TNFα. The TNF superfamily member TNFSF14/LIGHT induces a pro-inflammatory fibroblast phenotype that induces eosinophil tethering via ICAM-1 via both LIGHT receptors, herpes simplex virus (HSV) viral entry mediator, and lymphotoxin-beta receptor (LTβR). LIGHT deficient mice are protected from EoE remodeling with reduced collagen deposition and decreased muscle hypertrophy.[36] Consistent with an altered EoE phenotype, fibroblasts from patients with severe active EoE secrete a unique extracellular matrix proteome that reflects their in vivo state and induces collagen I and α-smooth muscle actin protein expression from normal fibroblasts. Proteome analysis of fibroblasts from patients with EoE identified thrombospondin-1 as a potential profibrotic mediator in EoE.[41]

Vascular remodeling in eosinophilic esophagitis

Subepithelial angiogenesis is present in EoE.[7,23,42,43] Consistent with this, there are elevated levels of pro-angiogenic factors including VEGF and angiotensin in the esophagus of pediatric EoE subjects.[42] Increased vascularity provides elevated numbers of conduits for the transport of inflammatory cells into the esophagus. Elevated levels of vascular activation factors described in EoE, such as vascular cell adhesion protein 1 (VCAM-1), allow vessels to have increased tethering and transmigration of inflammatory cells.[23,42] Indeed, mice deficient in eosinophils have diminished levels of angiogenesis.[7] In addition, vascular tetraspanin 12 (TSPAN12) is decreased in response to Il-13 and, via interactions with fibroblasts, can induce esophageal remodeling.[44]

Fibrostenotic Phenotype and Transcriptome

Fibrostenotic EoE is a phenotype that has been characterized in the literature and refers to patients with EoE who have either notable esophageal rings and/or esophageal narrowing or stricture.[3,4] This term forces an assumption that excess deposition of extracellular matrix components and fibrosis is the main driving force for stenosis. Although these changes occur in EoE, this assumption has not been rigorously proven and other processes may be contributing to stenosis such as muscular hypertrophy.[45] Importantly, the excessive subepithelial collagen described as lamina propria fibrosis in biopsies alone does not define this phenotype. This term however helps to distinguish patients with more severe narrowing and this phenotype has been shown to be more refractory to currently available treatments, require more dilation, and have more food impactions.[46,47]

It has been proposed that the fibrostenotic phenotype is a result of chronic inflammation. There are now multiple studies from the United States and Europe that conclude that during the natural course of EoE, there is progression from an inflammatory to a fibrostenotic phenotype.[3,4,48,49] With each additional year of undiagnosed EoE, the risk of stricture presence increases by approximately 10%.[48,50]

Recent molecular data show fibrostenotic patients have a distinct gene expression pattern compared with EoE without fibrostenosis lending support that predominant cellular pathways are propagating this phenotype or there is a progression in the molecular phenotype as a person progresses from primarily inflammatory to stenotic disease.[51] Studies that assess EoE bulk transcriptomics by severity identified that the transcriptome of EoE patients with endoscopic features of esophageal remodeling has enrichment of differentially expressed genes implicated in cellular proliferation, extracellular matrix organization, and inflammatory processes.[52,53] A study that assessed targeted gene expression by the presence or absence of food impaction showed decreased gene markers of inflammation and decreased markers of motility.[54] Additional study of pathways of interest will ideally lead to targeted treatment of esophageal remodeling in EoE.

Repeated esophageal biopsy sampling is routine in the clinical management of EoE. EoE therefore provides a unique opportunity to understand the clinical complications, natural history, and reversibility of eosinophil-associated tissue remodeling. In younger patients in particular, this allows us to investigate the long-term effects of tissue architectural changes on esophageal function and EoE progression. If EoE is akin to asthma, a person's phenotype may be defined very early in life.

Clinical Assessment of Remodeling and Fibrosis

Tissue remodeling leads to rigidity, narrowing, and motility disturbances. A variety of methods have been used in clinical practice and investigative studies to identify and measure esophageal remodeling in EoE. Whereas biopsies provide histologic evidence for tissue remodeling in EoE but gauge a very small portion (about 1/5000) of the esophagus, endoscopy and the other methods discussed allow for a global assessment of esophageal remodeling. Endoscopy and barium radiography are used most commonly in clinical practice to evaluate for stricture. In addition, endoscopic ultrasound, manometry, and endoluminal functional luminal imaging probe (FLIP) provide evidence for the remodeling that occurs in EoE.

Barium radiography: One of the oldest methods to evaluate the structure of the gastrointestinal tract is barium radiography. Early case series demonstrated the association of marked restriction of the esophageal lumen caliber with EoE, characterized as a narrow caliber or small caliber esophagus.[55] The multiple, ring-like stenoses spanning lengths of the esophagus were initially confused with congenital esophageal stenosis but were subsequently recognized to be a characteristic feature of EoE.[56] Lee and colleagues characterized restriction of the esophageal diameter in a cohort of adults with EoE, demonstrating a reduction in both the maximum and minimum diameters compared with controls. Esophageal diameter increased in some patients after treatment.[57] Radiologic assessment of esophageal remodeling is clinically feasible but does not assess for variations in diameter as a function of intraluminal distension forces. For example, a small volume of barium with low intrabolus distension pressure will tend to provide falsely low estimates of the diameter of an esophageal stricture because the stiffness of the esophageal wall limits the ability of the wall to expand. The use of a dissolvable barium tablet (13 mm) swallowed during fluoroscopic imaging can provide a helpful assessment of functional luminal narrowing if an obvious stricture or narrowing is suspected but not observed.[58]

Endoscopy: Endoscopy with biopsy is the mainstay of diagnosing and monitoring EoE. Prospective studies in EoE have identified endoscopic abnormalities in 93% of patients with EoE.[59] A validated classification and grading system to assess the endoscopic findings in EoE was developed to standardize and communicate visual findings during endoscopy.[60] The acronym for the Endoscopic REFerence Scoring system, EREFS, designates the five major features of EoE (edema, rings, exudates, furrows, and stricture). Rings and strictures have been characterized as fibrotic features and the others as inflammatory features.[3,4] EREFS features such as ring severity can associate with the occurrence of food impaction in adults.[47] Although endoscopy can detect stricture and long segment narrowing, careful inspection is required to appreciate narrowing that does not preclude passage of the endoscope and subtle narrowing can be missed. In a study of 70 adult patients with both radiographic upper GI series and upper endoscopy within 6 months of each other, upper GI fluoroscopy suggested EoE in 10% to 39%, whereas endoscopy identified characteristic abnormalities in 93%. The greatest difference in detection was in respect to identifying inflammatory features where EGD, not surprisingly, was better at detecting inflammatory features.[61]

Like symptoms, endoscopic findings in patients with EoE vary by age. Younger patients are more likely to have exudates, furrows, edema, or a normal appearing esophagus, whereas adult patients are more likely to have either mixed or fibrostenotic features strictures, rings, narrow caliber esophagus, and crepe-paper mucosa.[49,62] The presence of furrows and edema is similar between age groups but the presence of furrows can associate with histologic subepithelial fibrosis in children.[63] This variability in endoscopic features is in alignment with the observation of the prevalence of fibrostenotic consequences of esophageal eosinophilia in different age groups and the concept of progressive remodeling with duration of disease.

Additional measures to assess remodeling: In addition to epithelial and lamina propria remodeling, muscularis propria expansion has also been described. Human studies using endoscopic ultrasound demonstrate increased esophageal thickness including the concentric and longitudinal muscle layers in pediatric and adult EoE subjects.[64–66] Functional ultrasound can reveal dis-coordinated contraction between the concentric and longitudinal muscle layers.[67] The remodeling demonstrated by this tool allows a unique look below the epithelium; however, the technical challenges and time involved in capturing these measurements relegate it to investigative studies.

The expansion of the muscularis propria as well as reports of dysphagia in EoE in the absence of identified stricture have led to the concept that esophageal motor function and wall stiffness may be affected in EoE. Esophageal motility studies in adults with EoE have demonstrated both hypertensive or weak peristaltic function in a subset of EoE patients.[68,69] An investigation of adults using high-resolution esophageal manometry systematically compared a cohort of 50 patients with EoE, 50 patients with gastroesophageal reflux disease (GERD), and 50 healthy controls and demonstrated that 36% of EoE subjects had nonspecific esophageal motor patterns dominated by weak and failed peristalsis.[70] While of interest, the frequency of these abnormal patterns was not significantly different from the motility abnormalities in the cohort of patients with GERD. Another study from Spain demonstrated the manometric finding of pan esophageal pressurization in 48% of EoE patients as compared with a healthy control group.[71] The esophageal pressurization events in EoE may reflect reduced esophageal mural compliance secondary to transmural remodeling or alterations in motility that may occur secondary to associated inflammation and remodeling. The presence of either hypertensive or weak esophageal peristaltic abnormalities could impair esophageal bolus transport, especially when combined with luminal narrowing.

It should be acknowledged, however, that the manometric patterns identified are nonspecific and do not meet criteria for accepted, major esophageal motility disorders.

For most adults, dysphagia is the result of a combination of reduced luminal caliber, decreased esophageal compliance, and increased esophageal stiffness due to tissue remodeling. The FLIP provides an opportunity to study the physical mechanics of the esophageal lumen. The FLIP technology incorporates a multichannel electrical imped-ance catheter and manometric sensor surrounded by an infinitely compliant bag that is filled with an electrode conducting solution. As the bag is filled with the solution, the probe simultaneously ascertains the esophageal luminal diameter and pressure at multiple points along the catheter assembly. The resulting pressure–volume curves provide a detailed interrogation of the distensibility of the esophageal wall. A param-eter called the distension plateau characterizes the maximum ability of the esophagus to expand in spite of increasing intraluminal pressure at the point of minimal luminal diameter of the esophageal body.

An initial study of FLIP in patients with EoE demonstrated a significant reduction in distensibility in EoE compared with control subjects.[72] In an initial adult study, disten-sion plateau was reduced by 50% in EoE compared with controls. Although symptom duration and diagnostic delay correlate with lower distensibility,[73] our studies in chil-dren and adolescents demonstrate that distensibility is decreased and pre-stricture changes can be detected by FLIP even in these younger patients.[5,6] Unlike pediatric studies, studies in adults have not found a correlation with distensibility and epithelial eosinophil density. This is in contrast to studies in children and adolescents where distensibility seems to correlate with degree of eosinophilic inflammation.[5,6] This dif-ference in observation may point at the role of inflammation to promote esophageal remodeling early on and the progressive nature of fibrostenotic remodeling. Although epithelial eosinophilic inflammation is used to define one parameter of disease activity, it does not alone reflect the degree of remodeling and submucosal disease activity. FLIP may allow us to evaluate remodeling that is occurring below the mucosal surface. It is possible that lower grade esophageal stenosis is underreported in the literature due to a lack of sensitivity using the currently available endoscopic and radiographic techniques. FLIP may be a means of detecting lower grade stenosis.

In support of its role as a functional outcome, distensibility has been associated with endoscopic rings, symptom severity, and risk of esophageal food impaction.[47,74] Nic-odème and colleagues reported on the prospective assessment of 70 patients with EoE with a history of food impactions and found that baseline decreased esophageal distensibility predicted an increased risk of food impaction and need for dilation during a 12 month follow-up period. Other parameters that are derived from FLIP data can point to additional function of the esophagus in EoE.[75] For example, FLIP can catego-rize adult patients with EoE into several subcategories that account for both lumen distensibility and secondary peristalsis.[76,77] Future studies may help us know if these observed patterns explain disease severity or patient symptoms.

Treatment of Eosinophilic Esophagitis Remodeling and Impact on Fibrosis

Effectiveness of available therapies for remodeling in eosinophilic esophagitis

There is supportive evidence from multiple studies that effective control of inflammation can improve histologic and endoscopic features of remodeling. Short duration therapy can be effective in some patients. For example, esophageal rings and strictures improved after treatment with PPI or swallowed topical steroids and improvement was associated with deep remission of inflammation (eosinophil [eos]$\leq$5 per hpf).[78]

The largest body of evidence for therapeutic efficacy on remodeling has been demon-strated with the use of topical, swallowed corticosteroids. The benefits of these agents have been convincing in terms of resolving tissue inflammation and histologic evidence of remodeling including basal zone hyperplasia and lamina propria fibrosis.[25,79–81] There is, however, heterogeneity regarding the ability for topical steroids to improve esophageal subepithelial fibrosis in EoE. Aceves and colleagues first described significant reduction in severity of lamina propria fibrosis using topical budesonide in children with EoE.[82] This observation was confirmed by two subsequent pediatric series that used diet, topical fluticasone, or both, as well as in one adult study using topical budesonide.[25,83,84] It is important to note that in all of these studies, fibrosis improvement paralleled epithelial inflammatory improvement. In those patients who either did not improve with therapy or who were receiving placebo, both inflammation and fibrosis persisted.[25,82] The impact of treatment on subepithelial fibrosis in adults has been less consistent.[25] In a prospective uncontrolled study following a year of topical fluticasone used in a nonconventional formulation, fibrosis histology score was reduced but did not reach statistical significance after treatment.[85]

Several prospective studies in adults with EoE treated with topical steroids have demonstrated improvement in histologic remodeling and endoscopic features such as linear furrows but less impact on endoscopically detected fibrostenotic features including rings and strictures.[25,86] These differences in results suggest several possibilities such as an inability of topical corticosteroids to penetrate the deeper esophageal layers, difference in degree or irreversibility of fibrosis at different disease stages, or phenotypic distinctions among subjects who have concordance versus discordance between epithelial inflammation and subepithelial fibrosis.

Biologics impact on remodeling

Biologics may provide greater opportunity for targeting remodeling and fibrosis directly depending on the pathway impacted. Biologics studied to date have targeted the IL-13 pathway and eosinophils. IL-5 cytokine and receptor blockade have had limited efficacy in reversing remodeling. In contrast, dupilumab, the first approved EoE therapy, inhibits signaling through the common α chain of the IL-4/IL-13 receptors. Phase 2 adult data demonstrated improved distensibility after treatment with dupilumab compared with placebo.[15] Since the approval of dupilumab for EoE, there have been case series and reports of adults and adolescents with EoE and stricture refractory to other treatments that have been effectively treated with dupilumab.[87,88] A case series of adult and adolescent patients with fibrostenotic EoE refractory to swallowed topical steroids treated with dupilumab demonstrated 80% histologic treatment response for eosinophils less than 15 eosinophils per high power field and significant improvement in EREFS pre- and posttreatment. Although the proportion with esophageal stricture was stable, there was a significant increase in pre-dilation diameter from about 14 to 16 mm in this cohort. Whether this reflects true reversal of fibrosis or other factors of remodeling, it provides evidence that the degree of functional narrowing can be improved even in traditionally refractory patients.[87]

Impact of remodeling on treatment response

Later stages of remodeling and fibrosis are more challenging to impact with medical therapy. Patients with narrow caliber esophagus are generally more treatment resistant to current therapies even when looking at impact on eosinophil density.[46] Disease duration and/or progression of remodeling may be a factor in treatment response to currently available therapies. This may be influenced by the rigidity of the physical environment which can induce smooth muscle hypertrophy and fibroblast to myofibroblast transformation independently of inflammation.[26,30] As an example, treatment of adults with elemental formula for 4 weeks demonstrated improvements in inflammatory endoscopic features (furrows, plaques) but not in the features of rings or strictures.[89] Whether this is due to participant severity of disease, duration of disease or shorter treatment duration is unclear. Together, the current therapeutic trials suggest that less severely remodeled esophagi may be more likely to demonstrate reversal of both endoscopic and histologic remodeling.

Esophageal dilation

The most rapidly effective treatment for symptomatic strictures is esophageal dilation with either through-the-scope balloon or bougie systems.[90] Dilation leads to mechanical disruption of strictures but does not address the underlying remodeling or inflammatory process responsible. Although relief of dysphagia can continue for over a year following esophageal dilation, EoE is a chronic disease and symptomatic recurrence is expected in most patients[91–93] The control of inflammation can lessen the need for dilation.[94] As such, a reduction in esophageal inflammation and/or remodeling is a goal of effective management strategies.

Regardless of therapeutic agent used, clinical follow-up with patients is an important factor in preventing stricture formation and avoiding complications such as food impactions. EoE is a chronic disease and deserves follow-up. The interval needed however is not defined. Bon and colleagues retrospectively evaluated data from a long-term follow-up clinic for patients with EoE. Closer follow-up defined as follow-up within 18 months was associated with fewer stricture developments than those without close follow-up.[95] Although this dataset was limited by the number of follow-up visits per patients, the suggestion that patients should have follow-up within a 1- to 2-year interval is not unreasonable.

EoE therapies are rapidly evolving as the mechanisms underlying the disease become further understood. Several drugs are in the early stages of development. The primary endpoints used to judge the efficacy of therapies are symptoms and esophageal eosinophilic infiltration and to date have not accounted for effects on esophageal remodeling.[96] As measures of remodeling associate with patient outcomes such as food impaction and need for dilation and there continues to be some understood discrepancy between histologic remission and symptom improvement, measures that assess for remodeling may prove important in demonstrating efficacy in the future.

SUMMARY

In conclusion, tissue remodeling seems to be responsible for the major clinical symptoms and complications of EoE. Ongoing studies are investigating the mechanisms behind the chronic inflammation that drives the remodeling process. A variety of existing and novel biomarkers and tests provide important information on remodeling activity in patients with EoE. Clinical trials should account for the presence and reversibility of esophageal remodeling to fully elucidate the potential benefits and limitations of therapeutic interventions.

Although epithelial eosinophilic inflammation is used to define one parameter of disease activity, it may not reflect the degree of mucosal or submucosal disease activity. This is of particular relevance since the pathogenesis of remodeling lies largely below the mucosal surface. Mucosal eosinophilia travels in conjunction with other inflammatory cells and mediators that drive fibrosis, angiogenesis, stenosis, and smooth muscle changes. As such, it seems that although fibrostenosis is an important determinant of clinically relevant symptoms and complications, the persistence of eosinophilic inflammation is likely to be the most relevant determinant for the future risk of fibrostenosis.

CLINICS CARE POINTS

- Remodeling changes in eosinophilic esophagitis include epithelial basal zone hyperplasia, lamina propria fibrosis, increased vascularity, expansion of the muscularis propria, and increased stiffness of the esophageal lumen.
- Inflammation drives the remodeling process with mediators that include IL-5, IL-13, transforming growth factor beta as well as mast cells, fibroblasts, and eosinophils.
- Esophageal remodeling in eosinophilic esophagitis can be demonstrated using widely available tests including upper endoscopy, barium esophagram, and functional luminal imaging probe.
- Aspects of remodeling can improve with directed treatment but later stages of remodeling are often more refractory to current treatments.
- Clinical trials should account for the presence of esophageal remodeling as to ideally clarify the potential benefits and limitations of therapeutic interventions.

DISCLOSURE

None.

REFERENCES

1. Liacouras CA, Furuta GT, Hirano I, et al. Eosinophilic esophagitis: updated consensus recommendations for children and adults. J Allergy Clin Immunol 2011;128:3–20, e6; quiz 21-2.
2. Dellon ES, Gonsalves N, Hirano I, et al. ACG clinical guideline: Evidenced based approach to the diagnosis and management of esophageal eosinophilia and eosinophilic esophagitis (EoE). Am J Gastroenterol 2013;108:679–92 [quiz: 693].
3. Schoepfer AM, Safroneeva E, Bussmann C, et al. Delay in diagnosis of eosinophilic esophagitis increases risk for stricture formation in a time-dependent manner. Gastroenterology 2013;145:1230–1236 e1, 2.
4. Dellon ES, Kim HP, Sperry SL, et al. A phenotypic analysis shows that eosinophilic esophagitis is a progressive fibrostenotic disease. Gastrointest Endosc 2014;79:577–585 e4.
5. Menard-Katcher C, Benitez AJ, Pan Z, et al. Influence of Age and Eosinophilic Esophagitis on Esophageal Distensibility in a Pediatric Cohort. Am J Gastroenterol 2017;112:1466–73.
6. Hassan M, Aceves S, Dohil R, et al. Esophageal Compliance Quantifies Epithelial Remodeling in Pediatric Patients With Eosinophilic Esophagitis. J Pediatr Gastroenterol Nutr 2019;68:559–65.
7. Rubinstein E, Cho JY, Rosenthal P, et al. Siglec-F inhibition reduces esophageal eosinophilia and angiogenesis in a mouse model of eosinophilic esophagitis. J Pediatr Gastroenterol Nutr 2011;53:409–16.
8. Blanchard C, Wang N, Stringer KF, et al. Eotaxin-3 and a uniquely conserved gene-expression profile in eosinophilic esophagitis. J Clin Invest 2006;116:536–47.
9. Mavi P, Rajavelu P, Rayapudi M, et al. Esophageal functional impairments in experimental eosinophilic esophagitis. Am J Physiol Gastrointest Liver Physiol 2012;302:G1347–55.
10. Straumann A, Conus S, Grzonka P, et al. Anti-interleukin-5 antibody treatment (mepolizumab) in active eosinophilic oesophagitis: a randomised, placebo-controlled, double-blind trial. Gut 2010;59:21–30.

11. Assa'ad AH, Gupta SK, Collins MH, et al. An antibody against IL-5 reduces numbers of esophageal Intraepithelial eosinophils in children with eosinophilic esophagitis. Gastroenterology 2011;141:1593–604.

12. Dellon ES, Peterson KA, Mitlyng BL, et al. Mepolizumab for treatment of adolescents and adults with eosinophilic oesophagitis: a multicentre, randomised, double-blind, placebo-controlled clinical trial. Gut 2023;72:1828–37.

13. Spergel JM, Rothenberg ME, Collins MH, et al. Reslizumab in children and adolescents with eosinophilic esophagitis: results of a double-blind, randomized, placebo-controlled trial. J Allergy Clin Immunol 2012;129:456–63, 463 e1-3.

14. Blanchard C, Mingler MK, McBride M, et al. Periostin facilitates eosinophil tissue infiltration in allergic lung and esophageal responses. Mucosal Immunol 2008;1: 289–96.

15. Hirano I, Dellon ES, Hamilton JD, et al. Efficacy of Dupilumab in a Phase 2 Randomized Trial of Adults With Active Eosinophilic Esophagitis. Gastroenterology 2020;158:111–122 e10.

16. Gann PH, Deaton RJ, McMahon N, et al. An anti-IL-13 antibody reverses epithelial-mesenchymal transition biomarkers in eosinophilic esophagitis: Phase 2 trial results. J Allergy Clin Immunol 2020;146:367–376 e3.

17. Aceves SS, Chen D, Newbury RO, et al. Mast cells infiltrate the esophageal smooth muscle in patients with eosinophilic esophagitis, express TGF-beta1, and increase esophageal smooth muscle contraction. J Allergy Clin Immunol 2010;126: 1198–11204 e4.

18. Hsu Blatman KS, Gonsalves N, Hirano I, et al. Expression of mast cell-associated genes is upregulated in adult eosinophilic esophagitis and responds to steroid or dietary therapy. J Allergy Clin Immunol 2011;127:1307–1308 e3.

19. Janarthanam R, Bolton SM, Wechsler JB. Role of mast cells in eosinophilic esophagitis. Curr Opin Gastroenterol 2022;38:541–8.

20. Otani IM, Anilkumar AA, Newbury RO, et al. Anti-IL-5 therapy reduces mast cell and IL-9 cell numbers in pediatric patients with eosinophilic esophagitis. J Allergy Clin Immunol 2013;131:1576–82.

21. Niranjan R, Mavi P, Rayapudi M, et al. Pathogenic role of mast cells in experimental eosinophilic esophagitis. Am J Physiol Gastrointest Liver Physiol 2013; 304:G1087–94.

22. Noti M, Wojno ED, Kim BS, et al. Thymic stromal lymphopoietin-elicited basophil responses promote eosinophilic esophagitis. Nat Med 2013;19:1005–13.

23. Aceves SS, Newbury RO, Dohil R, et al. Esophageal remodeling in pediatric eosinophilic esophagitis. J Allergy Clin Immunol 2007;119:206–12.

24. Mishra A, Wang M, Pemmaraju VR, et al. Esophageal remodeling develops as a consequence of tissue specific IL-5-induced eosinophilia. Gastroenterology 2008;134:204–14.

25. Straumann A, Conus S, Degen L, et al. Budesonide is effective in adolescent and adult patients with active eosinophilic esophagitis. Gastroenterology 2010;139: 1526–37, 1537 e1.

26. Rawson R, Yang T, Newbury RO, et al. TGF-beta1-induced PAI-1 contributes to a profibrotic network in patients with eosinophilic esophagitis. J Allergy Clin Immunol 2016;138:791–800 e4.

27. Rawson R, Anilkumar A, Newbury RO, et al. The TGFbeta1 Promoter SNP C-509T and Food Sensitization Promote Esophageal Remodeling in Pediatric Eosinophilic Esophagitis. PLoS One 2015;10:e0144651.

28. Duong LD, Rawson R, Bezryadina A, et al. TGFbeta1 single-nucleotide polymorphism C-509T alters mucosal cell function in pediatric eosinophilic esophagitis. Mucosal Immunol 2020;13:110-7.

29. Cho JY, Doshi A, Rosenthal P, et al. Smad3-deficient mice have reduced esophageal fibrosis and angiogenesis in a model of egg-induced eosinophilic esophagitis. J Pediatr Gastroenterol Nutr 2014;59:10-6.

30. Muir AB, Dods K, Henry SJ, et al. Eosinophilic Esophagitis-Associated Chemical and Mechanical Microenvironment Shapes Esophageal Fibroblast Behavior. J Pediatr Gastroenterol Nutr 2016;63:200-9.

31. Beppu LY, Anilkumar AA, Newbury RO, et al. TGF-beta1-induced phospholamban expression alters esophageal smooth muscle cell contraction in patients with eosinophilic esophagitis. J Allergy Clin Immunol 2014,134.1100-1107 e4.

32. Kagalwalla AF, Akhtar N, Woodruff SA, et al. Eosinophilic esophagitis: epithelial mesenchymal transition contributes to esophageal remodeling and reverses with treatment. J Allergy Clin Immunol 2012;129:1387-1396 e7.

33. Nguyen N, Fernando SD, Biette KA, et al. TGF-beta1 alters esophageal epithelial barrier function by attenuation of claudin-7 in eosinophilic esophagitis. Mucosal Immunol 2018;11:415-26.

34. Kasagi Y, Dods K, Wang JX, et al. Fibrostenotic eosinophilic esophagitis might reflect epithelial lysyl oxidase induction by fibroblast-derived TNF-alpha. J Allergy Clin Immunol 2019;144:171-82.

35. Manresa MC, Chiang AWT, Kurten RC, et al. Increased Production of LIGHT by T Cells in Eosinophilic Esophagitis Promotes Differentiation of Esophageal Fibroblasts Toward an Inflammatory Phenotype. Gastroenterology 2020;159:1778-1792 e13.

36. Manresa MC, Miki H, Miller J, et al. A Deficiency in the Cytokine TNFSF14/LIGHT Limits Inflammation and Remodeling in Murine Eosinophilic Esophagitis. J Immunol 2022;209(12):2341-51.

37. Manresa MC, Wu A, Nhu QM, et al. LIGHT controls distinct homeostatic and inflammatory gene expression profiles in esophageal fibroblasts via differential HVEM and LTbetaR-mediated mechanisms. Mucosal Immunol 2022;15:327-37.

38. Muir A, Ackerman SJ, Pan Z, et al. Esophageal remodeling in Eosinophilic Esophagitis: Relationships to luminal captured biomarkers of inflammation and periostin. J Allergy Clin Immunol 2022;150(3):649-56 .e5.

39. Buechler MB, Pradhan RN, Krishnamurty AT, et al. Cross-tissue organization of the fibroblast lineage. Nature 2021;593:575-9.

40. Friscic J, Bottcher M, Reinwald C, et al. The complement system drives local inflammatory tissue priming by metabolic reprogramming of synovial fibroblasts. Immunity 2021;54:1002-1021 e10.

41. Hsieh LY, Chiang AWT, Duong LD, et al. A unique esophageal extracellular matrix proteome alters normal fibroblast function in severe eosinophilic esophagitis. J Allergy Clin Immunol 2021;148:486-94.

42. Persad R, Huynh HQ, Hao L, et al. Angiogenic remodeling in pediatric EoE is associated with increased levels of VEGF-A, angiogenin, IL-8, and activation of the TNF-alpha-NFkappaB pathway. J Pediatr Gastroenterol Nutr 2012;55:251-60.

43. McNamee EN, Biette KA, Hammer J, et al. Targeting granulocyte-macrophage colony-stimulating factor in epithelial and vascular remodeling in experimental eosinophilic esophagitis. Allergy 2017;72:1232-42.

44. Shoda T, Wen T, Caldwell JM, et al. Loss of Endothelial TSPAN12 Promotes Fibrostenotic Eosinophilic Esophagitis via Endothelial Cell-Fibroblast Crosstalk. Gastroenterology 2022;162:439-53.

45. Read AJ, Pandolfino JE. Biomechanics of esophageal function in eosinophilic esophagitis. J Neurogastroenterol Motil 2012;18.357–04.

46. Eluri S, Runge TM, Cotton CC, et al. The extremely narrow-caliber esophagus is a treatment-resistant subphenotype of eosinophilic esophagitis. Gastrointest Endosc 2016;83:1142–8.

47. Nicodeme F, Hirano I, Chen J, et al. Esophageal distensibility as a measure of disease severity in patients with eosinophilic esophagitis. Clin Gastroenterol Hepatol 2013;11:1101–1107 e1.

48. Warners MJ, Oude Nijhuis RAB, de Wijkerslooth LRH, et al. The natural course of eosinophilic esophagitis and long-term consequences of undiagnosed disease in a large cohort. Am J Gastroenterol 2018;113:836–44.

49. Straumann A, Aceves SS, Blanchard C, et al. Pediatric and adult eosinophilic esophagitis: similarities and differences. Allergy 2012;67:477–90.

50. Koutlas NT, Dellon ES. Progression from an Inflammatory to a Fibrostenotic Phenotype in Eosinophilic Esophagitis. Case Rep Gastroenterol 2017;11:382–8.

51. Shoda T, Wen T, Aceves SS, et al. Eosinophilic oesophagitis endotype classification by molecular, clinical, and histopathological analyses: a cross-sectional study. Lancet Gastroenterol Hepatol 2018;3:477–88.

52. Jacobse J, Brown R, Revetta F, et al. A synthesis and subgroup analysis of the eosinophilic esophagitis tissue transcriptome. J Allergy Clin Immunol 2023. in press.

53. Menard-Katcher C, Liu C, Galbraith MD, et al. Fibrostenotic eosinophilic esophagitis phenotype is defined by a proliferative gene signature. Allergy 2023;78: 579–83.

54. Sallis BF, Acar U, Hawthorne K, et al. A Distinct Esophageal mRNA Pattern Identifies Eosinophilic Esophagitis Patients With Food Impactions. Front Immunol 2018;9:2059.

55. Vasilopoulos S, Murphy P, Auerbach A, et al. The small-caliber esophagus: an unappreciated cause of dysphagia for solids in patients with eosinophilic esophagitis. Gastrointest Endosc 2002;55:99–106.

56. Zimmerman SL, Levine MS, Rubesin SE, et al. Idiopathic eosinophilic esophagitis in adults: the ringed esophagus. Radiology 2005;236:159–65.

57. Lee J, Huprich J, Kujath C, et al. Esophageal diameter is decreased in some patients with eosinophilic esophagitis and might increase with topical corticosteroid therapy. Clin Gastroenterol Hepatol 2012;10:481–6.

58. Nguyen N, Hayes K, Fenton L, et al. Case Series: Role of Pill Esophagram to Identify Pediatric Patients With Eosinophilic Esophagitis Amenable to Therapeutic Dilation. J Pediatr Gastroenterol Nutr 2020;71:530–2.

59. Kim HP, Vance RB, Shaheen NJ, et al. The prevalence and diagnostic utility of endoscopic features of eosinophilic esophagitis: a meta-analysis. Clin Gastroenterol Hepatol 2012;10:988–996 e5.

60. Hirano I, Moy N, Heckman MG, et al. Endoscopic assessment of the oesophageal features of eosinophilic oesophagitis: validation of a novel classification and grading system. Gut 2013;62:489–95.

61. Nelson MJ, Miller FH, Moy N, et al. Comparison of endoscopy and radiographic imaging for detection of esophageal inflammation and remodeling in adults with eosinophilic esophagitis. Gastrointest Endosc 2018;87:962–8.

62. Wechsler JB, Bolton SM, Amsden K, et al. Eosinophilic Esophagitis Reference Score Accurately Identifies Disease Activity and Treatment Effects in Children. Clin Gastroenterol Hepatol 2017;16(7):1056–63.

63. Aceves SS, Newbury RO, Dohil MA, et al. A symptom scoring tool for identifying pediatric patients with eosinophilic esophagitis and correlating symptoms with inflammation. Ann Allergy Asthma Immunol 2009;103:401–6.
64. Fox VL, Nurko S, Teitelbaum JE, et al. High-resolution EUS in children with eosinophilic "allergic" esophagitis. Gastrointest Endosc 2003;57:30–6.
65. Straumann A, Conus S, Degen L, et al. Long-term budesonide maintenance treatment is partially effective for patients with eosinophilic esophagitis. Clin Gastroenterol Hepatol 2011;9:400–409 e1.
66. Muroi K, Kakushima N, Furukawa K, et al. Subjective Symptoms in Patients with Eosinophilic Esophagitis Are Related to Esophageal Wall Thickness and Esophageal Body Pressure. Dig Dis Sci 2021;66:2291–300.
67. Korsapati H, Babaei A, Bhargava V, et al. Dysfunction of the longitudinal muscle of the oesophagus in eosinophilic oesophagitis. Gut 2009;58:1056–62.
68. Moawad FJ, Maydonovitch CL, Veerappan GR, et al. Esophageal motor disorders in adults with eosinophilic esophagitis. Dig Dis Sci 2011;56:1427–31.
69. Lucendo AJ, Castillo P, Martin-Chavarri S, et al. Manometric findings in adult eosinophilic oesophagitis: a study of 12 cases. Eur J Gastroenterol Hepatol 2007;19:417–24.
70. Roman S, Hirano I, Kwiatek MA, et al. Manometric features of eosinophilic esophagitis in esophageal pressure topography. Neuro Gastroenterol Motil 2011;23: 208–14.e111.
71. Martin Martin L, Santander C, Lopez Martin MC, et al. Esophageal motor abnormalities in eosinophilic esophagitis identified by high-resolution manometry. J Gastroenterol Hepatol 2011;26:1447–50.
72. Kwiatek MA, Hirano I, Kahrilas PJ, et al. Mechanical properties of the esophagus in eosinophilic esophagitis. Gastroenterology 2011;140:82–90.
73. Araujo I.K., Shehata C., Hirano I., et al., The Severity of Reduced Esophageal Distensibility Parallels Eosinophilic Esophagitis Disease Duration, *Clin Gastroenterol Hepatol*, 2023. in press.
74. Chen JW, Pandolfino JE, Lin Z, et al. Severity of endoscopically identified esophageal rings correlates with reduced esophageal distensibility in eosinophilic esophagitis. Endoscopy 2016;48:794–801.
75. Moosavi S, Shehata C, Kou W, et al. Measuring esophageal compliance using functional lumen imaging probe to assess remodeling in eosinophilic esophagitis. Neuro Gastroenterol Motil 2023;35:e14525.
76. Carlson DA, Shehata C, Gonsalves N, et al. Esophageal Dysmotility Is Associated With Disease Severity in Eosinophilic Esophagitis. Clin Gastroenterol Hepatol 2021;20(8):1719–28.
77. Carlson DA, Hirano I, Gonsalves N, et al. A Physiomechanical Model of Esophageal Function in Eosinophilic Esophagitis. Gastroenterology 2023;165(3):552–63.
78. Navarro P, Laserna-Mendieta EJ, Guagnozzi D, et al. Proton pump inhibitor therapy reverses endoscopic features of fibrosis in eosinophilic esophagitis. Dig Liver Dis 2021;53:1479–85.
79. Konikoff MR, Noel RJ, Blanchard C, et al. A randomized, double-blind, placebo-controlled trial of fluticasone propionate for pediatric eosinophilic esophagitis. Gastroenterology 2006;131:1381–91.
80. Dohil R, Newbury R, Fox L, et al. Oral viscous budesonide is effective in children with eosinophilic esophagitis in a randomized, placebo-controlled trial. Gastroenterology 2010;139:418–29.
81. Schroeder S, Fleischer DM, Masterson JC, et al. Successful treatment of eosinophilic esophagitis with ciclesonide. J Allergy Clin Immunol 2012;129:1419–21.

82. Aceves SS, Newbury RO, Chen D, et al. Resolution of remodeling in eosinophilic esophagitis correlates with epithelial response to topical corticosteroids. Allergy 2010;65:109–16.
83. Abu-Sultaneh SM, Durst P, Maynard V, et al. Fluticasone and food allergen elimination reverse sub-epithelial fibrosis in children with eosinophilic esophagitis. Dig Dis Sci 2011;56:97–102.
84. Chehade M, Sampson HA, Morotti RA, et al. Esophageal subepithelial fibrosis in children with eosinophilic esophagitis. J Pediatr Gastroenterol Nutr 2007;45: 319–28.
85. Lucendo AJ, Arias A, De Rezende LC, et al. Subepithelial collagen deposition, profibrogenic cytokine gene expression, and changes after prolonged fluticasone propionate treatment in adult eosinophilic esophagitis: a prospective study. J Allergy Clin Immunol 2011;128:1037–46.
86. Alexander JA, Jung KW, Arora AS, et al. Swallowed fluticasone improves histologic but not symptomatic response of adults with eosinophilic esophagitis. Clin Gastroenterol Hepatol 2012;10:742–749 e1.
87. Lee C.J. and Dellon E.S., Real-World Efficacy of Dupilumab in Severe, Treatment-Refractory, and Fibrostenotic Patients With Eosinophilic Esophagitis, *Clin Gastroenterol Hepatol*, 2023. in press.
88. Gangadharan Nambiar G, Rahhal R, Davis BP, et al. Refractory Pediatric Fibrostenotic Eosinophilic Esophagitis Treated With Dupilumab. ACG Case Rep J 2022; 9:e00887.
89. Peterson KA, Byrne KR, Vinson LA, et al. Elemental diet induces histologic response in adult eosinophilic esophagitis. Am J Gastroenterol 2013;108:759–66.
90. Dougherty M, Runge TM, Eluri S, et al. Esophageal dilation with either bougie or balloon technique as a treatment for eosinophilic esophagitis: a systematic review and meta-analysis. Gastrointest Endosc 2017;86:581–591 e3.
91. Safroneeva E, Pan Z, King E, et al. Long-Lasting Dissociation of Esophageal Eosinophilia and Symptoms After Dilation in Adults With Eosinophilic Esophagitis. Clin Gastroenterol Hepatol 2022;20:766–775 e4.
92. Assa'ad AH, Putnam PE, Collins MH, et al. Pediatric patients with eosinophilic esophagitis: an 8-year follow-up. J Allergy Clin Immunol 2007;119:731–8.
93. Dellon ES, Woosley JT, Arrington A, et al. Rapid Recurrence of Eosinophilic Esophagitis Activity After Successful Treatment in the Observation Phase of a Randomized, Double-blind, Double-dummy Trial. Clin Gastroenterol Hepatol 2019;18(7): 1483–92.
94. Runge TM, Eluri S, Woosley JT, et al. Control of inflammation decreases the need for subsequent esophageal dilation in patients with eosinophilic esophagitis. Dis Esophagus 2017;30:1–7.
95. Bon L, Safroneeva E, Bussmann C, et al. Close follow-up is associated with fewer stricture formation and results in earlier detection of histological relapse in the long-term management of eosinophilic esophagitis. United European Gastroenterol J 2022;10:308–18.
96. Hirano I. Therapeutic end points in eosinophilic esophagitis: is elimination of esophageal eosinophils enough? Clin Gastroenterol Hepatol 2012;10:750–2.

Epidemiologic and Clinical Clues to the Etiology of Eosinophilic Esophagitis

Joy W. Chang, MD, MS[a],*, Elizabeth T. Jensen, MPH, PhD[b]

KEYWORDS

- Eosinophilic esophagitis • Epidemiology • Early life • Environmental factors

KEY POINTS

- The incidence of eosinophilic esophagitis (EoE) is rising and understanding the epidemiology of EoE may provide clues into possible etiologic factors.
- EoE is a result of complex interactions between genetic and environmental factors.
- Early life factors that contribute to dysbiosis of the microbiome are associated with other atopic diseases and could be important clues to the etiology and development of EoE.

INTRODUCTION

Eosinophilic esophagitis (EoE) is a chronic immune-mediated inflammatory disease characterized by symptoms of esophageal dysfunction and esophageal eosinophilia, affecting both children and adults. Since it was first described 30 years ago, EoE has rapidly increased in prevalence and incidence, accounting for substantial health care costs (up to $1.36 billion annually) from emergency room visits, endoscopic procedures, outpatient visits, and pharmacologic therapy.[1,2] On an individual level, patients experience chronic symptoms, delayed diagnoses, and challenging treatment regimens. Despite these system and individual burdens, the etiology and pathophysiology of EoE are unknown, which hinders attempts at preventing and mitigating disease, and the development of targeted therapies or a cure.

Our understanding of potential underlying etiologies and risk factors for development of EoE stems from epidemiologic clues and observed clinical patterns. As a new and relatively rare disease affecting people across the lifespan, many challenges exist in studying the etiology of EoE. Diagnostic case definitions have evolved over time, and a variety of factors affect access to care, and diagnosis of EoE requires

[a] Division of Gastroenterology, Department of Internal Medicine, 3912 Taubman Center, 1500 East Medical Center Drive, SPC 5362, Ann Arbor, MI 48109, USA; [b] Department of Epidemiology and Prevention, Wake Forest University School of Medicine, 475 Vine Street, Winston-Salem, NC 27101, USA
* Corresponding author.
E-mail address: CHJOY@med.umich.edu

Immunol Allergy Clin N Am 44 (2024) 145–155
https://doi.org/10.1016/j.iac.2023.12.003
immunology.theclinics.com
0889-8561/24/© 2023 The Author(s). Published by Elsevier Inc. This is an open access article under the CC BY-NC-ND license (http://creativecommons.org/licenses/by-nc-nd/4.0/).

endoscopy with biopsies, current descriptive epidemiologic data likely reflects missed identification of cases or misclassification of non-cases.[3-6] Another challenge is that given EoE is a relatively uncommon disease, prospective cohort studies to measure true temporal risk factors are generally impractical or unfeasible. Despite these challenges and limitations, examining patterns and co-occurring conditions can provide clues to generate hypotheses about the etiology and factors that contribute to the development of EoE.

EPIDEMIOLOGIC CLUES

To untangle causes of risk factors for developing EoE, we first look to the disease incidence or the proportion or rate of newly developed disease during a time period. To date, epidemiologic studies report varying incidence of EoE—from 0.7 cases/100,000 up to 10 cases/100,000.[7] We can hypothesize that these inconsistent estimates may be due to bias in ascertainment, varying definitions of cases by diagnostic criteria, differences in source population or time periods examined. A review of regional trends shows a higher incidence in North America compared with Europe and Asia, which may be explained by these same factors or could suggest differences in environmental exposures that contribute to disease pathogenesis.[8] Although EoE has been reported in Latin America, Middle East, and South Asian countries, the estimated prevalence is comparatively lower due to unclear or possibly multifactorial causes. Temporal patterns of EoE can also provide insight on the development of EoE. Since the disease was described nearly 30 years ago, the incidence has dramatically increased, shown in multiple studies to outpace the increase in endoscopies with biopsies, suggesting a true increase in environmental risk factors and/or improved diagnosis.[9] Recent studies in both Europe and North America show that the incidence may be leveling off, potentially offering new clues for understanding disease pathogenesis.[10-12]

GENETIC RISK FACTORS

Studies examining the heritability of EoE and intrinsic genetic risk factors point at the development of disease as a multifactorial process. In genome wide association and candidate gene studies, EoE has been associated with susceptibility variants related to type 2 immunity (CCL26, TSLP, POSTN) and epithelial barrier dysfunction (CPN14, FLP, DSG1, SPINK5, SPINK7).[13] However, genetics alone do not explain the development of EoE, which does not follow a Mendelian inheritance pattern. In comparison to other immune-mediated chronic conditions, heritability estimate for EoE is relatively low. In a study of family clustering among twins, heritability among twins was 14.5% with the common environment accounting for 81.0% of the variation.[14] In addition, concordance for EoE among dizygotic twins (22.0%) was stronger compared with non-twin siblings (2.5%, $P < .001$), suggesting that not only are environmental factors implicated but also shared early life factors may be important in understanding disease risk. As such, it is posited that genetic factors interact with environmental factors to result in disease development. This concept was affirmed in a study demonstrating a protective effect of breastfeeding to the development of EoE in infants with a single-nucleotide polymorphism in CAPN14 (adjusted odds ratio [OR] 0.08, 95% CI 0.01–0.59) compared with those who were not breastfed.[15] There was no impact on EoE risk regardless of breastfeeding when the single nucleotide polymorphism (SNP) was absent, affirming this concept that among genetically susceptible people, environmental factors not only contribute but may be necessary for the development of EoE.

EARLY LIFE

Of environmental factors, early life factors are perhaps the most studied to date and provide the most evidence for the development of EoE. Early life exposures or those impacting fetal development and exposures within the first 3 years of life—including delivery, infant feeding, medication use, and maternal factors—likely influence the developing gut microbiome, promote dysbiosis, and inform the developing immune systems are associated risk factors for developing EoE.

Prenatal Period

Prenatal factors including maternal complications and medication use have been associated with an increased risk of EoE. In the only study that explored the association of maternal fever to the later development of EoE in children, maternal fever conferred an increased risk (adjusted odds ratio [aOR] 3.18, 95% CI 1.27–7.98), limited by potential recall bias of the mothers and case patients.[16] Leveraging a nationwide population-based database of Danish EoE cases, pregnancy complications (eg, infections, hypertensive disorders, gestational diabetes, preterm labor) were associated with EoE (aOR 1.4, 95% CI: 1.0–1.9) and maternal antibiotic use was associated with developing EoE (aOR 1.5, 95% CI 1.2–1.9) with increased risk with more frequent use (1 prescription aOR 1.4, 95% CI 1.0–1.8 ; 3+ prescriptions aOR 2.1, 95% CI 1.4–3.2) and timing closer to delivery (third trimester aOR 1.5, 95% CI 1.0–2.1).[17] Similarly, in this population, maternal use of acid suppression use was associated with an increased risk of developing EoE (aOR 1.7, 95% CI 1.0–2.8) in a dose–response manner (3+ prescription aOR 5.1; 95% CI: 1.8–14.8), supporting a relationship between medications that alter the microbiome as early as the in utero period and the development of EoE.[18]

Intrapartum Period

Intrapartum period factors associated with pediatric onset of EoE include preterm birth and cesarean delivery. In a landmark study of this relationship in cases in North Carolina, Jensen and colleagues reported preterm birth (OR 4.2, 95% CI 0.7–43.4) and cesarean section delivery (OR 2.2, 95% CI 0.8–6.4) associated with the development of EoE in childhood.[19] These findings of preterm labor (Ohio aOR 2.18, 95% CI 1.06–4.48) and cesarean delivery (Ohio aOR 1.77, 95% CI 1.01–3.09; Massachusetts aOR 3.21, 95% CI 1.20–8.60) are supported in distinct cohorts.[16,20] Similarly, within the recent population-based Danish cohort, preterm infants with gestational age between 32 and 34 weeks had the highest rate of EoE (32-week aOR 3.2, 95% 1.5–7.1; 33-week aOR 3.6, 95% CI 1.8–7.4; 34-week aOR 2.8, 95% CI 1.7–7.6).[17] However, in this recent large study, no association was observed between mode of delivery and EoE, once other confounding factors were accounted for in the analyses.

Infancy

During infancy, risk factors including neonatal intensive care unit (NICU) admission, infant medication use and feeding can potentially influence the developing microbiome and, thus, the risk of EoE. The risk of NICU admission on EoE development trended toward significance (aOR 1.92, 95% CI 0.95–3.89) when controlling for potential mediators of medication use.[16] This is supported by the highest rate of EoE observed in Danish infants who spent 2 to 3 weeks in the NICU (aOR 2.8, 95% CI 1.2–6.6).[17] In addition to maternal antibiotic and acid suppressant use, early antibiotic and acid suppression during infancy have been associated with EoE, further reinforcing dysbiosis and alterations in the gut microbiome as a potential mechanism in EoE. Of these medication exposures, the most robust evidence to date is in antibiotic use in infancy, first described by Jensen and colleagues (OR 6.0, 95% CI 1.7–20.8) and supported by separate cohorts (Ohio aOR 2.3, 95% CI 1.21–4.38; Massachusetts OR 3.61, 95% CI 1.11–11.74; North Carolina OR 4.64, 95% CI 1.63–13.2; Denmark aOR 1.4, 95% CI: 1.1–1.7), and reflected in insurance claims data (aOR 1.31; 95% CI 1.10–1.56).[16,18–22]

Although acid suppressants such as proton pump inhibitors (PPIs) are commonly used to treat EoE, their impact during the early life period is not clearly elucidated. Observational data show a strong association of acid suppression therapy in infancy (aOR 6.05, 95% 2.55–14.40) and are echoed by a large database study (PPI aOR 2.73, 95% CI 1.93–3.88; histamine type-2 receptor antagonist (H2RA) aOR 1.64, 95% CI 1.27–2.13).[16,22] Another study revealed a strong association between infant acid suppression and risk of EoE (aOR 16.0, 05% CI 9.1–27.7) and increased odds of EoE in a dose–response manner (1 prescription aOR 11.4, 95% CI 5.1–25.6; 3+ prescriptions aOR 23.5, 95% CI 9.1–60.7).[18] The role of breastfeeding in EoE is less clear with nonexclusive breastfeeding trending toward increased odds of EoE (OR 3.5, 95% CI 0.6–19.5) in one study, but nonsignificant association in others.[16,19,20,23] Complementing these data in pediatric-onset EoE, one study assessed these early life factors on the development of EoE in adulthood, demonstrating similarly strong associations between preterm delivery (OR 2.92, 95% CI 0.71–12.0), cesarean delivery (OR 3.08, 95% 0.75–12.6), NICU admission (OR 4.0, 95% CI 1.01–15.9), and antibiotic use in infancy (OR 4.64, 95% CI 1.63–13.2).[21]

LATER LIFE AND ENVIRONMENTAL EXPOSURES
Seasonality and Aeroallergens

Moving beyond the early life period, studies of environmental exposures demonstrate associations with and potential relationships with EoE. Studies of seasonality on EoE diagnosis and symptoms show trends and differences according to climate, suggesting a potential role of aeroallergens or ingestion of specific seasonally available foods. For example, a study of EoE cases from a national database reported an increased risk for EoE among those living in a cold climate zone (aOR 1.4, 95% CI 13.5–1.5) compared with temperate.[24] From this same database, seasonal variation was observed in EoE in temperate and cold climates with higher EoE diagnosis in the summer months and differing peak diagnoses by climate zones.[25] Despite these patterns, conflicting findings from several single-center studies report association between season and EoE, whereas others do not, signaling that aeroallergens do not universally cause or exacerbate EoE. Similarly, among studies describing disease recrudescence, no significant seasonal differences were observed (27.1% spring diagnosis vs 21.5% winter, $P = .70$).[26,27] Limitations of these studies to date include heterogeneity in defining seasonal exposure, geographic variations in aeroallergens, and retrospective designs. These findings are also likely biased by a temporal gap between initial symptom onset, report of symptoms, diagnosis, and using the time diagnosis or clinical presentation as a proxy for disease activity.

Environmental Quality

Recent investigation on air and water quality on EoE suggests potential modifiable environmental exposures, although findings from this early work remain inconclusive. Emergency room visits for indications of chest pain, dysphagia, and food impaction in the state of Utah were associated with high particulate pollution levels above environmental protection agency (EPA) standards.[28] However, a recent nationwide pathology database study reported increased odds of EoE in regions of the worst Environmental

Quality Index (OR 1.25, 95% CI 1.04–1.50), driven by poor water quality, but decreased odds of EoE in regions with poor air (OR 0.87, 95% 0.74–1.03) or land (OR 0.87, 95% CI 0.76–0.99) quality.[29] Using data collected from private well sampling in North Carolina, metal contaminants in drinking water (inorganic mercury OR 1.22, 95% CI 1.15–1.28; beryllium OR 1.35, 95% CI 1.30–1.39; thallium OR 1.25, 95% CI 1.21–1.29) has been associated with EoE.[30]

Other posited exposure risk factors associated with EoE include proximity to swine farming operations (aOR 2.56, 95% CI 1.33–4.95) and housing components (brick exterior aOR 1.83, 95% CI 1.11–3.02; gas heating 14% EoE vs 8% controls, $P = .06$; forced air 57% EoE vs 45% controls, $P = .009$).[31,32] Early in vitro and in vivo mouse studies demonstrating impaired esophageal epithelial barrier dysfunction and esophageal eosinophilia with detergent exposure may also explain evolving trends in EoE.[33] The absolute impact of these exposures on the development or exacerbation of EoE is unknown and calls for further investigation.

Prior Infections

With the rise in allergic disease coinciding with the decrease in *Helicobacter pylori* in the last few decades, specifically in Westernized countries, an inverse association between *H pylori* and atopic conditions is observed in studies to date.[34] The role of infectious agents in the development or protection against EoE has been theorized, but with conflicting findings. In a systematic review and meta-analysis of 11 adult and pediatric observational studies, *H pylori* exposure was inversely associated with EoE (OR 0.63, 95% CI 0.51–0.78) and esophageal eosinophilia (OR 0.62, 95% CI 0.52–76), suggesting a protective effect of *H pylori* infection.[35] Conversely, a large multicenter case-control study of European adults and children reported the prevalence of *H pylori* was not different between EoE (OR 0.97, 95% CI 0.73–1.30) and control cases.[36] In a recent nationwide case-control study of Swedish histopathology, antecedent infections conferred with an increased risk of EoE (OR 2.01, 95% CI 1.78–2.27), with further increased odds of sepsis with a diagnosis of EoE.[37]

CLINICAL CLUES
Comorbidity with Other Atopic Disorders

Clues about the etiology of EoE can also be found by examining its co-occurrence with other diseases. EoE is frequently comorbid with atopic diseases such as allergic rhinitis (OR 5.09, 95% CI 2.91–8.90), asthma (OR 3.01, 95% CI 1.96–4.62), eczema (OR 2.85, 95% CI 1.87–4.34), and food allergies (aOR 1.3, 95% CI 1.23–1.32), which share several clinical and epidemiologic similarities.[38–42] Much like EoE, the prevalence and incidence of atopic diseases has risen in recent decades, in part due to factors that may be explained by the hygiene hypothesis and alterations in the microbiome. Early life exposures shaping the gut microbiome and immune homeostasis are also posited in the development of atopic conditions, and similarly, observational studies of atopic conditions report a relationship between disease development and early life use of medications (acid suppressants, antibiotics) and environmental risk factors (eg, aeroallergens).[43]

Eosinophilic Esophagitis and Gastroesophageal Reflux Disease

Although EoE was initially thought to be a variant of gastroesophageal reflux disease (GERD), it is now recognized as a clinically distinct disease. As symptoms can be shared between the two disease states—EoE can precipitate symptoms of heartburn and regurgitation and GERD can cause dysphagia—differentiating the two disease states and determining the role of PPI in the treatment of both has been challenging and evolved over the last 2 decades. Despite the understanding of GERD as a separate entity from EoE, it has been hypothesized that one could contribute to the development of the other.[44] Acid damage and GERD are hypothesized to increase mucosal permeability of the esophagus, increasing antigenic exposure of food groups. Conversely, the infiltration of eosinophils and associated immune products can cause acid reflux through impaired esophageal motility (decreased acid clearance) and the anti-reflux barrier (relaxation of the lower esophageal sphincter). However, there is a lack of evidence to support these pathways as the sole etiology or predominant risk factor for developing EoE. In reality, EoE and GERD likely coexist in certain patients but the interaction of the two disease processes is not well characterized.

Eosinophilic Esophagitis and Inflammatory Bowel Disease

In searching for etiologic clues in EoE, parallels to inflammatory bowel disease (IBD) (Crohn's disease, in particular) are often drawn as both conditions are immune-mediated inflammatory states which can progress to fibrostenotic complications. Not only are there clinical analogies between the diseases but also several studies demonstrate disease co-occurrence. The initial single-center cohort study using diagnostic codes reported the prevalence of esophageal eosinophilia in IBD cases (0.25%) and prevalence of confirmed EoE in IBD (0.10%) but without significant differences between EoE patients with or without IBD.[45] Despite these low prevalence rates, concurrent EoE is two times higher in IBD than in the general population (0.05%). In a population-based analysis of insurance claims in the United States, the risk of EoE was higher among patients with Crohn's disease or ulcerative colitis, and the risk of IBD was higher among those with EoE compared with people without either disease.[46] The risk of EoE was higher among those with IBD and vice versa. In contrast, an inverse relationship between EoE and Crohn's disease (aOR 0.64, 95% CI 0.51–0.78), but not ulcerative colitis (aOR 0.97, 95% CI 0.75–1.24) using a national repository of histologic records from largely adult patients.[47] Focused cohort studies of pediatric EoE report heterogeneous prevalence from 0.35% in Italian children to 2.2% in American children from two tertiary centers.[48–50]

The reason for the observed overlap between EoE and IBD remains elusive, and when observed in the same patient, it is unclear whether these represent two distinct diseases. Eosinophilic infiltration of the gastrointestinal mucosa has been observed in Crohn's disease and ulcerative colitis. Still, EoE and IBD are currently thought of as distinct diseases with potentially shared mucosal immune dysregulation. Currently, clinical guidelines recommend excluding IBD as a secondary cause when making a diagnosis of EoE.[4] Despite being unique chronic inflammatory diseases of the GI tract, several similarities include epidemiologic trends (eg, rising incidence, disease enrichment in Westernized countries, early life risk factors), diagnostic challenges (eg, endoscopic assessment, poor reliance on symptoms), and management goals (eg, induction and maintenance therapies, long-term disease remission, chronic disease control) exist between EoE and IBD. Similar to EoE, the etiology of IBD remains unknown, and interactions between genetic, environmental, microbial, and lifestyle factors are thought to be necessary for disease development.

Eosinophilic Esophagitis and Celiac Disease

As another chronic immune-mediated gastrointestinal disorder, celiac disease (CD) has been hypothesized to be etiologically similar to EoE. Both likely arise from environmental, genetic, and immunologic factors, and are more prevalent in Westernized countries, induced by consuming food triggers, and treated by dietary avoidance strategies. Although some case reports and observational single-center studies, predominantly in children, demonstrate potential co-occurrence with prevalence of EoE in CD up to 4%, others report conflicting findings that patients with CD are not more likely to have esophageal eosinophilia on endoscopy and a diagnosis of CD is not associated with an increased risk of EoE.[51-61] In a cohort of adult EoE patients, Johnson and colleagues reported an increased rate of potential CD (13.6%), higher than the expected prevalence in the general population, and whose EoE resolved with gluten avoidance.[62] Using a national pathology database, Jensen and colleagues demonstrated that although the odds of EoE were 26% higher among those with CD compared with those without (aOR 1.26, 95% CI 0.98–1.60), there was only a weakly positive association when a more stringent case definition was applied.[63]

The potential association between EoE and CD remains uncertain due to or current understanding of EoE as a Th2-mediated disease versus CD as a Th2-mediated process, and conflicting findings, potentially due to heterogeneity in biopsy sampling, defining a diagnosis of EoE instead of esophageal eosinophilia in CD, and limited small studies to date.

SUMMARY/FUTURE DIRECTIONS

Over the last 2 decades, the incidence and prevalence of EoE has dramatically increased, with recent evidence of potential tapering. Along with these epidemiologic trends, studying early life and later life environmental factors provides clues about the etiology of EoE. Of these, the most consistent and compelling support is for early life factors such as antibiotic use. Although epidemiologic studies have been and will continue to be critical for hypothesis generation and evaluation of potential etiologic factors in the development of EoE, caution must be taken in interpretation and clinical application. Identifying and distinguishing pattern from "noise" that can contribute to bias and incorrect inferences remains a significant challenge. As such, applying casual inference methods to better discern associative versus causal effects, recognizing mediators in associations, and disentangling confounder factors are crucial. In addition, future studies probing additional mechanisms for how environmental factors contribute (eg, dysbiosis, epigenetic modifications) are needed.

CLINICS CARE POINTS

- Importance of obtaining a detailed history of atopy or environmental exposures in the care of individuals with eosinophilic esophagitis (EoE). Although prevention of EoE may not be possible in established cases, establishing comorbid exposures/allergic disease may play a role in the management of EoE.

- The development of EoE is multifactorial, a result of complex interactions between environmental exposures in genetically susceptible individuals.

- The most compelling and strong evidence for risk factors to developing EoE is in early life factors. However, studying environmental risk factors is encumbered by numerous threats to validity. Future studies with comprehensive exposure assessment are needed.

DISCLOSURE

Study concept and design: J.W. Chang and E.T. Jensen. Drafting of the article: J.W. Chang and E.T. Jensen. Critical revision of the article: J.W. Chang and E.T. Jensen. This work was supported by funding in part by NIH, United States awards

K23DK129784 (J.W. Chang), R01AI139126 (E.T. Jensen), and R01ES031940 (E.T. Jensen).

REFERENCES

1. Jensen ET, Kappelman MD, Martin CF, et al. Health-care utilization, costs, and the burden of disease related to eosinophilic esophagitis in the United States. Am J Gastroenterol 2015;110:626–32.
2. Lam AY, Lee JK, Coward S, et al. Epidemiologic Burden and Projections for Eosinophilic Esophagitis-Associated Emergency Department Visits in the United States: 2009-2030. Clin Gastroenterol Hepatol 2023;21(12):3041–50.
3. McGowan EC, Keller JP, Muir AB, et al. Distance to pediatric gastroenterology providers is associated with decreased diagnosis of eosinophilic esophagitis in rural populations. J Allergy Clin Immunol Pract 2021;9:4489–4492 e2.
4. Dellon ES, Gonsalves N, Hirano I, et al. ACG clinical guideline: Evidenced based approach to the diagnosis and management of esophageal eosinophilia and eosinophilic esophagitis (EoE). Am J Gastroenterol 2013;108:679–92.
5. Lenti MV, Savarino E, Mauro A, et al. Diagnostic delay and misdiagnosis in eosinophilic oesophagitis. Dig Liver Dis 2021;53:1632–9.
6. Murray FR, Kreienbuehl AS, Greuter T, et al. Diagnostic Delay in Patients With Eosinophilic Esophagitis Has Not Changed Since the First Description 30 Years Ago: Diagnostic Delay in Eosinophilic Esophagitis. Am J Gastroenterol 2022;117(11):1772–9.
7. Arias A, Perez-Martinez I, Tenias JM, et al. Systematic review with meta-analysis: the incidence and prevalence of eosinophilic oesophagitis in children and adults in population-based studies. Aliment Pharmacol Ther 2016;43:3–15.
8. Hahn JW, Lee K, Shin JI, et al. Global Incidence and Prevalence of Eosinophilic Esophagitis, 1976-2022: A Systematic Review and Meta-analysis. Clin Gastroenterol Hepatol 2023;21(13):3270–84.
9. Dellon ES, Erichsen R, Baron JA, et al. The increasing incidence and prevalence of eosinophilic oesophagitis outpaces changes in endoscopic and biopsy practice: national population-based estimates from Denmark. Aliment Pharmacol Ther 2015;41:662–70.
10. de Rooij WE, Barendsen ME, Warners MJ, et al. Emerging incidence trends of eosinophilic esophagitis over 25 years: Results of a nationwide register-based pathology cohort. Neuro Gastroenterol Motil 2021;33:e14072.
11. Hommeida S, Grothe RM, Hafed Y, et al. Assessing the incidence trend and characteristics of eosinophilic esophagitis in children in Olmsted County, Minnesota. Dis Esophagus 2018;31.
12. Robson J, O'Gorman M, McClain A, et al. Incidence and Prevalence of Pediatric Eosinophilic Esophagitis in Utah Based on a 5-Year Population-Based Study. Clin Gastroenterol Hepatol 2019;17:107–114 e1.
13. Sherrill JD, Rothenberg ME. Genetic dissection of eosinophilic esophagitis provides insight into disease pathogenesis and treatment strategies. J Allergy Clin Immunol 2011;128:23–32.
14. Alexander ES, Martin LJ, Collins MH, et al. Twin and family studies reveal strong environmental and weaker genetic cues explaining heritability of eosinophilic esophagitis. J Allergy Clin Immunol 2014;134:1084–1092 e1.
15. Jensen ET, Kuhl JT, Martin LJ, et al. Early-life environmental exposures interact with genetic susceptibility variants in pediatric patients with eosinophilic esophagitis. J Allergy Clin Immunol 2018;141:632–637 e5.

16. Jensen ET, Kuhl JT, Martin LJ, et al. Prenatal, intrapartum, and postnatal factors are associated with pediatric eosinophilic esophagitis. J Allorgy Clin Immunol 2018;141:214–22.
17. Kurt G, Svane HML, Erichsen R, et al. Prenatal, Intrapartum, and Neonatal Factors Increase the Risk of Eosinophilic Esophagitis. Am J Gastroenterol 2023; 118(9):1558–65.
18. Jensen ET, Svane HM, Erichsen R, et al. Maternal and infant antibiotic and acid suppressant use and risk of eosinophilic esophagitis: results from a population-based nationwide study. JAMA Pediatr 2023;177(12):1285–93.
19. Jensen ET, Kappelman MD, Kim HP, et al. Early life exposures as risk factors for pediatric eosinophilic esophagitis. J Pediatr Gastroenterol Nutr 2013;57:67–71.
20. Radano MC, Yuan Q, Katz A, et al. Cesarean section and antibiotic use found to be associated with eosinophilic esophagitis. J Allergy Clin Immunol Pract 2014;2: 475–477 e1.
21. Dellon ES, Shaheen O, Koutlas NT, et al. Early life factors are associated with risk for eosinophilic esophagitis diagnosed in adulthood. Dis Esophagus 2021;34.
22. Witmer CP, Susi A, Min SB, et al. Early Infant Risk Factors for Pediatric Eosinophilic Esophagitis. J Pediatr Gastroenterol Nutr 2018;67:610–5.
23. Slae M, Persad R, Leung AJ, et al. Role of Environmental Factors in the Development of Pediatric Eosinophilic Esophagitis. Dig Dis Sci 2015;60:3364–72.
24. Hurrell JM, Genta RM, Dellon ES. Prevalence of esophageal eosinophilia varies by climate zone in the United States. Am J Gastroenterol 2012;107:698–706.
25. Jensen ET, Shah ND, Hoffman K, et al. Seasonal variation in detection of oesophageal eosinophilia and eosinophilic oesophagitis. Aliment Pharmacol Ther 2015;42:461–9.
26. Lucendo AJ, Arias A, Redondo-Gonzalez O, et al. Seasonal distribution of initial diagnosis and clinical recrudescence of eosinophilic esophagitis: a systematic review and meta-analysis. Allergy 2015;70:1640–50.
27. Reed CC, Iglesia EGA, Commins SP, et al. Seasonal exacerbation of eosinophilic esophagitis histologic activity in adults and children implicates role of aeroallergens. Ann Allergy Asthma Immunol 2019;122:296–301.
28. May Maestas M, Perry KD, Smith K, et al. Food impactions in Eosinophilic esophagitis and acute exposures to fine particulate pollution. Allergy 2019;74:2529–30.
29. Nance D, Rappazzo KM, Jensen ET, et al. Increased risk of eosinophilic esophagitis with poor environmental quality as measured by the Environmental Quality Index. Dis Esophagus 2021;34.
30. Siebrasse A, Cotton CC, Gaber C, et al. Metal contamination in drinking water is associated with eosinophilic esophagitis, Digestive disease week. Gastroenterology 2022;162(7):S-538.
31. Jensen ET, Hoffman K, Cotton CC, et al. Assessment of proximity to swine farming operations as a risk factor for eosinophilic esophagitis. Gastroenterology 2017;152:S861.
32. Corder SR, Tappata M, Shaheen O, et al. Relationship Between Housing Components and Development of Eosinophilic Esophagitis. Dig Dis Sci 2020;65: 3624–30.
33. Doyle AD, Masuda MY, Pyon GC, et al. Detergent exposure induces epithelial barrier dysfunction and eosinophilic inflammation in the esophagus. Allergy 2022;78(1):192–201.
34. Taye B, Enquselassie F, Tsegaye A, et al. Is Helicobacter Pylori infection inversely associated with atopy? A systematic review and meta-analysis. Clin Exp Allergy 2015;45:882–90.

35. Shah SC, Tepler A, Peek RM Jr, et al. Association Between Helicobacter pylori Exposure and Decreased Odds of Eosinophilic Esophagitis-A Systematic Review and Meta-analysis. Clin Gastroenterol Hepatol 2019;17:2185–2198 e3.

36. Molina-Infante J, Gutierrez-Junquera C, Savarino E, et al. Helicobacter pylori infection does not protect against eosinophilic esophagitis: results from a large multicenter case-control study. Am J Gastroenterol 2018;113:972–9.

37. Uchida AM, Ro G, Garber JJ, et al. Prior hospital-based infection and risk of eosinophilic esophagitis in a Swedish nationwide case-control study. United European Gastroenterol J 2022;10:999–1007.

38. Benninger MS, Strohl M, Holy CE, et al. Prevalence of atopic disease in patients with eosinophilic esophagitis. Int Forum Allergy Rhinol 2017;7:757–62.

39. Gonzalez Cervera J, Arias A, Redondo-Gonzalez O, et al. Association between atopic manifestations and eosinophilic esophagitis: A systematic review and meta-analysis. Ann Allergy Asthma Immunol 2017;118:582–590 e2.

40. Guarnieri KM, Saba NK, Schwartz JT, et al. Food Allergy Characteristics Associated With Coexisting Eosinophilic Esophagitis in FARE Registry Participants. J Allergy Clin Immunol Pract 2023;11:1509–1521 e6.

41. Hill DA, Dudley JW, Spergel JM. The Prevalence of Eosinophilic Esophagitis in Pediatric Patients with IgE-Mediated Food Allergy. J Allergy Clin Immunol Pract 2017;5:369–75.

42. Mubanga M, Lundholm C, D'Onofrio BM, et al. Association of Early Life Exposure to Antibiotics With Risk of Atopic Dermatitis in Sweden. JAMA Netw Open 2021;4: e215245.

43. Muir AB, Benitez AJ, Dods K, et al. Microbiome and its impact on gastrointestinal atopy. Allergy 2016;71:1256–63.

44. Spechler SJ, Genta RM, Souza RF. Thoughts on the complex relationship between gastroesophageal reflux disease and eosinophilic esophagitis. Am J Gastroenterol 2007;102:1301–6.

45. Fan YC, Steele D, Kochar B, et al. Increased Prevalence of Esophageal Eosinophilia in Patients with Inflammatory Bowel Disease. Inflamm Intest Dis 2019;3: 180–6.

46. Limketkai BN, Shah SC, Hirano I, et al. Epidemiology and implications of concurrent diagnosis of eosinophilic oesophagitis and IBD based on a prospective population-based analysis. Gut 2019;68:2152–60.

47. Sonnenberg A, Turner KO, Genta RM. Comorbid Occurrence of Eosinophilic Esophagitis and Inflammatory Bowel Disease. Clin Gastroenterol Hepatol 2021; 19:613–615 e1.

48. Aloi M, D'Arcangelo G, Rossetti D, et al. Occurrence and Clinical Impact of Eosinophilic Esophagitis in a Large Cohort of Children With Inflammatory Bowel Disease. Inflamm Bowel Dis 2023;29:1057–64.

49. Eid R, Noonan E, Borish L, et al. High prevalence of gastrointestinal symptoms and undiagnosed eosino-philic esophagitis among allergic adults. J Allergy Clin Immunol Pract 2022;10:3325–3327 e1.

50. Moore H, Wechsler J, Frost C, et al. Comorbid Diagnosis of Eosinophilic Esophagitis and Inflammatory Bowel Disease in the Pediatric Population. J Pediatr Gastroenterol Nutr 2021;72:398–403.

51. Abraham JR, Persad R, Turner JM, et al. Gluten-free diet does not appear to induce endoscopic remission of eosinophilic esophagitis in children with coexistent celiac disease. Can J Gastroenterol 2012;26:521–4.

52. Ahmed OI, Qasem SA, Abdulsattar JA, et al. Esophageal eosinophilia in pediatric patients with celiac disease: is it a causal or an incidental association? J Pediatr Gastroenterol Nutr 2015;60:493–7.
53. Cristofori F, D'Abramo FS, Rutigliano V, et al. Esophageal Eosinophilia and Eosinophilic Esophagitis in Celiac Children: A Ten Year Prospective Observational Study. Nutrients 2021;13.
54. Leslie C, Mews C, Charles A, et al. Celiac disease and eosinophilic esophagitis: a true association. J Pediatr Gastroenterol Nutr 2010;50:397–9.
55. Ooi CY, Day AS, Jackson R, et al. Eosinophilic esophagitis in children with celiac disease. J Gastroenterol Hepatol 2008;23:1144–8.
56. Quaglietta L, Coccorullo P, Miele E, et al. Eosinophilic oesophagitis and coeliac disease: is there an association? Aliment Pharmacol Ther 2007;26:487–93.
57. Stewart MJ, Shaffer E, Urbanski SJ, et al. The association between celiac disease and eosinophilic esophagitis in children and adults. BMC Gastroenterol 2013; 13:96.
58. Thompson JS, Lebwohl B, Reilly NR, et al. Increased incidence of eosinophilic esophagitis in children and adults with celiac disease. J Clin Gastroenterol 2012;46:e6–11.
59. Verzegnassi F, Bua J, De Angelis P, et al. Eosinophilic oesophagitis and coeliac disease: is it just a casual association? Gut 2007;56:1029–30.
60. Dharmaraj R, Hagglund K, Lyons H. Eosinophilic esophagitis associated with celiac disease in children. BMC Res Notes 2015;8:263.
61. Hommeida S, Alsawas M, Murad MH, et al. The Association Between Celiac Disease and Eosinophilic Esophagitis: Mayo Experience and Meta-analysis of the Literature. J Pediatr Gastroenterol Nutr 2017;65:58–63.
62. Johnson JB, Boynton KK, Peterson KA. Co-occurrence of eosinophilic esophagitis and potential/probable celiac disease in an adult cohort: a possible association with implications for clinical practice. Dis Esophagus 2016;29:977–82.
63. Jensen ET, Eluri S, Lebwohl B, et al. Increased Risk of Esophageal Eosinophilia and Eosinophilic Esophagitis in Patients With Active Celiac Disease on Biopsy. Clin Gastroenterol Hepatol 2015;13:1426–31.

Clinical Evaluation of the Child with Eosinophilic Esophagitis

Maureen Bauer, MD[a],*, Nathalie Nguyen, MD[b],
Chris A. Liacouras, MD[c]

KEYWORDS

- Eosinophilic esophagitis • Pediatric eosinophilic esophagitis
- Transnasal endoscopy

KEY POINTS

- Clinical symptoms of eosinophilic esophagitis (EoE) vary based on age with feeding difficulties, vomiting, and/or abdominal pain as common presenting symptoms in children and with dysphagia and food impactions being more common in adolescents and adults.
- Histologic evidence of an eosinophil predominant esophageal inflammation is required for diagnosis. Less-invasive monitoring methods without the requirement for anesthesia such as transnasal endoscopy have emerged to monitor disease or response to therapies.
- First-line treatments for EoE include medications (proton pump inhibitors and swallowed topical steroids) dietary therapy and esophageal dilation. As esophageal dilation does not address underlying inflammation, it is not recommended as monotherapy in children.
- Dupilumab, a monoclonal antibody that blocks IL-4 receptor alpha, is approved for treatment of EoE in patients ≥12 years of age and ≥40 kg. At present, it is typically used in specific clinical scenarios.

INTRODUCTION

Eosinophilic esophagitis (EoE) is a chronic, immune/antigen-mediated disease characterized clinically by symptoms related to esophageal dysfunction and histologically

Funding: No funding sources were utilized.
[a] Department of Pediatric Allergy & Immunology, Gastrointestinal Eosinophilic Diseases Program, Children's Hospital Colorado, University of Colorado School of Medicine, 13123 East 16th Avenue, Box 518, Aurora, CO 80045, USA; [b] Department of Pediatric Gastroenterology, Hepatology and Nutrition, Gastrointestinal Eosinophilic Diseases Program, Digestive Health Institute, Children's Hospital Colorado, University of Colorado School of Medicine, 13123 East 16th Avenue, Box 518, Aurora, CO 80045, USA; [c] Department of Gastroenterology, Hepatology and Nutrition, Perelman School of Medicine, University of Pennsylvania, The Children's Hospital of Philadelphia, 3401 Civic Center Boulevard, Philadelphia, PA 19104, USA
* Corresponding author.
E-mail address: Maureen.Bauer@childrenscolorado.org

Immunol Allergy Clin N Am 44 (2024) 157–171
https://doi.org/10.1016/j.iac.2023.12.004
0889-8561/24/© 2023 Elsevier Inc. All rights reserved.

by eosinophil-predominant esophageal inflammation.[1] The prevalence in Western countries is estimated to be 0.4% among children and adults.[2] The pathophysiology is multifaceted and likely due to a complex interplay of genetic, heritable, environmental, and cellular factors.[3] Patients with EoE are more often male and frequently have comorbid atopic conditions, such as immunoglobulin E (IgE)-mediated food allergies, atopic dermatitis, asthma, and/or allergic rhinitis.[2]

Symptoms differ depending on age with feeding difficulties, vomiting and/or abdominal pain, and reflux symptoms as common presenting symptoms in children and with dysphagia and food impactions being more common in adolescents and adults.[2] In addition to clinical symptoms, pathologic evidence on esophageal biopsies is also required for diagnosis, defined as ≥ 15 eosinophils per high powered field in the esophageal mucosa after ruling out other causes of esophageal eosinophilia.[1,2] Previous diagnostic criteria for EoE required demonstrating persistent esophageal eosinophilia following treatment with high-dose proton pump inhibitor (PPI) therapy, theoretically ruling out gastroesophageal reflux disease (GERD).[1] However, more recent studies demonstrate that PPIs may treat EoE based on their anti-inflammatory properties in a subset of patients.[4] Therefore, guidelines for EoE were recently updated to list PPIs as a treatment option for EoE.[4] Complications of untreated EoE include malnutrition, feeding difficulties, esophageal stricture formation, and food impaction.[2] EoE is unfortunately rarely outgrown, and thus requires chronic treatment.[2]

EPIDEMIOLOGY

Since the initial descriptions of EoE as it is known today in the mid-1990s,[5] EoE has emerged from an initially rare disease to one that is increasing in incidence and prevalence[6–8] which seems to outpace increased knowledge about EoE.[9] A recent systematic review and meta-analysis identified a pooled prevalence rate of 22.7/100,000 persons with a higher prevalence in adults (43.4/100,000) than in children (29.5/100,000).[10] However, significant heterogeneity among included studies existed, particularly due to the difference in definition based on responsiveness to PPIs.[10] Prevalence of EoE also varies based on location as it is more commonly reported in North America, Western Europe, and Australia and less often reported in other areas of the world.[9]

EoE has a clear male predominance with a male-to-female ratio of nearly 3:1[11] and a strong familial pattern as evidenced by concordance of 58% in monozygotic twins.[12] However, a concordance of 36% in dizygotic twins and 2.4% in non-twin siblings[12] demonstrates the effects of genetic and environmental influences.[3] Additionally identified risk factors include genetic variants, cellular pathology (ie, impaired epithelial barrier), atopic status, and environmental factors such as cesarean birth and antibiotics.[3]

Children diagnosed with EoE are more likely to be White, non-Hispanic[11] and from English-speaking, socioeconomically advantaged neighborhoods.[13,14] However, as this is not the case in other atopic diseases, it is unclear if this reflects the true epidemiology of EoE or results from discrepant health care access and other barriers.[13]

CLINICAL SYMPTOMS

The clinical symptoms of EoE are due to esophageal dysfunction, vary according to patient age and can often be nonspecific such as abdominal pain and/or vomiting.[2] Food refusal, vomiting, and failure to thrive are common in the infant population. Vomiting, abdominal pain, heartburn, regurgitation, and feeding refusal/aversion are often reported in school age children with dysphagia, food impactions, and heartburn being more prevalent in older children, adolescent, and adult patients.[15,16] Patients often develop compensatory mechanisms such as avoiding certain foods with denser textures, taking smaller bites, chewing foods for a prolonged period and using sauces or liquids to lubricate food.[17] Clinical symptoms often do not correlate with histologic findings.[18]

EoE is frequently associated with other atopic diseases as 68% of patients also have another allergic disease such as rhinitis, asthma, and/or atopic dermatitis. In addition, other food allergies have been reported including oral allergy syndrome, urticaria, or diarrhea. Many patients also have a high frequency of aero-allergen sensitization and more than 50% have IgE-mediated food allergen sensitization. Allergic airway diseases often precede the development of EoE suggesting that the initial sensitization might take place in the airways.[19]

A few studies suggest that ethnicity may also impact presenting symptoms. Recent literature has demonstrated that pediatric Black patients are more likely to present with multiple atopic comorbidities and failure to thrive/poor growth while non-Black patients were more likely to present with abdominal pain.[20] Similarly, a recent retrospective chart review demonstrated that Black children when compared with White children were younger at diagnosis and at first dilation, arguing for greater disease severity at diagnosis.[13] However, these results have not been confirmed and may reflect discrepancies in access to care as opposed to inherent differences in symptomatology.[13]

Clinical scoring systems for EoE have been difficult to create. Owing to the differing clinical symptoms based on age, the Pediatric Eosinophilic Esophagitis System Score, the only validated outcome measure of pediatric patients with EoE, incorporates symptoms such as nausea and abdominal pain which differ from adult outcome measures that focus more on dysphagia.[21,22] A recently proposed Index of Severity for Eosinophilic Esophagitis for patients with known EoE incorporates 3 domains: symptoms, endoscopy, and histology to assess EoE as inactive, mild active, moderate active, or severe active.[22] Although specific symptoms are not specified due to the variance based on age, the severity is based on frequency (ie, weekly to multiple times/day) and complications such as malnutrition with body mass < 5% or decreased growth trajectory indicating severe disease.[22]

PHYSICAL EXAMINATION

There are no pathognomonic clinical examination findings that are diagnostic of EoE. In the pediatric population, particular attention to growth is needed as up to 30% of children have evidence of failure to thrive secondary to malnutrition.[23,24] As most patients with EoE will have comorbid conditions, it is also prudent to assess for evidence of atopic comorbidities on examination as their presence may impact management of EoE (discussed in more detail in the next section).[25]

ENDOSCOPIC FINDINGS

Esophagogastroduodenoscopy (EGD) with biopsy is required for the diagnosis of EoE.[26] In pediatrics, EGD is typically done under general anesthesia or conscious sedation. Although there are no pathognomonic endoscopic markers to make the diagnosis of EoE, several endoscopic findings have been associated with EoE including longitudinal furrows, edema, white exudate, esophageal rings, esophageal stricture or narrow caliber esophagus, and crepe paper mucosa. Longitudinal furrows, edema and exudate reflect acute inflammatory changes in the esophagus, whereas the features of esophageal rings, stricture and crepe paper mucosa reflect chronic fibrotic features. The Endoscopic Reference Score (EREFS Score) is a standardized assessment tool that provides a numerical score at the time of EGD to grade the presence and severity of endoscopic findings including Edema, Rings, Exudate, Furrows and Stricture.[27] The EREFS has been shown to correlate with histologic features in order to be used with histology as an outcome measure to assess treatment response.[28,29]

HISTOLOGIC FEATURES AND DIAGNOSTIC CRITERIA

The diagnosis of EoE requires both symptoms of esophageal dysfunction and histologic confirmation.[26] Esophageal mucosal biopsies are obtained from the esophagus at multiple levels for histologic evaluation. Normally, the esophagus is devoid of eosinophils. In EoE, esophageal eosinophilia is present in the esophageal mucosa (defined as $\geq$ 15 eosinophils per high powered field), but other histologic changes can also be seen in EoE including basal cell hyperplasia, rete peg elongation, lamina propria fibrosis, eosinophilic microabscesses, and dilated intercellular spaces.[26,30] The EoE Histologic Severity Score is a histologic scoring system that has been developed to provide a broad assessment of histologic features in addition to peak eosinophil count.[30,31] The histologic features are given a grade for degree of activity and stage for degree of the specimen involved.[30,31] This scoring system has been shown to correlate with peak eosinophil count.[30]

COMPLICATIONS OF EOSINOPHILIC ESOPHAGITIS

EoE is a chronic disease that requires long-term management.[2] The goal of treatment of EoE is to improve symptoms, quality of life, and prevent disease progression and potential complications. The delay in the diagnosis of EoE or untreated EoE can lead to remodeling of the esophagus and increase the risk for development of esophageal stricture.[32] One study noted that with each additional year of undiagnosed EoE, the risk of stricture increased by 9%.[33] Potential complications of EoE include esophageal strictures that may require endoscopic dilation and acute food impactions that may require urgent endoscopic removal. In the pediatric population, additional complications of untreated EoE include malnutrition/failure to thrive and persistent feeding difficulties.[2,34]

TREATMENT

Treatment of EoE includes medications (ie, PPI or swallowed topical corticosteroid [TCS]), dietary therapy, or esophageal dilation. Dupilumab, a monoclonal antibody, has been recently approved for patients $\geq$12 years and at least 40 kg.[35-37] Although some current guidelines recommend selecting one therapy among PPI therapy, TCS, and dietary therapy as an initial treatment, a significant number of clinicians continue to follow the recommendations adopted from the original guidelines that suggest initial therapy should utilize aggressive PPI therapy as a first-line treatment.[38,39] These guidelines were written before the approval of dupilumab which is the only FDA-approved therapy for EoE. Despite its FDA approval, currently most clinicians generally consider dupilumab as either a step up therapy for patients who fail other treatment options or as first-line therapy in specific clinical contexts (discussed in the next section).[40]

Multidisciplinary care in EoE has been associated with high patient satisfaction and high quality care.[41] In addition to a gastroenterologist and allergist, comprehensive multidisciplinary care in pediatric EoE may include a dietician and an occupational/speech therapist with an expertise in feeding dysfunction. Dieticians with an expertise in EoE are instrumental in implementation of dietary therapy and evaluation of potential nutritional deficiencies.[24] Similarly, feeding specialists can assist with maladaptive feeding behaviors commonly encountered in pediatric EoE.[42]

Proton Pump Inhibitors

PPIs are a class of medications commonly used in the treatment of GERD. In 2007, because GERD had been demonstrated to be a cause for esophageal eosinophilia, the original consensus guidelines for the definition of EoE recommended to rule out GERD with a trial of PPI.[26] If esophageal eosinophilia persisted despite PPI therapy, the etiology was then likely related to food antigens. There is substantial evidence that PPIs decrease esophageal eosinophilia in children, adolescents, and adults.[43] Patients with esophageal eosinophilia who respond to PPI have similar clinical, histologic, and molecular features as those with food-driven EoE.[43] Therefore, in 2018, consensus guidelines were updated to recommend that PPIs be considered a treatment of esophageal eosinophilia rather than part of the diagnostic criteria.[43] A meta-analysis including both pediatric and adult studies showed a 61% clinical response and 50% histologic response to PPI.[44]

Swallowed Topical Corticosteroids

TCSs have been shown to reduce esophageal eosinophilia in patients with EoE. They are typically administered either as an oral viscous budesonide slurry or by using a metered dose inhaler, such as fluticasone or ciclesonide that is swallowed. When topical steroids are given by metered dose inhaler, patients are instructed to puff the medication into their mouth and swallow rather than inhale it. When given as a viscous solution, patients mix the budesonide liquid with a mixing agent, typically sucralose (Splenda), to make a viscous slurry that they then swallow.[45] They then do not eat or drink for at least 30 minutes. These medications are provided to coat the esophagus to achieve a topical anti-inflammatory effect. The efficacy of TCS ranges from 60% to 90%.[46–52]

Esophageal Dilation

Esophageal dilation is an important therapeutic modality in the treatment of EoE.[53] It is used when patients have esophageal strictures or narrowing.[53,54] Esophageal dilation is typically performed via bougie dilators or through the scope balloon dilators.[53,55–57] Medications and diet elimination reduce or eliminate esophageal eosinophilia, whereas esophageal dilation does not, and is typically used concomitantly with medical therapy. Chest pain is the most common complication post esophageal dilation and complications of bleeding and perforation are exceedingly rare.[53,55–57]

Dietary Therapy

Dietary therapy was the first therapy utilized for EoE and has been shown to decrease esophageal eosinophilia. Standard elimination diets for EoE include elemental diets utilizing amino acid-based formulas, directed diets based on allergy testing, or empiric dietary elimination diets.[34] The elemental diet consists of exclusive feeding with an amino acid-based formula with high success rates, up to 90% in children and 94% in adults[58]; however, this diet is highly restrictive due to poor palatability, social implications, and often requiring placement of a gastrostomy tube, limiting its practical use for treatment of EoE.[34]

Targeted allergy testing-directed diets, include diets in which foods are removed based on positive IgE-mediated and/or atopy patch allergy testing. This method of food removal has generally been unsuccessful in identifying EoE triggers with an efficacy of approximately 45%.[39,58,59]

Empiric elimination diets consist of avoiding foods that are deemed the most likely cause of food allergens in EoE without allergy testing.[34] Commonly recommended empiric elimination diets are the 6-food elimination diet (6FED) consisting of avoidance of cow's milk, wheat, egg, soy, peanut/tree nuts and fish/shellfish; 4 food elimination diet (4FED) with avoidance of cow's milk, egg, wheat, and soy/legumes; 2 food elimination diet (2FED) with avoidance of cow's milk and wheat; and the 1 food elimination diet (1FED) with avoidance of cow's milk. In general, the more restrictive the diet the more successful with efficacy of the 6FED reported as high as 74%,[34] the 4FED up to 64%,[60] the 2FED 43%,[61] and 51% in the 1FED.[62] However, the success rate of empiric elimination diets varies greatly based on the study and, in general, is more efficacious in pediatric patients than adult patients.[58,59] For example, a recent prospective observational study of 41 pediatric patients who underwent the 1FED demonstrated histologic remission in 51%,[62] whereas a recent randomized multicenter open label trial of adult patients demonstrated success in 34% of patients on the 1FED.[63]

The decision about which diet to select is based on shared decision making between the physician and patient/family. Because a dissociation between clinical symptoms and histologic findings is common,[18] it is almost always essential that mucosal biopsies be obtained after introduction or change in any therapy or food elimination or reintroduction to assess histology and treatment success.[34] Therefore, extensive elimination diets are typically accompanied by an increased number of EGDs with subsequent food reintroductions. As the majority of patients with EoE only has 1 to 2 food triggers, beginning with a less restrictive diet may be a reasonable approach.[64] Molina-Infante et al. noted a 20% reduction in endoscopies when using a step-up approach as opposed to a step-down approach to dietary therapy.[61] Other factors such as the age, nutritional status and social/financial factors may weigh into the decision on selecting dietary therapy as a treatment and the specific type of diet.[34]

Biologic Therapy/Dupilumab

Dupilumab is a monoclonal antibody that blocks IL-4 receptor alpha, thereby inhibiting IL-4 and IL-13, two key cytokines in allergic inflammation. As of June 2022, dupilumab was approved for treatment of EoE in patients $\geq$12 years of age and $\geq$40 kg due to improvement in clinical symptoms, histologic inflammation and endoscopic findings in pivotal clinical studies.[35–37] More specifically, in the phase 3 randomized placebo-controlled trial by Dellon and colleagues, 60% of patients who received dupilumab 300 mg every week achieved histologic remission as defined by the primary endpoint ($\leq$6 eos/hpf) compared to 5% in the placebo group ($P < .001$) with a secondary endpoint (<15 eos/hpf) noted in?? 75% increase compared to placebo. Similar histologic findings were noted in every other week dosing. Clinical symptoms were assessed by the Dysphagia Symptom Questionnaire with a significant improvement in symptoms with weekly dupilumab dosing but not every other week dosing.[37] The most common reported adverse event in the dupilumab group was injection-site reactions with conjunctivitis being rare (a common adverse event of dupilumab in other conditions). Of note, a majority of this cohort (70%) had previously tried additional therapeutic options for EoE such as dietary therapy or TCS and 89% had a comorbid atopic condition.[37] Clinical trials in a younger age group for EoE are currently ongoing.[65]

Although dupilumab is the only FDA-approved therapy for EoE, there is strong evidence to support the initial use of either dietary therapy or medical therapy (PPI or TCS).[39] Given the refractory nature of the population studied that lead to dupilumab's approval and the cost of the therapy, the initial use of dupilumab in specific clinical scenarios may be reasonable. Following its approval, Aceves and colleagues suggested consideration of dupilumab as a first-line agent in patients with comorbid atopic conditions that would qualify them for dupilumab, or patients with a strong preference to avoid diet therapy or swallowed topical steroid therapy.[40] They otherwise recommended dupilumab as a step up therapy for patients who are difficult to treat, exhibiting poor growth, on severe dietary restriction/elemental diet, with significant esophageal stricture, refractory to current therapy, or experiencing adverse effects (ie, iatrogenic adrenal insufficiency) to current therapy.[40]

EVALUATION OF ATOPIC COMORBIDITIES

The majority of patients with EoE has atopic comorbidities with EoE being a late manifestation of the atopic march.[66] Evaluation of comorbidities is necessary in providing comprehensive care as their presence may impact management decisions regarding EoE. Patients with EoE have a higher prevalence of IgE-mediated food allergy than the general population (10%–60% compared with 8%[25,67–71]). Additionally, up to 4% of patients have biopsy-confirmed EoE to the same foods that they outgrew as an IgE-mediated allergy.[72] Oral immunotherapy (OIT), a treatment of IgE-mediated food allergy which is discussed further sections, has also been associated with development of EoE in 3% to 5% of cases.[73,74] Knowledge of comorbid IgE-mediated food allergies may impact the treatment decision for EoE. For example, if many common EoE trigger foods are already avoided, an empiric elimination may be less successful[34] or may render dietary therapy difficult due to concerns for further nutritional compromise and quality of life.[34]

Allergic rhinitis is similarly more common in pediatric patients with EoE compared with those without (30%–93%[25,71,75,76] compared with 13%[77]). Although food allergens are the culprit in the majority of patients with EoE, aeroallergens are a trigger in a small subset of patients[78] with rare case reports of patients with primarily aeroallergen-driven EoE.[79] Aeroallergen-exacerbated EoE has been noted to occur in approximately 3% to 5% of patients,[80,81] characterized by patients who respond to typical treatment for EoE but have clinical and histologic flares coinciding with the pollen season. In these cases, knowledge of their aeroallergen-sensitization profile may impact decisions on timing of endoscopies.[78] Pesek and colleagues noted that pediatric patients sensitized to perennial aeroallergens are less likely to respond to traditional therapies,[82] highlighting that perennial aeroallergen exposure may contribute to disease in treatment refractory patients. Therefore, a comprehensive evaluation and management of allergic rhinitis is essential in providing care to patients with EoE.

Atopic dermatitis and/or asthma both have an increased prevalence in EoE compared with the general population (20%–55% vs[25,71,76,83] 12.5%,[84] and 35%–60%[25,71,76] compared with 7%[85] respectively). Knowledge of the severity of any associated atopic disease may aid in the treatment decision of patients with EoE. As previously discussed, dupilumab is currently approved for EoE ($\geq$12 years of age and $\geq$40 kg),[37] atopic dermatitis ($\geq$6 months with moderate-to-severe atopic dermatitis whose disease is not controlled on topical therapies[86]), asthma (patients $\geq$ 6 years of age with moderate-to-severe eosinophilic asthma[87]), chronic rhinosinusitis with nasal polyposis ($\geq$18 years) and prurigo nodularis ($\geq$18 years).[40] Therefore, pediatric patients with EoE who also have comorbid atopic dermatitis and/or asthma which require biologic therapy may be ideal candidates for dupilumab.[40] Given dupilumab's approval in patients younger than 12 years for other atopic indications, patients with comorbid EoE < 12 years of age have received it with associated clinical and histologic remission.[88]

NOVEL METHODS FOR DISEASE MONITORING IN EOSINOPHILIC ESOPHAGITIS

Performing an EGD to obtain esophageal biopsies is an important tool in assessing response to treatment.[26] Of note, as already discussed, symptom improvement reported by patients do not correlate with histologic improvement.[89] As a result, EGD to obtain biopsies continues to be the gold standard to assess for response to treatment. In pediatrics, EGD is time consuming, expensive, and has risks associated with general anesthesia. To date, no serum biomarkers exist that accurately depict disease activity. This has led to the development of less invasive methods of disease monitoring, such as unsedated transnasal endoscopy (TNE).[90,91] In pediatrics, unsedated TNE uses an ultra-thin endoscope introduced through the nasal cavity and into the esophagus to perform endoscopic examination and obtain biopsies while utilizing distraction techniques such as virtual reality to improve tolerability of the procedure.[90,91] The advantages to unsedated TNE are that it requires no anesthesia or sedation, is lower cost, requires less time for recovery and less time away from school or work.[90] Innovative methods of disease monitoring that do not require endoscopy include the esophageal string test (EST), Cytosponge, and blind esophageal brushings.[92–96] These techniques obtain esophageal luminal effluents to assess the esophagus without the need for endoscopy. The EST is a weighted gelatin capsule with nylon string attached.[92,93] Patients swallow the capsule allowing the string to unwind in the esophagus and after 1 hour the string is retrieved and the esophageal eluate is evaluated.[92,93] The Cytosponge is a capsule that dissolves in the stomach after being swallowed and releases an expandable sponge.[94,95] The sponge is retrieved from the esophagus with the attached cord and as it is being retrieved, the sponge collects cells from the esophageal mucosa.[94,95] Blind esophageal brushings obtain esophageal effluent from a cytology brush inserted through a nasogastric tube.[96] Of these less-invasive techniques, TNE is the first to be used more commonly in clinical practice while the others are currently being used in the research setting. Finally, the disadvantages of these techniques include the inability of visualizing the esophagus or detecting the presence of an esophageal stricture, the possibility of not obtaining enough esophageal tissue, and the inability of evaluating the stomach and duodenum.

RELATIONSHIP WITH ORAL IMMUNOTHERAPY

EoE is a known side effect of OIT, a treatment for IgE-mediated food allergy, with a prevalence of biopsy-confirmed EoE after initiation in approximately 3% to 5% of cases.[73,74] Because gastrointestinal symptoms are a common occurrence after OIT, and patients are not routinely biopsied, prevalence estimates based on symptoms characteristic of EoE and/or biopsy findings may be as high as 8% to 14%.[74,97] EoE in the setting of OIT typically resolves with cessation of therapy[73]; however, there are cases of patients whose EoE persists despite discontinuation of OIT.[98]

Much is still unknown about the use of OIT and the development of EoE. Because patients with IgE-mediated food allergies are at increased risk of EoE,[97] and because patients are not routinely biopsied prior to initiation of OIT, it is not fully understood whether there is subclinical esophageal disease before the initiation of OIT. Thus, it may be impossible to know whether EoE would have developed irrespective of OIT or if EoE is induced by OIT. To further investigate this relationship, Wright and colleagues performed baseline endoscopies on 21 adults before initiation of peanut OIT and noted that while all patients were clinically asymptomatic (thus not meeting diagnostic criteria for EoE), 24% had $\geq$5 eos/hpf and 14% had $\geq$ 15 eos/hpf.[99] Those patients underwent serial endoscopic biopsies following dose escalation and on maintenance therapy, noted that OIT-induced or exacerbated esophageal eosinophilia was common in the treatment group, but was typically transient and not correlated with gastrointestinal symptoms.[100] However, one patient did develop EoE (dysphagia accompanied by esophageal eosinophilia) and OIT was discontinued.[100]

At present, the optimal management of EoE during OIT or pursuing OIT in patients with known EoE is unknown.[101] However, particularly given the recent approval of dupilumab, shared decision making may be a reasonable approach based on balancing the risks the patient/family attributes to IgE-mediated food allergy (ie, anaphylaxis, quality of life) compared with risks of management of EoE (ie, chronic disease requiring medications and endoscopic evaluation).[101]

SUMMARY

EoE is a chronic antigen-mediated condition of increasing prevalence characterized by clinical symptoms of esophageal dysfunction and histologic findings of eosinophilic predominant inflammation on endoscopy.[1] In the pediatric population, particular attention to symptoms such as chronic vomiting, feeding difficulties, abdominal pain, reflux, and poor growth is needed as characteristic symptoms such as dysphagia and food impaction are not common until adolescence/adulthood.[2] Recent advances in treatment of EoE include approval of dupilumab for treatment in patients $\geq$12 years of age and $\geq$40 kg.[37] Novel methods for monitoring EoE, such as the TNE and EST, allow for a less-invasive approach to assess responses to treatment without the requirement for general anesthesia, addressing a long-term need in EoE.[102] These less-invasive methods may additionally aid in future efforts to better understand questions such as the relationship between OIT and EoE, identification of patients at risk for fibrostenotic disease and optimal management of clinically symptomatic patients.

DISCLOSURE

M. Bauer, has served as a consult for Sanofi. N. Nguyen, has served as a consultant for Regeneron/Sanofi and is on the advisory board for EvoEndo. C.A. Liacouras, has served a speaker and consultant for Abbott; a speaker for Regeneron and a speaker for Sanofi.

REFERENCES

1. Liacouras CA, Furuta GT, Hirano I, et al. Eosinophilic esophagitis: updated consensus recommendations for children and adults. J Allergy Clin Immunol 2011;128(1):3–20, e26; quiz 21-22.

2. Furuta GT, Katzka DA. Eosinophilic esophagitis. N Engl J Med 2015;373(17): 1640–8.

3. O'Shea KM, Aceves SS, Dellon ES, et al. Pathophysiology of eosinophilic esophagitis. Gastroenterology 2018;154(2):333–45.

4. Dellon ES, Liacouras CA, Molina-Infante J, et al. Updated international consensus diagnostic criteria for eosinophilic esophagitis: proceedings of the AGREE conference. Gastroenterology 2018;155(4):1022–33.e1010.

5. Kelly KJ, Lazenby AJ, Rowe PC, et al. Eosinophilic esophagitis attributed to gastroesophageal reflux: improvement with an amino acid-based formula. Gastroenterology 1995;109(5):1503–12.

6. Straumann A, Simon HU. Eosinophilic esophagitis: escalating epidemiology? J Allergy Clin Immunol 2005;115(2):418–9.

7. Prasad GA, Alexander JA, Schleck CD, et al. Epidemiology of eosinophilic esophagitis over three decades in Olmsted County, Minnesota. Clin Gastroenterol Hepatol 2009;7(10):1055–61.

8. van Rhijn BD, Verheij J, Smout AJ, et al. Rapidly increasing incidence of eosinophilic esophagitis in a large cohort. Neuro Gastroenterol Motil 2013;25(1): 47–52.e45.

9. Dellon ES, Hirano I. Epidemiology and natural history of eosinophilic esophagitis. Gastroenterology 2018;154(2):319–32.e313.

10. Arias Á, Pérez-Martínez I, Tenías JM, et al. Systematic review with meta-analysis: the incidence and prevalence of eosinophilic oesophagitis in children and adults in population-based studies. Aliment Pharmacol Ther 2016;43(1):3–15.

11. Mansoor E, Cooper GS. The 2010-2015 Prevalence of eosinophilic esophagitis in the USA: a population-based study. Dig Dis Sci 2016;61(10):2928–34.

12. Alexander ES, Martin LJ, Collins MH, et al. Twin and family studies reveal strong environmental and weaker genetic cues explaining heritability of eosinophilic esophagitis. J Allergy Clin Immunol 2014;134(5):1084–92.e1081.

13. Mehta P, Pan Z, Zhou W, et al. Examining disparities in pediatric eosinophilic esophagitis. J Allergy Clin Immunol Pract 2023;11(9):2855–9.

14. McGowan EC, Keller JP, Dellon ES, et al. Prevalence and geographic distribution of pediatric eosinophilic esophagitis in the 2012 US Medicaid population. J Allergy Clin Immunol Pract 2020;8(8):2796–8.e2794.

15. Barni S, Arasi S, Mastrorilli C, et al. Pediatric eosinophilic esophagitis: a review for the clinician. Ital J Pediatr 2021;47(1):230.

16. Spergel JM, Brown-Whitehorn TA, Muir A, et al. Medical algorithm: Diagnosis and treatment of eosinophilic esophagitis in children. Allergy 2020;75(6): 1522–4.

17. Hirano I, Furuta GT. Approaches and challenges to management of pediatric and adult patients with eosinophilic esophagitis. Gastroenterology 2020; 158(4):840–51.

18. Pentiuk S, Putnam PE, Collins MH, et al. Dissociation between symptoms and histological severity in pediatric eosinophilic esophagitis. J Pediatr Gastroenterol Nutr 2009;48(2):152–60.

19. Spergel JM, Brown-Whitehorn TF, Beausoleil JL, et al. 14 years of eosinophilic esophagitis: clinical features and prognosis. J Pediatr Gastroenterol Nutr 2009;48(1):30–6.

20. Edwards-Salmon S, Moraczewski J, Offerle T, et al. Comparing Eosinophilic Esophagitis in a Black and Non-Black Pediatric Cohort. J Pediatr Gastroenterol Nutr 2022;75(4):485–90.

21. Collins MH, Martin LJ, Wen T, et al. Eosinophilic esophagitis histology remission score: significant relations to measures of disease activity and symptoms. J Pediatr Gastroenterol Nutr 2020;70(5):598–603.

22. Dellon ES, Khoury P, Muir AB, et al. A clinical severity index for eosinophilic esophagitis: development, consensus, and future directions. Gastroenterology 2022;163(1):59–76.

23. Chehade M, Sampson HA, Morotti RA, et al. Esophageal subepithelial fibrosis in children with eosinophilic esophagitis. J Pediatr Gastroenterol Nutr 2007;45(3): 319–28.
24. Groetch M, Venter C, Skypala I, et al. Dietary therapy and nutrition management of eosinophilic esophagitis: a work group report of the american academy of allergy, asthma, and immunology. J Allergy Clin Immunol Pract 2017;5(2): 312–24.e329.
25. Cianferoni A, Warren CM, Brown-Whitehorn T, et al. Eosinophilic esophagitis and allergic comorbidities in a US-population-based study. Allergy 2020;75(6): 1466–9.
26. Furuta GT, Liacouras CA, Collins MH, et al. Eosinophilic esophagitis in children and adults: a systematic review and consensus recommendations for diagnosis and treatment. Gastroenterology 2007;133(4):1342–63.
27. Hirano I, Moy N, Heckman MG, et al. Endoscopic assessment of the oesophageal features of eosinophilic oesophagitis: validation of a novel classification and grading system. Gut 2013;62(4):489–95.
28. Wechsler JB, Bolton SM, Amsden K, et al. Eosinophilic esophagitis reference score accurately identifies disease activity and treatment effects in children. Clin Gastroenterol Hepatol 2018;16(7):1056–63.
29. Hiremath G, Correa H, Acra S, et al. Correlation of endoscopic signs and mucosal alterations in children with eosinophilic esophagitis. Gastrointest Endosc 2020;91(4):785–794 e781.
30. Collins MH, Martin LJ, Alexander ES, et al. Newly developed and validated eosinophilic esophagitis histology scoring system and evidence that it outperforms peak eosinophil count for disease diagnosis and monitoring. Dis Esophagus 2017;30(3):1–8.
31. Warners MJ, Ambarus CA, Bredenoord AJ, et al. Reliability of histologic assessment in patients with eosinophilic oesophagitis. Aliment Pharmacol Ther 2018; 47(7):940–50.
32. Warners MJ, Oude Nijhuis RAB, de Wijkerslooth LRH, et al. The natural course of eosinophilic esophagitis and long-term consequences of undiagnosed disease in a large cohort. Am J Gastroenterol 2018;113(6):836–44.
33. Schoepfer AM, Safroneeva E, Bussmann C, et al. Delay in diagnosis of eosinophilic esophagitis increases risk for stricture formation in a time-dependent manner. Gastroenterology 2013;145(6):1230–6, e1231-1232.
34. Chehade M, Brown S. Elimination diets for eosinophilic esophagitis: making the best choice. Expet Rev Clin Immunol 2020;16(7):679–87.
35. Al-Horani RA, Chiles R. First therapeutic approval for eosinophilic esophagitis. Gastroenterol Insights 2022;13(3):238–44.
36. Hirano I, Dellon ES, Hamilton JD, et al. Efficacy of dupilumab in a phase 2 randomized trial of adults with active eosinophilic esophagitis. Gastroenterology 2020;158(1):111–22.e110.
37. Dellon ES, Rothenberg ME, Collins MH, et al. Dupilumab in adults and adolescents with eosinophilic esophagitis. N Engl J Med 2022;387(25):2317–30.
38. Lucendo AJ, Molina-Infante J, Arias Á, et al. Guidelines on eosinophilic esophagitis: evidence-based statements and recommendations for diagnosis and management in children and adults. United European Gastroenterol J 2017; 5(3):335–58.
39. Hirano I, Chan ES, Rank MA, et al. AGA institute and the joint task force on allergy-immunology practice parameters clinical guidelines for the management of eosinophilic esophagitis. Gastroenterology 2020;158(6):1776–86.

40. Aceves SS, Dellon ES, Greenhawt M, et al. Clinical guidance for the use of dupilumab in eosinophilic esophagitis: a yardstick. Ann Allergy Asthma Immunol 2023;130(3):371–8.

41. Sauer BG, West A, McGowan EC. Multidisciplinary eosinophilic esophagitis care: a model for comprehensive patient-centered care through shared decision making between gastroenterology, allergy, and nutrition. Clin Gastroenterol Hepatol 2021;19(11):2226–9.

42. Mehta P, Furuta GT, Brennan T, et al. Nutritional state and feeding behaviors of children with eosinophilic esophagitis and gastroesophageal reflux disease. J Pediatr Gastroenterol Nutr 2018;66(4):603–8.

43. Dellon ES, Liacouras CA, Molina-Infante J, et al. Updated international consensus diagnostic criteria for eosinophilic esophagitis: Proceedings of the AGREE conference. Gastroenterology 2018;155(4):1022–33, e10.

44. Lucendo AJ, Arias A, Molina-Infante J. Efficacy of proton pump inhibitor drugs for inducing clinical and histologic remission in patients with symptomatic esophageal eosinophilia: a systematic review and meta-analysis. Clin Gastroenterol Hepatol 2016;14(1):13–22 e11.

45. Aceves SS, Dohil R, Newbury RO, et al. Topical viscous budesonide suspension for treatment of eosinophilic esophagitis. J Allergy Clin Immunol 2005;116(3):705–6.

46. Konikoff MR, Noel RJ, Blanchard C, et al. A randomized, double-blind, placebo-controlled trial of fluticasone propionate for pediatric eosinophilic esophagitis. Gastroenterology 2006;131(5):1381–91.

47. Aceves SS, Bastian JF, Newbury RO, et al. Oral viscous budesonide: a potential new therapy for eosinophilic esophagitis in children. Am J Gastroenterol 2007;102(10):2271–9, quiz 2280.

48. Dohil R, Newbury R, Fox L, et al. Oral viscous budesonide is effective in children with eosinophilic esophagitis in a randomized, placebo-controlled trial. Gastroenterology 2010;139(2):418–29.

49. Straumann A, Conus S, Degen L, et al. Budesonide is effective in adolescent and adult patients with active eosinophilic esophagitis. Gastroenterology 2010;139(5):1526–37, 1537 e1521.

50. Gupta SK, Vitanza JM, Collins MH. Efficacy and safety of oral budesonide suspension in pediatric patients with eosinophilic esophagitis. Clin Gastroenterol Hepatol 2015;13(1):66–76 e63.

51. Dellon ES, Woosley JT, Arrington A, et al. Efficacy of budesonide vs fluticasone for initial treatment of eosinophilic esophagitis in a randomized controlled trial. Gastroenterology 2019;157(1):65–73 e65.

52. Dellon ES, Lucendo AJ, Schlag C, et al. Fluticasone propionate orally disintegrating tablet (APT-1011) for eosinophilic esophagitis: randomized controlled trial. Clin Gastroenterol Hepatol 2022;20(11):2485–2494 e2415.

53. Richter JE. Esophageal dilation in eosinophilic esophagitis. Best Pract Res Clin Gastroenterol 2015;29(5):815–28.

54. Gentile N, Katzka D, Ravi K, et al. Oesophageal narrowing is common and frequently under-appreciated at endoscopy in patients with oesophageal eosinophilia. Aliment Pharmacol Ther 2014;40(11–12):1333–40.

55. Runge TM, Eluri S, Cotton CC, et al. Outcomes of esophageal dilation in eosinophilic esophagitis: safety, efficacy, and persistence of the fibrostenotic phenotype. Am J Gastroenterol 2016;111(2):206–13.

56. Menard-Katcher C, Furuta GT, Kramer RE. Dilation of pediatric eosinophilic esophagitis: adverse events and short-term outcomes. J Pediatr Gastroenterol Nutr 2017;64(5):701–6.
57. Dougherty M, Runge TM, Eluri S, et al. Esophageal dilation with either bougie or balloon technique as a treatment for eosinophilic esophagitis: a systematic review and meta-analysis. Gastrointest Endosc 2017;86(4):581–591 e583.
58. Arias A, González-Cervera J, Tenias JM, et al. Efficacy of dietary interventions for inducing histologic remission in patients with eosinophilic esophagitis: a systematic review and meta-analysis. Gastroenterology 2014;146(7):1639–48.
59. Mayerhofer C, Kavallar AM, Aldrian D, et al. Efficacy of elimination diets in eosinophilic esophagitis: a systematic review and meta-analysis. Clin Gastroenterol Hepatol 2023;21(9):2197–210.e2193.
60. Kagalwalla AF, Wechsler JB, Amsden K, et al. Efficacy of a 4-food elimination diet for children with eosinophilic esophagitis. Clin Gastroenterol Hepatol 2017;15(11):1698–707.e1697.
61. Molina-Infante J, Arias Á, Alcedo J, et al. Step-up empiric elimination diet for pediatric and adult eosinophilic esophagitis: The 2-4-6 study. J Allergy Clin Immunol 2018;141(4):1365–72.
62. Wechsler JB, Schwartz S, Arva NC, et al. A single-food milk elimination diet is effective for treatment of eosinophilic esophagitis in children. Clin Gastroenterol Hepatol 2022;20(8):1748–56.e1711.
63. Kliewer KL, Gonsalves N, Dellon ES, et al. One-food versus six-food elimination diet therapy for the treatment of eosinophilic oesophagitis: a multicentre, randomised, open-label trial. Lancet Gastroenterol Hepatol 2023;8(5):408–21.
64. Spergel J, Aceves SS. Allergic components of eosinophilic esophagitis. J Allergy Clin Immunol 2018;142(1):1–8.
65. Available at: clinicaltrials.gov/study/NCT04394351.
66. Hill DA, Grundmeier RW, Ramos M, et al. Eosinophilic Esophagitis Is a Late Manifestation of the Allergic March. J Allergy Clin Immunol Pract 2018;6(5):1528–33.
67. Guajardo JR, Plotnick LM, Fende JM, et al. Eosinophil-associated gastrointestinal disorders: a world-wide-web based registry. J Pediatr 2002;141(4):576–81.
68. Liacouras CA, Spergel JM, Ruchelli E, et al. Eosinophilic esophagitis: a 10-year experience in 381 children. Clin Gastroenterol Hepatol 2005;3(12):1198–206.
69. Jyonouchi S, Brown-Whitehorn TA, Spergel JM. Association of eosinophilic gastrointestinal disorders with other atopic disorders. Immunol Allergy Clin 2009;29(1):85–97, x.
70. Gupta RS, Springston EE, Warrier MR, et al. The prevalence, severity, and distribution of childhood food allergy in the United States. Pediatrics 2011;128(1):e9–17.
71. Capucilli P, Cianferoni A, Grundmeier RW, et al. Comparison of comorbid diagnoses in children with and without eosinophilic esophagitis in a large population. Ann Allergy Asthma Immunol 2018;121(6):711–6.
72. Maggadottir SM, Hill DA, Ruymann K, et al. Resolution of acute IgE-mediated allergy with development of eosinophilic esophagitis triggered by the same food. J Allergy Clin Immunol 2014;133(5):1487–9, 1489.e1481.
73. Lucendo AJ, Arias A, Tenias JM. Relation between eosinophilic esophagitis and oral immunotherapy for food allergy: a systematic review with meta-analysis. Ann Allergy Asthma Immunol 2014;113(6):624–9.

74. Petroni D, Spergel JM. Eosinophilic esophagitis and symptoms possibly related to eosinophilic esophagitis in oral immunotherapy. Ann Allergy Asthma Immunol 2018;120(3):237–40.e234.
75. Assa'ad AH, Putnam PE, Collins MH, et al. Pediatric patients with eosinophilic esophagitis: an 8-year follow-up. J Allergy Clin Immunol 2007;119(3):731–8.
76. Sugnanam KK, Collins JT, Smith PK, et al. Dichotomy of food and inhalant allergen sensitization in eosinophilic esophagitis. Allergy 2007;62(11):1257–60.
77. Dykewicz MS, Wallace DV, Amrol DJ, et al. Rhinitis 2020: A practice parameter update. J Allergy Clin Immunol 2020;146(4):721–67.
78. Egan M, Atkins D. What is the relationship between eosinophilic esophagitis (EOE) and aeroallergens? implications for allergen immunotherapy. Curr Allergy Asthma Rep 2018;18(8):43.
79. Fogg MI, Ruchelli E, Spergel JM. Pollen and eosinophilic esophagitis. J Allergy Clin Immunol 2003;112(4):796–7.
80. Ram G, Lee J, Ott M, et al. Seasonal exacerbation of esophageal eosinophilia in children with eosinophilic esophagitis and allergic rhinitis. Ann Allergy Asthma Immunol 2015;115(3):224–8.e221.
81. Reed CC, Iglesia EGA, Commins SP, et al. Seasonal exacerbation of eosinophilic esophagitis histologic activity in adults and children implicates role of aeroallergens. Ann Allergy Asthma Immunol 2019;122(3):296–301.
82. Pesek RD, Rettiganti M, O'Brien E, et al. Effects of allergen sensitization on response to therapy in children with eosinophilic esophagitis. Ann Allergy Asthma Immunol 2017;119(2):177–83.
83. Brown-Whitehorn TF, Spergel JM. The link between allergies and eosinophilic esophagitis: implications for management strategies. Expet Rev Clin Immunol 2010;6(1):101–9.
84. Jackson KD, Howie LD, Akinbami LJ. Trends in allergic conditions among children: United States, 1997-2011. NCHS Data Brief 2013;121:1–8.
85. Pate CA, Zahran HS, Malilay J, et al. The shifting prevalence of asthma and allergic disease in US children. Ann Allergy Asthma Immunol 2022;129(4):481–9.
86. Paller AS, Simpson EL, Siegfried EC, et al. Dupilumab in children aged 6 months to younger than 6 years with uncontrolled atopic dermatitis: a randomised, double-blind, placebo-controlled, phase 3 trial. Lancet 2022;400(10356):908–19.
87. Bacharier LB, Maspero JF, Katelaris CH, et al. Dupilumab in Children with Uncontrolled Moderate-to-Severe Asthma. N Engl J Med 2021;385(24):2230–40.
88. Spergel BL, Ruffner MA, Godwin BC, et al. Improvement in eosinophilic esophagitis when using dupilumab for other indications or compassionate use. Ann Allergy Asthma Immunol 2022;128(5):589–93.
89. Safroneeva E, Straumann A, Coslovsky M, et al. Symptoms have modest accuracy in detecting endoscopic and histologic remission in adults with eosinophilic esophagitis. Gastroenterology 2016;150(3):581–590 e584.
90. Nguyen N, Lavery WJ, Capocelli KE, et al. Transnasal endoscopy in unsedated children with eosinophilic esophagitis using virtual reality video goggles. Clin Gastroenterol Hepatol 2019;17(12):2455–62.
91. Friedlander JA, DeBoer EM, Soden JS, et al. Unsedated transnasal esophagoscopy for monitoring therapy in pediatric eosinophilic esophagitis. Gastrointest Endosc 2016;83(2):299–306 e291.

92. Furuta GT, Kagalwalla AF, Lee JJ, et al. The oesophageal string test: a novel, minimally invasive method measures mucosal inflammation in eosinophilic oeso-phagitis. Gut 2013;62(10):1395–405.
93. Ackerman SJ, Kagalwalla AF, Hirano I, et al. One-hour esophageal string test: a nonendoscopic minimally invasive test that accurately detects disease activity in eosinophilic esophagitis. Am J Gastroenterol 2019;114(10):1614–25.
94. Katzka DA, Geno DM, Ravi A, et al. Accuracy, safety, and tolerability of tissue collection by Cytosponge vs endoscopy for evaluation of eosinophilic esopha-gitis. Clin Gastroenterol Hepatol 2015;13(1):77–83 e72.
95. Katzka DA, Smyrk TC, Alexander JA, et al. Accuracy and safety of the cyto-sponge for assessing histologic activity in eosinophilic esophagitis: a two-center study. Am J Gastroenterol 2017;112(10):1538–44.
96. Smadi Y, Deb C, Bornstein J, et al. Blind esophageal brushing offers a safe and accurate method to monitor inflammation in children and young adults with eosinophilic esophagitis. Dis Esophagus 2018;31(12). https://doi.org/10.1093/dote/doy056.
97. Hill DA, Dudley JW, Spergel JM. The prevalence of eosinophilic esophagitis in pediatric patients with ige-mediated food allergy. J Allergy Clin Immunol Pract 2017;5(2):369–75.
98. Hamant L, Freeman C, Garg S, et al. Eosinophilic esophagitis may persist after discontinuation of oral immunotherapy. Ann Allergy Asthma Immunol 2021; 126(3):299–302.
99. Wright BL, Fernandez-Becker NQ, Kambham N, et al. Baseline gastrointestinal eosinophilia is common in oral immunotherapy subjects with ige-mediated pea-nut allergy. Front Immunol 2018;9:2624.
100. Wright BL, Fernandez-Becker NQ, Kambham N, et al. Gastrointestinal eosino-phil responses in a longitudinal, randomized trial of peanut oral immunotherapy. Clin Gastroenterol Hepatol 2021;19(6):1151–9.e1114.
101. Chu DK, Spergel JM, Vickery BP. Management of eosinophilic esophagitis dur-ing oral immunotherapy. J Allergy Clin Immunol Pract 2021;9(9):3282–7.
102. Nguyen N, Mark J, Furuta GT. Emerging role of transnasal endoscopy in chil-dren and adults. Clin Gastroenterol Hepatol 2022;20(3):501–4.

Recognition and Management of Feeding Dysfunction in the Pediatric Patient with Eosinophilic Esophagitis

Angela M. Haas, MA, CCC-SLP[a],*, Rebecca J. Doidge, MS, CCC-SLP[a],
Girish Hiremath, MD, MPH[b]

KEYWORDS

- Feeding dysfunction • Dysphagia • Eosinophilic esophagitis • Food refusal
- Gagging • Vomiting • Compensatory strategies
- Maladaptive learned feeding difficulties

KEY POINTS

- Signs and symptoms of feeding dysfunction in children with EGIDs may present differently at different developmental stages and may change over time.
- Feeding dysfunction often persists after resolution of underlying esophageal inflammation.
- Feeding specialists play a significant role in the treatment of the pediatric patient with EGIDS: addressing challenges with expanding volume of intake, expanding diet variety and textures, facilitating compensatory strategies, improving medication acceptance, and reducing maladaptive feeding behaviors.

CLINICAL PRESENTATION OF FEEDING DYSFUNCTION IN CHILDREN WITH EOSINOPHILIC GASTROINTESTINAL DISORDERS

Eosinophilic gastrointestinal disorders (EGIDs) are a group of chronic, immune-mediated gastrointestinal (GI) conditions characterized by GI symptoms and pathologic infiltration of the eosinophils in specific locations within the GI tract in the absence of other causes of eosinophilia. Feeding dysfunction (FD) is the presenting complaint in almost half of children who eventually receive a diagnosis of eosinophilic esophagitis

[a] Department of Speech Language Pathology, Children's Hospital Colorado, Anschutz Medical Campus, 13123 East 16th Avenue, B030, Aurora, CO 80045, USA; [b] Department of Pediatrics, Monroe Carell Jr. Children's Hospital at Vanderbilt, Vanderbilt University, Gastroenterology, Hepatology and Nutrition, 2200 Children's Way, Nashville, TN 37232, USA
* Corresponding author. 13123 East 16th Avenue, B030, Aurora, CO 80045.
E-mail address: Angela.Haas@childrenscolorado.org

Immunol Allergy Clin N Am 44 (2024) 173–184
https://doi.org/10.1016/j.iac.2023.12.005
0889-8561/24/© 2024 Elsevier Inc. All rights reserved.
immunology.theclinics.com

(EoE). A feeding and swallowing specialist is often the first contact for children with feeding difficulties. FD may affect many aspects of a child's health, development, growth, nutrition, and overall well-being. No other activity of daily living consumes more time, attention, and energy in the life of a family than feeding and eating.[1] Food refusal, esophageal dysphagia, abdominal pain, loss of appetite, maladaptive learned feeding behaviors, reduced volume, and reduced variety of intake are common complaints associated with EGIDs in children.[2–9] Accurate diagnosis of EGID is frequently missed because many of its features parallel other GI diseases.[10] Gastroenterologists, allergists, feeding and swallowing specialists, dietitians, psychologists, and social workers are now collaborating to provide integrated comprehensive care for optimal diagnosis and treatment of children with EoE/EGIDs. In the general population, feeding difficulties are present in 25% of typically developing children and in 75% to 80% of children with developmental disabilities.[10–12] Although prevalence numbers for feeding issues in children with EGIDs are unknown, studies of EoE specifically place the prevalence at 16%, with the actual number suspected to be nearly double.[13]

There is a developmental continuum for the acquisition of feeding skills, which include motor skills, sensory systems, behavioral/emotional components, and communication.[14,15] With increasing experience in working with children with EGIDs, it has been recognized that feeding difficulties are common in children and may be associated with disruption of the typical developmental feeding continuum. This disruption can manifest in a variety of ways depending on the age of the child, the duration of the disease, and the unique family or social situation. Knowledge of the normal acquisition of feeding skills is critical to interpret the impact of the disease and plan appropriate intervention.

SYMPTOMS SUGGESTIVE OF FEEDING DYSFUNCTION

Frequently cited symptoms of EoE are: vomiting, abdominal pain, and dysphagia.[2–7,13] Symptoms promoting referral and evaluation have been grouped by age: vomiting and food refusal in infants and toddlers; coughing, abdominal pain, texture preferences, and vomiting in preschool and school-aged children; and abdominal pain, loss of appetite, coughing, throat clearing, food stuck sensation, and dysphagia in older children.[4,6,7,16] All age groups can exhibit maladaptive learned feeding behaviors, ranging from delayed texture advancement for age,[5] oral motor skill delay, altered oral sensory processing, food and texture selectivity, and prolonged mealtimes. Interoceptive differences and other comorbidities can also negatively impact the development of feeding skills and feeding/mealtime behavior (**Fig. 1**).[4,17]

Dysphagia

Swallow function is typically described as having three distinct phases: oral, pharyngeal, and esophageal.[15,18,19] The type of swallow dysfunction most associated with esophageal disease is intermittent esophageal dysphagia followed by oral phase dysphagia. Esophageal dysphagia is characterized by food impaction or the sensation of food "getting stuck."[20] This difficulty is in contrast to pharyngeal dysphagia, which is related to aspiration, laryngeal penetration, or compromised airway protection. Pharyngeal dysphagia is not commonly associated or reported in children. Management of food impaction, pharmacologic interventions, and esophageal dilation are often used for esophageal narrowing or strictures. A characteristic of children with EoE is avoidance of solid foods or higher textured foods, presumably a result of altered ability to pass the food comfortably through the esophagus. Prolonged mealtimes secondary to the use of compensatory strategies (liquid washes, small bites, prolonged chewing) is a

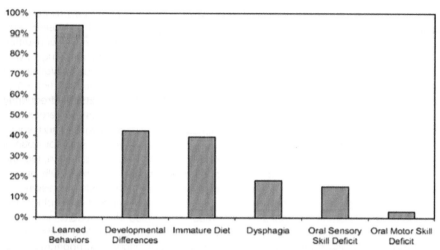

Fig. 1. Types of feeding dysfunction found in children with EoE.[13] (*Data from* Menard-Katcher C, Henry M, Furuta GT, Atkins D, Maune NC, Haas AM. Significance of feeding dysfunction in eosinophilic esophagitis. World J Gastroenterol. 2014 Aug 21;20(31):11019-22. https://doi.org/10.3748/wjg.v20.i31.11019. PMID: 25152606; PMCID: PMC4138483. https://www.ncbi.nlm.nih.gov/pmc/articles/PMC4138483/?report=reader).

feature often seen in toddlers, school-aged children, and teenagers because of esophageal dysphagia.[17] In some children who are refractory to feeding treatment, the question of esophageal dysphagia and esophageal remodeling may be a factor. Oral phase dysphagia, characterized by oral motor dysfunction, is less likely than oral motor immaturity.[5] Oral and pharyngeal dysphagia may be present in children who have concomitant neurologic and/or neuromotor disease, such as cerebral palsy.

Gagging, vomiting, and coughing
A child may gag and vomit for a variety of reasons. It is important to differentiate between gagging and choking, because caregivers often use these terms interchangeably. The gag response is a protective reflex, reflecting the sensation that a bolus is too big to be swallowed.[15] Gagging can also be caused by nausea or related to other GI disorders, such as gastroesophageal reflux. For a child who has a history of frequent vomiting, gagging may be more easily elicited and may more readily trigger vomiting. Gagging may occur secondary to altered oral motor and/or oral sensory skills. It may also be a learned response, as a strategy to avoid eating. Determining the cause of gagging and vomiting is critical to planning appropriate feeding treatment. Coughing may occur in response to the sensation of food sticking. Additionally, oral, pharyngeal, and esophageal discomfort may result in persistent coughing and throat clearing; often ignored by the pediatric patient and family given its subtle manifestation and commonality of occurrence.

Learned Behaviors and Food Refusal
Eating is a learned behavior with a predictable developmental sequence in the healthy child. When this sequence is interrupted by illness, discomfort, or environmental stressors, it can lead to altered patterns of mealtime behavior for the child and the caregiver. Operant and classical conditioning influence not only the variety of foods consumed but also the behaviors associated with mealtimes. A child who experiences

cycles of hunger, successful eating, satiety, and comfort is reinforced to continue eating. This experience is also rewarding and satisfying to the caregiver. Conversely, a child who repeatedly experiences hunger, followed by pain or discomfort with eating is reinforced to avoid eating. This experience is frustrating, confusing, and unsatisfying to the caregiver; and often results in well-intended, but ultimately unsuccessful altered feeding practices on the part of the caregiver in an effort to feed their child.[1,21,22] The child, in an effort to avoid pain, engages in avoidant, altered, and ultimately frustrating feeding behaviors, which combine to reinforce a cycle of unsuccessful and highly stressful feeding experiences, often several times a day. Maladaptive learned feeding behaviors often persist in children with EoE after they have been successfully treated pharmacologically, with diet elimination, or both. This is confusing to providers and caregivers alike, because the underlying cause of the disease has been addressed, yet the feeding difficulties remain, requiring skilled feeding treatment to improve.

Maladaptive learned FD in children with EoE commonly manifest as food refusal, grazing behaviors (small frequent snacks vs meals throughout the day), a need for distractions during mealtimes, preference for brand-specific foods, eating alone versus with family/peers, use of and persistence of compensatory strategies, and hyperfocus on preferred foods at the exclusion of others (**Table 1**).

Oral Motor

The sequence for the development of mature oral motor skills occurs between birth and 24 months of age.[14] There are critical windows in the developmental continuum related to the sensory and motor aspects of learning to eat, when the child's maturation and opportunities to learn a new skill coincide. If the opportunities to learn are not there at the same time, or the child does not experience feeding during a particular portion of the developmental sequence, it can become more difficult for the child to learn the skill at a later date.[23] Children who have EoE/EGIDs may not have had well-aligned maturation and opportunities to learn in terms of feeding and eating.

Table 1 Prevalence of learned feeding dysfunctions[13]	
Learned Feeding Dysfunction	**% of Patients**
Low variety intake	90.9
Food refusal	87.9
Requires prompting to eat	87.9
Poor acceptance of new foods	84.8
Low volume of intake	81.8
Unstructured mealtimes	81.8
Inconsistent patterns of eating	78.8
Grazing	78.8
Easily distracted from eating	60.6
Prolonged feeding times	57.6
Holding food in mouth	27.3
Spitting food	27.3

(*Data from* Menard-Katcher C, Henry M, Furuta GT, Atkins D, Maune NC, Haas AM. Significance of feeding dysfunction in eosinophilic esophagitis. World J Gastroenterol. 2014 Aug 21;20(31):11019-22. https://doi.org/10.3748/wjg.v20.i31.11019. PMID: 25152606; PMCID: PMC4138483. https://www.ncbi.nlm.nih.gov/pmc/articles/PMC4138483/?report=reader).

The influence of the disease on this process can be dramatic in that oral motor skill development may be interrupted because of conditioned food refusal because of discomfort or pain. In these cases, children may not progress their diet to include foods that require advanced oral motor skills, resulting in an immature oral motor skill set. Treatment itself may require children to be on a liquid elemental diet or significantly restrict the range of foods or textures, with a similar impact on skill development. These children present with issues of oral motor immaturity rather than oral motor dysfunction. Children may also have true oral motor dysfunction related to altered tone, strength, or coordination with coexisting diagnoses, such as cerebral palsy or Down syndrome.

Sensory Processing and Development

Oral sensory development is not as easily observed and measured as oral motor development. It is more reliant on children's behavior to assess. As part of successful feeding, children must have appropriate perception of tactile input and the ability to adaptively respond.[15] The motor system is reliant on the sensory system to supply accurate information regarding food properties for the most efficient motor response. Oral sensory dysfunction may present as food refusal, gagging in response to a particular taste or texture, or inability to manage certain foods. These difficulties may be related to lack of experience and exposure, which may be self-imposed or because of treatment. Frequent discomfort related to food and eating may lead to reduced motivation for oral exploration and play in younger children, which may negatively impact oral sensory development. Children may present with food aversion, oral aversion, or global sensory processing disorders, all of which have distinct characteristics. Food aversion, or specific refusal to bring food items to the mouth, is the most common oral sensory disturbance the authors have encountered in children with EGIDs. The impact of visceral hyperalgesia in the esophagus and stomach should also be considered as a possible limiting factor in children's ability to overcome maladaptive learned feeding behaviors.[4–7]

Developmental Differences

In addition to the previously discussed characteristics, feeding can also be impacted by the psychosocial behaviors associated with chronic discomfort. The authors have observed children with the following: decreased social, communicative, and motor initiation; low energy; decreased motivation; flat affect; altered pragmatics (social/language skills); and emotional lability. Following appropriate treatment of their disease, many of these behaviors improve without the need for additional interventions. These children can be mislabeled as having developmental differences, when it is the chronic disease process that seems to be responsible.

ASSESSMENT

Understanding the role of EGID is a critical first step in the assessment of children's feeding difficulties. Collaboration with a team of treating professionals in gastroenterology, allergy, and nutrition may be helpful to determine the baseline status of the patient. This baseline information, combined with a patient's history, provides the feeding specialist with a foundation to analyze the feeding behaviors of the child and the caregiver, and to form hypotheses regarding developmental function, experiences, and learning. Assessment must include an observation of a meal or snack that replicates home mealtimes as closely as possible. The meal should include preferred and challenging food items. A child's oral motor patterns, oral sensory responses, mealtime behaviors, and child/caregiver mealtime dynamics are carefully observed. Assessment should also include the impact of overall development, muscle tone, postural alignment, and stability, breathing, global sensory processing, and communication on feeding and the mealtime dynamic.

FEEDING TREATMENT

Given prevalence of FD in pediatric patients, feeding specialists can play a significant role in treatment.[8] Various interventions may be used, including teaching compensatory strategies, establishing mealtime schedules, decreasing maladaptive behaviors, encouraging acceptance of new diets or recommended nutritious beverages, aiding with necessary increased volumes, medication acceptance, teaching pill swallowing, and assisting with allergio food trials to promote success. Caregiver and patient education are paramount in treating pediatric patients. During treatment, the therapist should be cognizant of tertiary services that the patient may benefit from, such as psychology, social work, physical therapy, or occupational therapy when available. A comprehensive approach underscores the importance of addressing not only the immediate FD but also considers the broader context of the child's and caregiver's needs. It should be noted that feeding treatment targeting texture advancement is most effective in the context of histologic remission of underlying esophageal inflammation.

Gastrostomy (Feeding) Tubes

In select cases, a feeding tube may be a consideration.[5,24,25] It can provide relief from the stress and anxiety that often surrounds insufficient intake, help diffuse difficult mealtime dynamics, and discourage the temptation to force feed. Feeding tubes can provide energy and nutrition for health and development, and in most cases, do not need to replace oral feeding but supplement diet to ensure growth. Children can remain oral feeders and develop oral motor skills, appropriate mealtime behaviors, and opportunities for positive learning about eating with those foods that are identified as safe. It is important that a feeding tube not be presented or viewed as a failure on the part of the child or caregiver but rather a temporary therapeutic bridge to consider for a child who needs additional support during the treatment process.

General Treatment Strategies

Feeding treatment has been found to be effective[26] and can take many forms, from weekly outpatient in person or by telehealth, in intensive one-on-one daily sessions to weekly group treatment sessions with peer models. Early diagnosis and timely intervention can minimize or avoid maladaptive feeding practices. When feeding treatment is recommended, commitment to the treatment regime from a child's caregivers is critical for a successful outcome. Parent education regarding mealtime schedules and routines, reinforcement (physiologic and behavioral), and systematic interaction with food is a cornerstone to success. Anticipatory guidance is recommended to support the developmental progression of feeding when a child is on an exclusive elemental diet. Success is also dependent on the treatment of underlying disease.[27] It is important to appreciate that feeding difficulties can require a great deal of energy, effort, and time to change in response to treatment.

For the anxious patient that presents with feeding difficulties because of fear of aversive consequences,[28] a confrontation versus avoidance approach is used to increase oral intake and confidence in navigating situations previously avoided. A common reaction to anxiety-producing stimuli is avoidance, which often brings short-term fear reduction; however, it may ultimately increase anxiety. Exposure in treatment is a highly effective intervention for targeting mealtime fears. Exposures should be implemented through education, systematic desensitization, and encouraging the patient to confront fear with success. Exposure is external (feared foods situations) or internal (interceptive exposures).[28] Given the nature of the anxious patient, feeding treatment may include collaboration or cotreating with a psychologist.[6,28]

CASE STUDIES

The following case studies illustrate the role of the feeding specialist in the management of children with EGID at varied ages.

Case Study #1: LD, a 3-Year-Old Boy

LD presented with a long-standing history of poor oral intake, poor weight gain, food allergy, atopic disease, and selective eating. Allergy testing revealed multiple food allergies at 12 months, and an endoscopy with biopsy resulted in diagnosis of EoE. Treatment included medication management, supplemental formula, and food elimination. He started a strict elimination diet and course of topical steroid with continued proton pump inhibitor treatment. LD persisted with low volume of intake, selective eating, and maladaptive mealtime behaviors. He required consistent prompting to eat resulting in caregivers feeding him. LD became reliant on distractions to decrease length of meal and increase oral volume. At 29 months of age, LD was referred to a multidisciplinary clinic to address persistent eczema, allergies, EoE, and feeding difficulties despite adherence to medications. The appointment included evaluations by a gastroenterologist, allergist, dietician, and feeding specialist. Feeding evaluation results indicated extremely selective eating characterized by a limited variety of foods, poor appetite, preference for soft textures, and refusals of meats/breads. LD was brand specific within his preferred foods. Although LD preferred soft textures and purees, he was found to have age-appropriate oral motor skills. His weight was found to be in the fourth percentile. The team agreed to continue with diet elimination of allergic foods, wean current medications, and switch to biologics given his eczema. Direct feeding therapy was initiated via telehealth once weekly.

Treatment plan

LD's treatment plan was created collaboratively with his parents. Feeding therapy goals emphasized building a foundation for relearning positive mealtime behaviors; teaching compensatory strategies; rewarding participation; redirecting maladaptive behaviors; and providing parent education regarding developing a meal-time schedule, structure, and routine. Other goals of therapy were to increase his daily volume of formula per Registered Dietitian recommendations and to establish mealtime schedule encouraging hunger. He was encouraged to remain seated in a supportive chair for meals and provided with opportunities to have positive interactions with new foods using small successful bites with token rewards. Mealtimes were limited to 30 minutes with the majority focusing on eating and the remaining 5 to 10 minutes prioritizing formula. LD benefitted from a mealtime visual schedule to fade persistent verbal prompting from parents. Treatment also included expanding accepted food textures.

Progress

LD received 16 telehealth individual feeding treatment sessions. After 16 sessions over 4 months, LD had met all established goals including eating age-appropriate servings of three foods in a mealtime, interacting with new foods, and consuming recommended volumes of formula. LD was now found to be in the 12th percentile for growth. Diet included harder to chew and swallow foods including meats, breads, raw vegetables, rice, quinoa, and ground beef. His parents were able to create a mealtime schedule for him that was age-appropriate, with five to six scheduled daily mealtimes versus grazing. His daily formula intake increased, meeting the established goal set by the RD. The need for verbal prompting was decreased. LD benefited from modeling, gestural cues, foods cut into small bite sizes, preloaded fork bites, and dips to aid with swallowing.

Case Study #2: MH, a 9-Year-Old Girl

MH presented with an initial complaint of a choking incident while eating chips. She was brought to a hospital and was diagnosed with "suspected strep throat." MH was treated with a course of antibiotics. Despite treatment, complaints of throat and abdominal pain persisted. MH began losing weight. She relied on drinking milk and eating ice cream as her primary source of nutrition. Given her oral intake refusals and fear of choking, MH's mother brought her to the emergency department. She presented with complaints of sore throat and generalized abdominal pain. Evaluation by the attending physician indicated lethargy and mild oropharyngeal erythema. Ear, nose, throat was consulted and recommended upper GI. A feeding therapy referral was made.

During subsequent individual feeding evaluation via telehealth, the feeding specialist completed a comprehensive feeding history intake with MH and her mother, which indicated long-standing feeding difficulties beginning early in life, including picky eating and vomiting. MH was reported to "never eat meat well." They also reported multiple incidents in which MH perceived she was choking. Frequent coughing and throat clearing were also reported with a reliance on liquid washes at all meals. During direct observation, coughing and throat clearing was noted with milk and applesauce. MH was noted to use her fingers to press on her throat near larynx when swallowing purees. MH refused all other foods. Given results of the evaluation including loss of weight, an RD and GI consultation was scheduled to identify a nutritional supplement and to determine additional testing warranted. MH underwent an esophagogastroduodenoscopy with biopsy, revealing significant EoE with 100+ eosinophils per high power field in the proximal and distal esophagus. MH was prescribed a topical steroid and formula supplementation. A multidisciplinary team recommended continued feeding therapy to support MH in accepting supplemental formula, expanding diet, and eventual expansion of accepted textures as her underlying inflammation decreased.

Treatment

Feeding treatment was established for weekly visits working in concert with the treating gastroenterologist and dietician. Direct therapy sessions targeted acceptance of recommended formula, establishing mealtime schedule, increasing variety of safe comfortable foods, and parent education. MH initially presented with increased anxiety on telehealth visits, often hiding from camera, but with encouragement was able to participate in feeding sessions. MH was taught compensatory strategies of small bites, dipping in sauces for moisture, and liquid washes to aid with esophageal discomfort and dysphagia. Caregiver teaching was provided to establish a predicable mealtime and snack schedule to limit grazing on recommended formula. Foods were presented before formula, and all intake was presented during a meal or snack time while sitting at the table. MH was allowed to drink free water throughout the day between meals and snacks. Ongoing consultations with an RD occurred to adjust formula needs as oral intake increased. Additional consultations with GI were necessary for reeducation regarding medication dosage. The family benefitted from a social worker to support the family with new demands including new costs, travel to appointments, filling prescriptions, and food insecurity.

Progress
MH was able to meet the goal of recommended formula volumes, regain lost weight from the previous month, going from the 22nd to 38th percentile. Avoidance behaviors of eating solids were reduced using a "confrontation with success versus avoidance" approach. MH benefitted from use of compensatory strategies for esophageal discomfort (liquid washed, dips for moisture and lubrication, and small bites). Although underlying esophageal inflammation was noted to be treated, MH persisted with continued complaints of abdominal pain. To address this, she was taught diaphragmatic breathing strategies surrounding mealtimes to aid with discomfort. Interoceptive exposures of liquid intake and awareness of hunger and satiety was taught to help MH differentiate between abdominal discomfort and hunger. A significant improvement in MH's mood and decreased anxiety were noted by all team members. Ongoing caregiver education was provided, which resulted in significantly fewer mealtime struggles. Continued outpatient feeding therapy was recommended to expand volume and variety supporting long-term health and eventual wean from recommended formula.

Case Study #3: TP, a 16-Year-Old-Boy

TP presented as a well-nourished 16 year old with an established diagnosis of EoE, food allergy, and mild eczema. EoE diagnosis came after a food impaction. A subsequent scope indicated EoE with stricture. During scope, he benefitted from dilation. He was referred to a multidisciplinary clinic to manage his EoE and was placed on a two-food elimination. During his team visit his pill swallowing and general feeding skills were assessed by a feeding specialist. He was not reported to be a selective eater but preferred to eat only "softer meats," refused most raw vegetables, and fruits with peels. TP was reported to be a slow eater. He was found to use compensatory strategies of liquid washes and preference for a softer textured diet. Oral feeding skills were found to be age appropriate; however, he was not able to swallow pills. On all pill swallow attempts, TP reported the pill remained anteriorly in his oral cavity, although he was able to swallow the surrounding water. Feeding therapy was recommended to target pill swallowing in the outpatient setting to proceed with additional diagnostic evaluation.

Treatment
TP was seen in the outpatient setting using an in-person and telehealth approach. His initial three sessions were held in person and then transitioned to telehealth for convenience of schedule and travel. Pill swallowing was taught through a step-up approach going from small to large candy, and puree to liquid with success. During sessions, he learned to swallow a 5- to 10-mL bolus of puree and liquid without chewing or lateralizing in mouth. He benefitted from a neutral head position (vs chin tuck or head back). Once consistent success was noted, a single candy piece starting with baking sprinkle was added to puree. With continued success, candy sizes were increased until he was able to swallow a tic tac–sized candy in 80% of attempts. Using a straw with liquids while bringing cup to mouth to facilitated an appropriate head position. He followed a weekly home program to practice specific candy sizes in either puree or

liquids, practicing 4 days a week. Caregivers were educated on specific strategies to support him throughout the week.

Progress

TP was able to successfully swallow tic tac–sized candy "pills" after eight total feeding sessions. With pill swallow capabilities, he is a candidate for participation in subsequent testing by a gastroenterologist to further assess EoE.

SUMMARY

Eating is a dynamic learning experience. EoE is associated with derailed development of oral feeding and may alter family dynamics at mealtimes. Despite effective medical treatment, the residual effects on feeding can persist and need to be addressed. Specific strategies may be required to help children move toward the goals of optimal intako, incroaεed variety in diet, developing appropriate oral motor and oral sensory skills, and addressing mealtime behaviors and environment. A multidisciplinary team approach affords the opportunity to provide comprehensive care for this unique population. Collaboration regarding the medical, nutritional, and developmental plan of care optimizes outcomes for the well-being of children and families affected by this disease.

CLINICS CARE POINTS

- Refer to a feeding and swallowing specialist for assessment when caregivers report concerns about stressful mealtimes or feeding difficulties.
- Feeding therapy is efficacious for pediatric patients with EGIDs and feeding dysfunction.
- Ongoing collaboration with medical specialists and feeding and swallowing specialists may be required to achieve optimal developmental, behavioral, and growth outcomes.

DISCLOSURE

None.

REFERENCES

1. Satter E. Child of mine: feeding with love and good sense. Palo Alto (CA): Bull Publishing Co; 1991. p. 406–27.
2. Furuta GT, Liacouras CA, Collins MH, et al. Eosinophilic esophagitis in children and adults: a systematic review and consensus recommendations for diagnosis and treatment. Gastroenterol 2007;133:1342–63.
3. Spergel JM. Eosinophilic esophagitis in adults and children: evidence for a food allergy component in many patients. Curr Opin Allergy Clin Immunol 2007;7:274–8.
4. Feo-Ortega Sara, Lucendo AJ. Evidence-based treatments for eosinophilic esophagitis: insights for the clinician. Therapeutic Advances in Gastroenterology 2022;15(Jan). 175628482110686.
5. Thomas Jennifer J, Eddy Kamryn. Cognitive-behavioral therapy for avoidant/restrictive food intake disorder: children, adolescents, and adults. Cambridge, United Kingdom ; New York, Ny: Cambridge University Press; 2019.
6. Atwood S, Epstein J. Frontline Gastroenterol 2021;12:644–9. https://doi.org/10.1136/flgastro-2019-101313.

7. Piller Aimee, Penning J, Bonsall A. Effectiveness of outpatient pediatric feeding interventions on increasing variety of foods consumed and adaptive mealtime behaviors.". Am J Occup Ther 2022;76(Supplement_1). https://doi.org/10.5014/ajot. 2022.76s1-po29. 7010505029p1. Accessed 21 November. 2022.

8. Mehta P, Furuta GT, Brennan T, et al. Nutritional state and feeding behaviors of children with eosinophilic esophagitis and gastroesophageal reflux disease. J Pediatr Gastroenterol Nutr 2018;66(4):603–8. PMID: 28906318. https:// journals.lww.com/jpgn/Fulltext/2018/04000/Nutritional_State_and_Feeding_Behaviors_of.10.aspx.

9. Knotowicz H, Haas A, Coe S, et al. Opportunities for innovation and improved care using telehealth for nutritional interventions. Gastroenterology 2019;157(3): 594–7. Epub 2019 Jun 13. PMID: 31376397. https://www.sciencedirect.com/science/article/pii/S0016508519410093?via%3Dihub.

10. Aceves SS, Furuta GT, Spechler SJ. Integrated approach to treatment of children and adults with eosinophilic esophagitis. Gastrointest Endosc Clin N Am 2008;18: 195–217.

11. Kerwin ME, Ahearn WH, Eicher PS, et al. The costs of eating: a behavioral economic analysis of food refusal. J Appl Behav Anal 1995;28:245–60.

12. Eicher PM. Feeding. In: Batshaw ML, editor. Children with disabilities. 4th edition. Baltimore (MD: Paul H. Brookes Publishing Co; 1997. p. 621–41.

13. Menard-Katcher C, Henry M, Furuta GT, et al. Significance of feeding dysfunction in eosinophilic esophagitis. World J Gastroenterol 2014;20(31):11019–22. PMID: 25152606; PMCID: PMC4138483. https://www.ncbi.nlm.nih.gov/pmc/articles/PMC4138483/?report=reader.

14. Morris SE, Klein MD. Pre-feeding skills: a comprehension resource for feeding development. 2nd edition. Tucson (AZ: Therapy Skill Builders; 1987. p. 59–94.

15. Wolf L, Glass RP. Feeding and swallowing disorders in infancy: assessment and management. Tucson (AZ): Therapy Skill Builders; 1992.

16. Putnam P. Eosinophilic esophagitis in children: clinical manifestations. Gastrointest Endosc Clin N Am 2008;18:11–23.

17. Pentiuk Scott, Putnam PE, Collins MH, et al. Dissociation between symptoms and histological severity in pediatric eosinophilic esophagitis.". J Pediatr Gastroenterol Nutr 2009;48(2):152–60.

18. Logemann JA. Evaluation and treatment of swallowing disorders. 2nd edition. San Diego (CA): College Hill Press; 1997.

19. Stevenson D, Allaire JH. The development of normal feeding and swallowing. Pediatr Clin 1991;38(6):1439–53.

20. Nurko S, Rosen R. Esophageal dismotility in patients who have eosinophilic esophagitis. Gastrointest Endosc Clin N Am 2008;18:73–89.

21. Kedesdy JL, Budd KS. Childhood feeding disorders: biobehavioral assessment and intervention. Baltimore (MD): Paul H. Brookes Publishing Co; 1998.

22. Iwata B, Riordan M, Wohl MK, et al. Pediatric feeding disorders: behavioral analysis and treatment. In: Accardo PJ, editor. Failure to thrive in infancy and early childhood. Baltimore (MD): University Park Press; 1982. p. 297–329.

23. Illingworth RS, Lister J. The critical or sensitive period, with special reference to certain feeding problems in infants and children. J Pediatr 1964;65:839–48.

24. Young C. Nutrition. In: Arvedson JC, Brodsky L, editors. Pediatric swallowing and feeding: assessment and management. Thousand Oaks (CA): Singular Publishing; 1985. p. 157–20817.

25. Pentiuk SP, Miller CK, Kaul A. Eosinophilic esophagitis in infants and toddlers. Dysphagia 2007;22:44–7.

26. Mukkada VA, Haas A, Maune NC, et al. Feeding dysfunction in children with eosinophilic gastrointestinal diseases. Pediatrics 2010;126(3):e672–7. Epub 2010 Aug 9. PMID: 20696733. https://publications.aap.org/pediatrics/article/126/3/e672/66170/Feeding-Dysfunction-in-Children-With-Eosinophilic?autologincheck=redirected.

27. Gunasekaran T, Prabhakar G, Schwartz A, et al. Eosinophilic esophagitis in children and adolescents with abdominal pain: comparison with EoE-dysphagia and functional abdominal pain. Canadian Journal of Gastroenterology and Hepatology 2016;2016:1–7.

28. Asthma and Allergy Foundation of America and American Partnership for Eosinophilic Disorders, (2023). Life with EoE: the patient experience and opportunities to improve care in the US. Retrieved from aafa.org/EoELife.

Clinical Evaluation of the Adult with Eosinophilic Esophagitis

Luc Biedermann, MD[a],*, Alex Straumann, MD[a]

KEYWORDS

- Eosinophilic esophagitis • Physical examination • Laboratory abnormalities
- Endoscopic signs • Histologic findings • Treatment modalities

KEY POINTS

- The hallmark symptom of eosinophilic esophagitis (EoE) is solid food dysphagia. However, some patients with EoE may only have reflux-like symptoms, retrosternal pain, a vague feeling of thoracic oppression and/or immediate reaction in the esophageal region on the ingestion of certain trigger foods.
- Eosinophil tissue infiltration is the current conditio sine qua non to make the diagnosis of EoE. However, EoE variants have recently been described—an immune-mediated chronic esophageal inflammation with dysphagia without a sufficient eosinophil count per high power field for classic EoE diagnosis.
- Proper history taking and a high index of suspicion in patients with atopic comorbidities and/or familial history of EoE remain key in the evaluation of EoE.
- Do not be satisfied with a simple "no" as an answer toward a superficial interrogation regarding dysphagia. A chronic and slowly evolving symptoms often may remain unrecognized by the patient.
- As EoE may be a patchy disease, it is crucial to profoundly observe the entire esophageal mucosa during endoscopy and perform targeted high-quality biopsies including submucosal tissue.

INTRODUCTION

Eosinophilic esophagitis (EoE) may affect individuals at any age and similar genotypic abnormalities are evoked in children and adults, thereby indicating that the disorder is one single entity. However, some phenotypic manifestations of EoE are highly age dependent and justify a different management. The clinical evaluation of adult patients with EoE entails the exceptional feature that treating physicians typically encounter

[a] Department of Gastroenterology and Hepatology, University Hospital Zurich, Raemistrassse 100, CH-8091 Zurich, Switzerland
* Corresponding author.
E-mail address: Luc.Biedermann@usz.ch

Immunol Allergy Clin N Am 44 (2024) 185–196
https://doi.org/10.1016/j.iac.2023.12.006
0889-8561/24/© 2023 Elsevier Inc. All rights reserved.
immunology.theclinics.com

apparently healthy individuals.[1–4] EoE cannot be described as an overt disease, nor is it, except for episodic complications, characterized by a spectacular or dramatic presentation. This characteristic is first due to the anatomic location of the esophagus, hidden deep within the chest cavity and, second, due to the fact that in adults, EoE rarely evokes systemic effects, such as fatigue, fever, wasting, or severe pain. This overall rather subtle presentation contrasts sharply to pediatric EoE where general symptoms such as food refusal, failure to thrive and pain, alert family members and physicians early during the course of the disease.[5–8] This unimpressive adult presentation may explain after symptoms commence in the adult, some 4 to 5 years pass on the average before EoE is finally diagnosed and may be considerably above 10 years in a fraction of patients.[9,10] Nevertheless, gastroenterologists are familiar with this pattern of clinical appearance from other chronic gastrointestinal inflammatory diseases. Of note, despite the absence of a dramatic appearance, EoE represents a relevant burden for the majority of affected individuals, substantially impairing the patient's quality of life[11–13] and being associated with several relevant risks.[14,15]

In summary, the clinical evaluation of EoE requires a deep probing into the matter, first, by taking a careful history and second, by using invasive examination methods, even beyond the frontiers of the endoscope.

DEFINITION

EoE is defined in adults, adolescents, and children, as a chronic, clinicopathologic disease characterized by symptoms of esophageal dysfunction in combination with a dense esophageal eosinophilia. As an eosinophilic infiltration per se is a nonspecific phenomenon other esophageal diseases leading to eosinophilia, in particular gastroesophageal reflux (GERD), must be ruled out before the diagnosis is confirmed.[2,4,16,17] In EoE, eosinophilic inflammation is absent in the stomach, small intestine, and colon.[2–4] Of note, the diagnosis of EoE is based on several clinical and pathologic features, but not on one single "all-or-nothing" marker, for example, number of eosinophils in the esophagus. This comprehensive definition constitutes a guideline for the diagnostic workup and for the proper selection of the diagnostic procedures and when to use or potentially repeat these in a given patient with suspected EoE.[18]

EPIDEMIOLOGIC FEATURES AND DEMOGRAPHIC CHARACTERISTICS

Previously considered a rare curiosity, the startling prevalence of adult EoE has reached almost epidemic proportions. One prospectively conducted, long-term study carried out in Switzerland showed that the prevalence of EoE in adult patients increased during a 19 years period from an initial 2, to a final 43, patients per 100,000 inhabitants.[19] These data illustrate that EoE is indeed of general relevance: about 1 individual in 2500 is affected.[20] In addition, while the average incidence in this area used to be 2.45, it increased to 4.4 to 7.4 newly diagnosed cases per 100,000 inhabitants per year presently. However, is this a true rise in the incidence or simply an increased awareness of the disease? As this study was conducted in a demographically stable, well-defined indicator area, under population-based conditions and unchanged recording practices, the data likely reflect a real increase in EoE cases, and not just an enhanced awareness of the disease.

EoE shows a strong predilection for the male gender: among the reported cases, more than 70% involve men.[20,21] Of note, in a national database analysis, Katzka and colleagues demonstrated that EoE occurs in all age groups; with a patient range between 1 and 98 years, yet a peak in the 5th decade of life.[22] Of interest, EoE affects mainly highly educated individuals.[23] Despite this multiple confirmed observation, the reason is currently not at all clear.

ASSESSMENT OF SYMPTOMS IN ADULTS WITH EOSINOPHILIC ESOPHAGITIS

When diagnosing EoE, important clues is found by taking a careful history that focuses on esophageal-related and upper abdominal symptoms, atopies, and family history. As in many other diseases, there are age-related differences in the presenting symptoms. In contrast to children who experience food refusal, failure to thrive and pain, EoE in adolescents and adults causes a rather narrow spectrum of symptoms, with the typical complaint being *dysphagia for solids.*[5–8]

Importantly, solid-food dysphagia is a hidden symptom. Some patients occasionally report difficulty with swallowing that then increases over time, whereas others report an abrupt onset. In general, symptoms are more prominent and the swallowing disturbances more pronounced when the ingested food's consistency is dry or rough, and/or when the patient eats quickly. Patients almost always adapt their eating habits to prevent food impactions. Questions focusing directly on reduced eating-speed, avoidance, and modification of critical foods are therefore important. However, owing to these adaptation mechanisms having slowly evolved over years and even decades, demasking esophageal dysfunction as a symptom may be challenging, which is why several technical measures in a detailed history taking may frequently be required to detect even subtle forms of dysphagia. For instance, an up-front "no" or "not really" to the question of whether a given patient experiences dysphagia for solid food items may simply be due to the fact, that the patient entirely and notoriously (not infrequently subconsciously) avoids certain food items, with a specifically solid, fibrous, or dense and therefore mechanically challenging consistency. We therefore always advocate inquiring, whether distinctive food items tend to be avoided, which most often is the case in the event of eating in a social environment (eg, business lunch or restaurant with friends and family). Also, it is not rare, that a patient-perceived absence of solid food dysphagia is directly rebutted by the patient's spouse or a family member. Therefore, presence of a close person during initial history taking may be helpful for demasking hidden dysphagia. We thus recommend continuously escalating the difficulty level of "presented" imaginary food items during an interview. For instance, a presumable absence of any problems to ingest a given meal may only be recognizable, if the patient is asked, whether he or she would also feel comfortable or be able to eat this dish, if the waiter would not yet have served the accompanying beverage. Potential further modifications in this direction include "Could you also eat this served meal, if the kitchen ran out of any sauce? What if you had to lead an agitated or complicated discussion during this meal, would you still feel comfortable to eat? If you were to catch a bus in 10 minutes and the large plate has just been served, could you wolf down this plate, considering that you are very hungry and knowing that this is your last meal for the next couple of hours today?"

According to our experience, it may also be helpful to challenge a given subject while exploring for the presence of dysphagia with an imaginary food challenge by precisely mentioning the characteristics of the food including the circumstances such as, for instance, an imaginary large plate of dry rice with strips of meat; no sauce, no beverage on the table and being in a rush for your next appointment.

In general, we recommend quantifying the severity of symptoms systematically during each visit, to assess the natural course or the effects of therapeutic interventions. Although for the purpose of clinical trials scoring systems, preferentially validated ones—such as EEsAI[24] or dysphagia days[25]—should be used, in clinical practice more user-friendly tools are often sufficient. A simple visual analog scale (VAS) might be appropriate for clinical purposes, that is, VAS from 0 (absolutely no trouble swallowing) to 10 (extreme difficult to swallow with a maximal impact on quality of life). According to our experience for an as much as possible quantitative inquiry of eating speed a comparison with driving your car may be even more illustrative for the patient and thus of superior accuracy. We recommend inquiring about this using a permitted driving speed of 100 km/h with an agile car on an empty road. Importantly, 100 km/h would be the equivalent of the patient's baseline normal eating velocity prior to the first occurrence of symptoms of EoE. According to our experience, this provides not only prompt and reliable quantitative estimation of the current eating speed under a given disease activity of EoE with or without additional impairment due to fibro-stenotic chronic esophageal remodeling but also represents an ideal way for longitudinal assessment of potential changes on medical and/or mechanical therapeutic interventions.

During the course of the disease, more than one-third of untreated patients with EoE will experience a *long-lasting food impaction* that will require endoscopic bolus removal.[26,27] In a report from a private practice setting, Desai and colleagues found that 17 of 31 (55%) adults presenting with food impaction were found to have EoE.[28] Currently EoE is likely the leading cause of food impaction, at least in younger male patients.[26]

A minority of adult patients with EoE experience retrosternal pain occurring immediately after the ingestion of a distinct food, such as nuts or alcoholic beverages. This phenomenon is referred to as food-induced immediate response of the esophagus, has similarities to pollen-food allergy syndrome or oral allergy syndrome while primarily being perceived at the esophageal/retrosternal and not oral cavity level, and may or may not response to successful anti-inflammatory treatment of EoE. A careful history is required to differentiate between the EoE-inherent solid-food dysphagia, heartburn due to coexisting GERD and oral-allergy syndrome.[29,30]

More than 70% of adults with EoE have a *history of atopy*, mainly allergic diseases of the airways, such as seasonal rhino-conjunctivitis and/or asthma.[31,32] Finally, a family history may provide further information: Noel and colleagues found that in their series of 103 patients with EoE, 73.5% had a positive family history for atopic diseases, 6.8% for EoE, and 9.7% had undergone esophageal dilation.[33]

PHYSICAL EXAMINATION OF ADULTS WITH EOSINOPHILIC ESOPHAGITIS

In contrast to the conspicuous medical history, the physical examination of adult patients with EoE is usually unremarkable.[1] This is due to the anatomic inaccessibility of the esophagus during the physical examination and because EoE in adults seldom evokes systemic manifestations. However, physical examination may be important to investigate for signs of 2 diseases that may present with esophageal manifestations mimicking EoE. First, scleroderma may potentially reveal sclerodactyly, telangiectasia, or Raynaud phenomenon on physical examination in a given patient evaluated for dysphagia or "refractory GERD" and thus represents a differential diagnosis. Another entity is lichen planus, which frequently leads to esophageal strictures or narrow caliber esophagus and sometimes also lymphocytic esophagitis.

LABORATORY ANALYSES

For the clinical evaluation of a patient with EoE, laboratory analyses have no more than a subsidiary value. Unfortunately, no noninvasive markers for establishing the diagnosis or monitoring the disease is currently available.[34–36] However, two routine laboratory methods may provide additional information: Between 5% and 50% of adults with EoE have a mild eosinophilia on their differential blood count,[35] though values seldom exceed 1500 eos/mm^3. A differential blood count may provide supporting evidence for the presence of EoE, but is not diagnostic. Whether the degree of eosinophilia correlates with the disease activity is not yet elucidated. Furthermore, approximately 70% of patients with EoE have elevated total immunoglobulin E (IgE) values.[37–39] To date, no studies have been able to document whether total IgE can serve as a surrogate marker for disease progression or resolution, but there is some evidence that, when compared with patients having normal levels, those with high total IgE levels respond less well to corticosteroid treatment.[40]

ENDOSCOPIC ASSESSMENT OF ADULTS WITH EOSINOPHILIC ESOPHAGITIS

Upper endoscopy is the first diagnostic step in the evaluation of an individual with dysphagia.[41] EoE-related endoscopic abnormalities include edema, rings, white exudates, longitudinal furrows, and strictures.[37,38] These 5 key features are summarized under the acronym EREFS (endoscopic reference score for EoE), graded and validated by Hirano and colleagues.[42] Edema (grading 0/1), white exudates (grading 0/1/2), and furrows (grading 0/1/2) likely reflect acute inflammation, whereas rings (grading 0/1/2/3) and strictures (grading 0/1) likely reflect remodeling of the esophagus due to the chronic eosinophilic inflammation (grading according to original EREFS score; alternative and collapsed version—modified EREFS[42]—currently more frequently used in clinical trials and clinical practice). All these signs are suggestive of the diagnosis of EoE, but the endoscopic suspicion requires histologic confirmation. Importantly, in patients with a history of solid-food dysphagia biopsies should be taken even in the absence of overt endoscopic signs.[2]

In adult patients, endoscopy is reliable for the assessment of the inflammatory disease activity. In contrast, assessment of the degree of underlying remodeling is difficult if not impossible solely based on standard endoscopy, but it allows estimation of the esophageal diameter. At the least, the inability to pass a standard adult endoscope is a clear sign of a high-grade stricture. An indirect approach of "measuring" the minimal luminal diameter involves the use of any of the established dilation methods, including bougie and balloon with stepwise determination of minimal device diameter needed to induce a mucosal tear. Recently, over-the-scope placement of a translucent cone-shaped device (BougieCap) has also been described as a simple single-use tool for both measuring luminal minimal diameter and performing dilation under direct endoscopic visualization.[43] Determination of the esophageal distensibility using EndoFlip is another option with increasing use in clinical trials as an exploratory endpoint and also in clinical practice to assess the degree of remodeling.[44–46] The latter might also be a promising tool to assess response to medical therapy beyond the rather narrow classical endpoint of tissue eosinophilia.[47]

PARTICULARITIES OF BIOPSY-SAMPLING IN EOSINOPHILIC ESOPHAGITIS

Considering that EoE represents a clinicopathologic entity and according to its definition, diagnosis not only requires histologic confirmation but histology is the genuine key to any diagnosis of EoE: the esophageal biopsy shows a marked eosinophilic infiltration.[2,37,38] Under healthy conditions, the human esophagus is devoid of eosinophils.[48] Despite an eosinophilic infiltration of the esophagus is a rather nonspecific sign that can be found in several other conditions,[2,16,17] finding a relevant number of eosinophils in the esophageal mucosa is highly suspicious for EoE. Because nature is never black or white, experts agree that diagnosis of EoE can be established if a peak infiltration of greater than 15 eosinophils per hpf is found in combination with other subsidiary histologic findings and typical symptoms.[2–4,17] Because the eosinophilic infiltration in EoE can be very patchy,[49] the question remains how many biopsies should be taken to prevent a false negative diagnosis. Using an arithmetical model, Gonsalves and colleagues have demonstrated that the selected threshold value (peak number of eos per hpf) and the number of biopsies taken for analysis determine the sensitivity of the combined "endoscopy-histology" method[50] and currently most experts recommend taking 3 to 4 biopsy samples from the proximal and the distal esophagus, respectively.[2–4,17,51]

Taking biopsies of the esophagus poses 2 technical problems for the endoscopist: first, the squamous epithelium is a quite solid and thick layer, and second, due to the tubular shape of the esophagus the tip of the biopsy forceps is placed almost always tangential to the esophageal surface. Routine biopsies frequently contain only epithelial material. However, EoE is not an exclusive epithelial disease and affects deeper layers of the esophageal wall as well.[52] Some of the histologic features—in particular fibrosis—are only present in the subepithelial layers of the wall. Furthermore, tissue eosinophilia might be even more pronounced in the subepithelial compartment than in the epithelium. A special biopsy technique is therefore needed to obtain a representative amount of lamina propria to enable the pathologist to reliably assess the inflammatory and fibrotic activity of the disease.[53]

IMAGING METHODS

The barium esophagram is a radiological tool sometimes used to assess strictures. It may additionally provide important information regarding potential differential diagnoses such as achalasia or esophageal diverticula including Zenker's diverticulum. However, the yield of the barium esophagram in evaluating EoE-induced strictures is limited, as the diameter frequently is underestimated. This limitation is likely due to the remodeling-associated reduced distensibility of the esophageal wall. Thus, direct endoscopic inspection and measurement using a classical dilation tool (Bougie, Balloon or BougieCap) or functional lumen imaging probe (FLIP) represent more reliable means. Whether a barium tablet might be superior compared with a liquid barium swallow remains to be determined.

ESOPHAGEAL STRESS TESTS—THE EMERGING "ERGOMETRY" FOR GASTROENTEROLOGISTS TO DEMASK AND QUANTIFY HIDDEN DYSPHAGIA?

As mentioned above, dysphagia may remain unrecognized, even after careful and dedicated history taking, mainly due to patients' considerable adaptive potential with regard to food intake. Therefore, in analogy with other medical fields, provocation or stress testing could be helpful to uncover dysphagia. For instance, the dysphagia stress test was developed by a group of experts from Chicago. This test, comprised of 5 bolus challenges (water, applesauce, rice, bread, barium tablet) with self-rated trouble swallowing and pain, revealed promising results.[54] In this study it was shown that 3 food items seem to have a sufficient diagnostic potency, simplifying this test to applesauce, rice, and bread. Another tool might be direct observation of patients with (suspected) EoE eating a sandwich. In the published research communication a standardized turkey sandwich was used in 10 patients with active and inactive EoE.[55] While such testing may increase in importance, currently it is hardly used in clinical practice due to the relatively high expense.

NATURAL HISTORY, COMPLICATIONS, AND INDICATIONS FOR TREATMENT OF ADULT EOSINOPHILIC ESOPHAGITIS

Despite our understanding of the natural history of EoE is still limited, it has become clear that this is a chronic disease whose course may be either chronic-persistent or chronic-relapsing.[14,15,56] So far, no case of EoE with a superimposed premalignant condition or with a malignancy has been reported, but long-term follow-up is required to confirm this observation. The main concern is that a long-standing, not or insufficiently treated eosinophilic inflammation would evoke irreversible structural alterations of the esophagus, leading to fibrosis and angiogenesis, and result in thickening of the wall with abnormal fragility and subsequent functional impairment.[15,57,58] Of note, strictures are rarely reported in children, suggesting that this complication requires years of unbridled eosinophilic inflammation.[15,59,60] This so-called esophageal remodeling may lead to several complications.

Acute *food impactions* are the leading complication of untreated EoE. Indeed, EoE was diagnosed in about 60% of adult patients referred for a diagnostic workup of food impaction[28,61] and during the course of their disease, more than one-third of adult patients experience long-lasting food impactions requiring endoscopic removal.[62] The risk of impaction primarily depends on the consistency of the food, and particularly problematic are dry rice and fibrous meat, for example, chicken or beef. This extremely disagreeable and frightening form of dysphagia is a sword of Damocles hanging permanently over almost all patients with EoE. Food impactions are often the trigger for patients to consult a physician to perform a diagnostic workup of long-lasting dysphagia. These unforeseeable events harbor several risks, such as retching-induced esophageal rupture (Boerhaave's syndrome) or procedure-related perforation.[63–65] This has the practical consequence that, in patients with a long history of dysphagia, invasive procedures (eg, removal of impacted food or dilations) must be performed most delicately.

In addition to dysphagia as the leading symptom, typical reflux symptoms which respond to acid-suppressive medication may appear during the long-term course of EoE. In their case series, Remedios and colleagues found that among 26 adult patients with EoE, 10 had coexisting reflux disease previously confirmed by pH monitoring.[66] Furthermore, based on motility studies, the authors found that 8 of the 10 patients with coexisting reflux also had a reduced pressure in the lower esophageal sphincter (LES). These findings suggest that, in EoE, the chronic inflammation can lead to an LES dysfunction, and thus to a clinically relevant, secondary reflux disease. However, we have to admit that our knowledge of the natural history of EoE is still fragmentary and further studies are urgently needed.

Finally, we would like to emphasize that a precise understanding of the natural course of EoE is of practical importance, because decisions for any therapeutic interventions are based primarily on the natural course, including its inherent complications. There are at least 3 crucial reasons to treat an adult patient presenting with clinically and histologically confirmed active EoE to (1) alleviate the diminished quality of life associated with continuous symptoms; (2) prevent acute food impactions and their associated risks; and (3) protect the esophagus from long-term sequelae, that is, fibrostenotic remodeling and subsequent functional impairment.

OUTLOOK

Even though our understanding of EoE has increased enormously during the last decades, many issues remain unresolved. Indeed, our understanding of EoE's natural history is still quite limited and we have no predictive factors to identify patients at highest risk of developing esophageal remodeling. Moreover, the appearance of EoE variants[67] and the shift among variants and the transition from variants to classical EoE illustrates that EoE is not a "single-cell" disease and other inflammatory cells may play an even more important role than eosinophils. Classical EoE and EoE variants are likely members of a bigger family of immune-mediated esophageal inflammatory diseases, best denominated with a cell-independent term such as inflammatory dysphagia syndrome.

CLINICS CARE POINTS

- Symptoms in EoE may be subtle and often are not recognized, neither by the physician nor the patient – at least in the early stages of the disease.
- It is not just all dysphagia in EoE. Indeed, dysphagia may be entirely absent (not just in kids but also adults) and retrosternal pain/discomfort may be the only presentation.
- The latter two points and escape strategies (chewing, avoiding certain foods, high-volume beverage consumption during meals etc.) are the foundation of a persistent long diagnostic delay – both patient's and doctor's diagnostic delay.
- A timely diagnosis is only possible with profound history taking, a high index of suspicion (specifically in younger male subjects with atopic comorbidities) and education of general practitioners.

ACKNOWLEDGMENTS

The authors would like to thank Professor Ikuo Hirano (Northwestern, Chicago) for his critical input and valuable comments on this study.

DISCLOSURE

L. Biedermann has consulting contracts with Abbvie, BMS, MSD, Vifor, Falk, Esocap, Calypso, Ferring, Pfizer, Takeda, Janssen, Sanofi. A. Straumann has consulting contracts with Astra-Zeneca, BMS, Calypso, EsoCap, Falk Pharma, GSK and Sanofi.

REFERENCES

1. Straumann A. Clinical evaluation of the adult who has eosinophilic esophagitis. Immunol Allergy Clin North Am 2009;29(1):11–8, vii.
2. Lucendo AJ, Molina-Infante J, Arias Á, et al. Guidelines on eosinophilic esophagitis: Evidence-based statements and recommendations for diagnosis and management in children and adults. United European Gastroenterology Journal 2017; 124. 205064061668952.
3. Dellon ES, Gonsalves N, Hirano I, et al. ACG clinical guideline: Evidenced based approach to the diagnosis and management of esophageal eosinophilia and eosinophilic esophagitis (EoE). Am J Gastroenterol 2013;108(5):679–92 [quiz: 693].
4. Dellon ES, Liacouras CA, Molina-Infante J, et al. Updated international consensus diagnostic criteria for eosinophilic esophagitis: Proceedings of the AGREE conference. Gastroenterology 2018. https://doi.org/10.1053/j.gastro.2018.07.009.
5. Orenstein SR, Shalaby TM, Di Lorenzo C, et al. The spectrum of pediatric eosinophilic esophagitis beyond infancy: a clinical series of 30 children. Am J Gastroenterol 2000;95(6):1422–30.

6. Gonsalves N. Distinct features in the clinical presentations of eosinophilic esophagitis in children and adults: is this the same disease? Dig Dis 2014;32(1–2): 89–92.

7. Lucendo AJ, Sánchez-Cazalllla M. Adult versus pediatric eosinophilic esophagitis: important differences and similarities for the clinician to understand. Expert Rev Clin Immunol 2012;8(8):733–45.

8. Straumann A, Aceves SS, Blanchard C, et al. Pediatric and adult eosinophilic esophagitis: similarities and differences. Allergy 2012;67(4):477–90.

9. Murray FR, Kreienbuehl AS, Greuter T, et al. Diagnostic Delay in Patients With Eosinophilic Esophagitis Has Not Changed Since the First Description 30 Years Ago: Diagnostic Delay in Eosinophilic Esophagitis. Am J Gastroenterol 2022; 117(11):1772–9.

10. Melgaard D, Westmark S, Laurberg PT, et al. A diagnostic delay of 10 years in the DanEoE cohort calls for focus on education - a population-based cross-sectional study of incidence, diagnostic process and complications of eosinophilic oesophagitis in the North Denmark Region. United European Gastroenterology Journal 2021;9(6):688–98.

11. Safroneeva E, Coslovsky M, Kuehni CE, et al. Eosinophilic oesophagitis: Relationship of quality of life with clinical, endoscopic and histological activity. Aliment Pharmacol Ther 2015;42(8):1000–10.

12. Frazzoni L, Tolone S. Eosinophilic esophagitis: definition, epidemiology and quality of life. Minerva Gastroenterol 2022;68(1):60–8.

13. Rooij WE de, Bennebroek Evertsz' F, Lei A, et al. Mental distress among adult patients with eosinophilic esophagitis. Neuro Gastroenterol Motil 2020;e14069. https://doi.org/10.1111/nmo.14069.

14. Dellon ES, Kim HP, Sperry SLW, et al. A phenotypic analysis shows that eosinophilic esophagitis is a progressive fibrostenotic disease. Gastrointest Endosc 2014;79(4):577–85.e4.

15. Warners MJ, Oude Nijhuis RAB, Wijkerslooth LRH de, et al. The natural course of eosinophilic esophagitis and long-term consequences of undiagnosed disease in a large cohort. Am J Gastroenterol 2018;113(6):836–44.

16. Dellon ES, Gibbs WB, Fritchie KJ, et al. Clinical, endoscopic, and histologic findings distinguish eosinophilic esophagitis from gastroesophageal reflux disease. Clin Gastroenterol Hepatol 2009;7(12):1305.

17. Liacouras CA, Furuta GT, Hirano I, et al. Eosinophilic esophagitis: updated consensus recommendations for children and adults. J Allergy Clin Immunol 2011;128(1):3–20.e6 [quiz: 21–2].

18. Dellon ES, Gonsalves N, Abonia JP, et al. International Consensus Recommendations for Eosinophilic Gastrointestinal Disease Nomenclature. Clin Gastroenterol Hepatol 2022;20(11):2474–84.e3.

19. Hruz P, Straumann A, Bussmann C, et al. Escalating incidence of eosinophilic esophagitis: a 20-year prospective, population-based study in Olten County, Switzerland. J Allergy Clin Immunol 2011;128(6):1349–50.e5.

20. Arias A, Perez-Martinez I, Tenias JM, et al. Systematic review with meta-analysis: the incidence and prevalence of eosinophilic oesophagitis in children and adults in population-based studies. Aliment Pharmacol Ther 2016;43(1):3–15.

21. Dellon ES, Hirano I. Epidemiology and Natural History of Eosinophilic Esophagitis. Gastroenterology 2018;154(2):319–32.e3.

22. Kapel RC, Miller JK, Torres C, et al. Eosinophilic esophagitis: a prevalent disease in the United States that affects all age groups. Gastroenterology 2008;134(5): 1316–21.

23. Roth R, Safroneeva E, Saner Zilian C, et al. Higher educational level in patients with eosinophilic esophagitis: a comparative analysis. Dis Esophagus 2021. https://doi.org/10.1093/dote/doab010.

24. Schoepfer AM, Straumann A, Panczak R, et al. Development and validation of a symptom-based activity index for adults with eosinophilic esophagitis. Gastroenterology 2014;147(6):1255–66.e21.

25. Hirano I, Rothenberg ME, Zhang S, et al. Dysphagia Days as an Assessment of Clinical Treatment Outcome in Eosinophilic Esophagitis. Am J Gastroenterol 2023;118(4):744–7.

26. Truskaite K, Dlugosz A. Prevalence of Eosinophilic Esophagitis and Lymphocytic Esophagitis in Adults with Esophageal Food Bolus Impaction. Gastroenterology Research and Practice 2016;2016:9303858.

27. Sengupta N, Tapper EB, Corban C, et al. The clinical predictors of aetiology and complications among 173 patients presenting to the Emergency Department with oesophageal food bolus impaction from 2004-2014. Aliment Pharmacol Ther 2015;42(1):91–8.

28. Desai TK, Stecevic V, Chang C-H, et al. Association of eosinophilic inflammation with esophageal food impaction in adults. Gastrointest Endosc 2005;61(7): 795–801.

29. Biedermann L, Holbreich M, Atkins D, et al. Food-induced immediate response of the esophagus-A newly identified syndrome in patients with eosinophilic esophagitis. Allergy 2021;76(1):339–47.

30. Holbreich M, Straumann A. Features of food-induced immediate response in the esophagus (FIRE) in a series of adult patients with eosinophilic esophagitis. Allergy 2021. https://doi.org/10.1111/all.14886.

31. González-Cervera J, Arias Á, Redondo-González O, et al. Association between atopic manifestations and eosinophilic esophagitis: A systematic review and meta-analysis. Ann Allergy Asthma Immunol 2017;118(5):582–90.e2.

32. Simon D, Marti H, Heer P, et al. Eosinophilic esophagitis is frequently associated with IgE-mediated allergic airway diseases. J Allergy Clin Immunol 2005;115(5): 1090–2.

33. Noel RJ, Putnam PE, Rothenberg ME. Eosinophilic esophagitis. N Engl J Med 2004;351(9):940–1.

34. Dellon ES, Rusin S, Gebhart JH, et al. Utility of a Noninvasive Serum Biomarker Panel for Diagnosis and Monitoring of Eosinophilic Esophagitis: A Prospective Study: A Prospective Study. Am J Gastroenterol 2015;110(6):821–7.

35. Votto M, Filippo M de, Castagnoli R, et al. Non-invasive biomarkers of eosinophilic esophagitis. Acta Biomed 2021;92(S7):e2021530.

36. Straumann A, Greuter T. Lifting the Veil: The Quest for Noninvasive Biomarkers for the Accurate Diagnosis of Eosinophilic Esophagitis. Dig Dis Sci 2020. https://doi.org/10.1007/s10620-020-06451-8.

37. Attwood SE, Smyrk TC, Demeester TR, et al. Esophageal eosinophilia with dysphagia. A distinct clinicopathologic syndrome. Dig Dis Sci 1993;38(1): 109–16.

38. Straumann A, Spichtin HP, Bernoulli R, et al. Idiopathic eosinophilic esophagitis: a frequently overlooked disease with typical clinical aspects and discrete endoscopic findings. Schweiz Med Wochenschr 1994;124(33):1419–29.

39. Furuta GT, Liacouras CA, Collins MH, et al. Eosinophilic esophagitis in children and adults: a systematic review and consensus recommendations for diagnosis and treatment. 2011 DDW Abstract Supplement. 2007;133(4):1342-1363.

40. Lee JJ, Fried AJ, Hait E, et al. Topical inhaled ciclesonide for treatment of eosinophilic esophagitis. J Allergy Clin Immunol 2012;130(4):1011 [author reply: 1011–2].

41. Varadarajulu S, Eloubeidi MA, Patel RS, et al. The yield and the predictors of esophageal pathology when upper endoscopy is used for the initial evaluation of dysphagia. Gastrointest Endosc 2005;61(7):804–8.

42. Hirano I, Moy N, Heckman MG, et al. Endoscopic assessment of the oesophageal features of eosinophilic oesophagitis: validation of a novel classification and grading system. Gut 2013;62(4):489–95.

43. Schoepfer AM, Henchoz S, Biedermann L, et al. Technical feasibility, clinical effectiveness, and safety of esophageal stricture dilation using a novel endoscopic attachment cap in adults with eosinophilic esophagitis. Gastrointest Endosc 2021;94(5):912–9.e2.

44. Savarino E, Di Pietro M, Bredenoord AJ, et al. Use of the Functional Lumen Imaging Probe in Clinical Esophagology. Am J Gastroenterol 2020. https://doi.org/10.14309/ajg.0000000000000773.

45. Kwiatek MA, Hirano I, Kahrilas PJ, et al. Mechanical Properties of the Esophagus in Eosinophilic Esophagitis. Gastroenterology 2011;140(1):82–90.

46. Lin Z, Kahrilas PJ, Xiao Y, et al. Functional luminal imaging probe topography: an improved method for characterizing esophageal distensibility in eosinophilic esophagitis. Therapeutic Advances in Gastroenterology 2013;6(2):97–107.

47. Carlson DA, Hirano I, Zalewski A, et al. Improvement in Esophageal Distensibility in Response to Medical and Diet Therapy in Eosinophilic Esophagitis. Clin Trans Gastroenterol 2017;8(10):e119.

48. Kato M, Kephart GM, Talley NJ, et al. Eosinophil infiltration and degranulation in normal human tissue. Anat Rec 1998;252(3):418–25.

49. Dellon ES, Speck O, Woodward K, et al. Distribution and variability of esophageal eosinophilia in patients undergoing upper endoscopy. Mod Pathol 2015;28(3):383–90.

50. Gonsalves N, Policarpio-Nicolas M, Zhang Q, et al. Histopathologic variability and endoscopic correlates in adults with eosinophilic esophagitis. Gastrointest Endosc 2006;64(3):313–9.

51. Dhar A, Haboubi HN, Attwood SE, et al. British Society of Gastroenterology (BSG) and British Society of Paediatric Gastroenterology, Hepatology and Nutrition (BSPGHAN) joint consensus guidelines on the diagnosis and management of eosinophilic oesophagitis in children and adults. Gut 2022. https://doi.org/10.1136/gutjnl-2022-327326.

52. Schoepfer AM, Simko A, Bussmann C, et al. Eosinophilic Esophagitis: Relationship of Subepithelial Eosinophilic Inflammation With Epithelial Histology, Endoscopy, Blood Eosinophils, and Symptoms. Am J Gastroenterol 2018. https://doi.org/10.1038/ajg.2017.493.

53. Bussmann C, Schoepfer AM, Safroneeva E, et al. Comparison of different biopsy forceps models for tissue sampling in eosinophilic esophagitis. Endoscopy 2016;48(12):1069–75.

54. Taft TH, Kern E, Starkey K, et al. The dysphagia stress test for rapid assessment of swallowing difficulties in esophageal conditions. Neuro Gastroenterol Motil 2019;31(3):e13512.

55. Alexander R, Alexander JA, Ravi K, et al. Measurement of Observed Eating Behaviors in Patients With Active and Inactive Eosinophilic Esophagitis. Clin Gastroenterol Hepatol 2019;17(11):2371–3.

56. Straumann A, Spichtin H-P, Grize L, et al. Natural history of primary eosinophilic esophagitis: a follow-up of 30 adult patients for up to 11.5 years. Gastroenterology 2003;125(6):1660–9.
57. van Rhijn BD, Oors JM, Smout AJPM, et al. Prevalence of esophageal motility abnormalities increases with longer disease duration in adult patients with eosinophilic esophagitis. Neuro Gastroenterol Motil 2014;26(9):1349–55.
58. Carlson DA, Shehata C, Gonsalves N, et al. Esophageal Dysmotility Is Associated With Disease Severity in Eosinophilic Esophagitis. Clin Gastroenterol Hepatol 2021. https://doi.org/10.1016/j.cgh.2021.11.002.
59. Greenberg SB, Ocampo AA, Xue Z, et al. Increasing Rates of Esophageal Stricture and Dilation Over 2 Decades in Eosinophilic Esophagitis. Gastro Hep Adv 2023;2(4):521–3.
60. Schoepfer AM, Safroneeva E, Bussmann C, et al. Delay in diagnosis of eosinophilic esophagitis increases risk for stricture formation in a time-dependent manner. Gastroenterology 2013;145(6):1230.
61. Sperry SLW, Crockett SD, Miller CB, et al. Esophageal foreign-body impactions: epidemiology, time trends, and the impact of the increasing prevalence of eosinophilic esophagitis. Gastrointest Endosc 2011;74(5):985–91.
62. Straumann A, Bussmann C, Zuber M, et al. Eosinophilic esophagitis: analysis of food impaction and perforation in 251 adolescent and adult patients. Clin Gastroenterol Hepatol 2008;6(5):598–600.
63. Arias-González L, Rey-Iborra E, Ruiz-Ponce M, et al. Esophageal perforation in eosinophilic esophagitis: A systematic review on clinical presentation, management and outcomes. Dig Liver Dis 2020;52(3):245–52.
64. Biedermann L, Straumann A, Hruz P. Defer No Time, Delays Have Dangerous Ends (William Shakespeare). Gastroenterology 2021;161(1):42–4.
65. Larsson H, Attwood S. Eosinophilic esophagitis (EoE); a disease that must not be neglected - implications of esophageal rupture and its management. BMC Gastroenterol 2020;20(1):185.
66. Remedios M, Campbell C, Jones DM, et al. Eosinophilic esophagitis in adults: clinical, endoscopic, histologic findings, and response to treatment with fluticasone propionate. Gastrointest Endosc 2006;63(1):3–12.
67. Greuter T, Straumann A, Fernandez-Marrero Y, et al. Characterization of eosinophilic esophagitis variants by clinical, histological, and molecular analyses: A cross-sectional multi-center study. Allergy 2022;77(8):2520–33.

Endoscopic Features of Eosinophilic Esophagitis

Alain M. Schoepfer, MD[a],*, Ekaterina Safroneeva, PhD[b],
Kathryn Peterson, MD[c]

KEYWORDS

- Eosinophilic esophagitis • Edema • Rings • Exudates • Furrows • Strictures

INTRODUCTION

What Are the Endoscopic Features in Patients with Eosinophilic Esophagitis?

Eosinophilic esophagitis (EoE) is a chronic type 2 allergic inflammatory disease characterized by an increasing incidence and prevalence in both children and adults.[1–3] The diagnosis of EoE is based on the presence of symptoms related to esophageal dysfunction, the presence of at least 15 eosinophils per high-power field (400-fold magnification under the microscope), and the exclusion of other diseases associated with esophageal eosinophilia (such as gastroesophageal reflux disease, esophageal infection, and so forth).[1–3] If left untreated, the majority of EoE patients will develop esophageal strictures that substantially increase the risk for food bolus impactions.[4–6] Food bolus impactions should be avoided, not only due to patient discomfort but also because food bolus impactions can be associated with esophageal perforations, either induced by retching or procedure-related.[7] Although the endoscopic presentations are not part of EoE's diagnostic pillars, knowledge regarding these features is key for several reasons. First, endoscopy with esophageal mucosal biopsy sampling is needed to diagnose EoE, and endoscopic appearances can identify areas of inflammation. Second, endoscopic activity, for example, the presence of esophageal strictures, drives therapeutic decisions beyond histologic severity. As such, endoscopic assessment is highly supportive of the diagnosis and critical for monitoring disease activity and the natural history of EoE patients.

In order to address an unmet need, the validated Endoscopic Reference System (EREFS; edema, rings, exudates, furrows, and strictures) was developed to describe

Funding sources: Work supported by a grant from the Swiss National Science Foundation (32003B_204751/1 to A.M. Schoepfer) and the Swiss EoE foundation (to A.M. Schoepfer). Specific author contributions: All authors contributed equally to this article.
[a] Department of Gastroenterology and Hepatology, Centre Hospitalier Universitaire Vaudois and University of Lausanne, Rue Du Bugnon 44, Lausanne 1011, Switzerland; [b] Institute of Social and Preventive Medicine, University of Bern, Mittelstrasse 43, Bern 3012, Switzerland; [c] Division of Gastroenterology and Hepatology, Department of Internal Medicine, University of Utah, 50 North Medical Drive, SOM 4R118, Salt Lake City, UT 84132, USA
* Corresponding author.
E-mail address: alain.schoepfer@chuv.ch

endoscopic features of EoE. In their landmark study, Hirano and colleagues[8] evaluated endoscopy videos from 25 EoE patients and controls reviewed by 21 gastroenterologists. Interobserver agreement of different endoscopic features was analyzed. The original grading system included the following major features of the EREFS scoring system: edema (also referred to as decreased vascular pattern; graded from 0 to 2), fixed rings (graded from 0 to 3), exudates (graded from 0 to 2), furrows (also referred to as vertical lines; graded from 0 to 2), and strictures (graded binary absent vs present). The *initial grading system* included the following minor features: feline esophagus (also referred to as transient concentric mucosal rings; graded binary as absent vs present), narrow caliber esophagus (reduced luminal diameter of the majority of the tubular esophagus; graded binary as absent vs present), and crepe paper esophagus (also referred to as mucosal fragility or laceration after passage of the diagnostic endoscope but not after esophageal dilation; graded binary as absent vs present).[8] The *final classification* and grading system is shown in **Box 1**. Typical endoscopic features of EoE are shown in **Fig. 1**. Of note, the EREFS system was developed as a grading system to document the type and severity of endoscopic features of EoE. The development and validation of EREFS as an endoscopic scoring system to document change of endoscopic severity following a therapeutic intervention were published in later studies.

The sensitivity of endoscopic features to diagnose EoE is reported with a considerable variability. An endoscopically normal esophagus has been described in 10% to 32% of both pediatric and adult patients with EoE.[9,10] These early studies that reported a high prevalence of endoscopically normal esophagus in EoE patients might

---

Box 1
Final classification and grading system for the endoscopic assessment of the esophageal features of eosinophilic esophagitis according to Hirano and colleagues[8]

Major Features
- *Fixed rings* (also referred to as concentric rings, corrugated esophagus, corrugated rings, ringed esophagus, trachealisation)
  - Grade 0: none
  - Grade 1: mild (subtle circumferential ridges)
  - Grade 2: moderate (distinct rings that do not impair passage of a standard diagnostic adult endoscope [outer diameter of 8–9.5 mm])
  - Grade 3: severe (distinct rings that do not permit passage of a diagnostic endoscope)
- *Exudates* (also referred to as white spots, plaques)
  - Grade 0: none
  - Grade 1: mild (lesions involving<10% of the esophageal surface area)
  - Grade 2: severe (lesions involving>10% of the esophageal surface area)
- *Furrows* (also referred to as vertical lines, longitudinal furrows)
  - Grade 0: absent
  - Grade 1: present
- *Edema* (also referred to as decreased vascular markings, mucosal pallor)
  - Grade 0: absent (distinct vascularity present)
  - Grade 1: present (loss of clarity of absence of vascular markings)
- *Stricture*
  - Grade 0: absent
  - Grade 1: present

Minor features
- Crepe paper esophagus (mucosal fragility or laceration after passage of the diagnostic endoscope but not after esophageal dilation)
  - Grade 0: absent
  - Grade 1: present

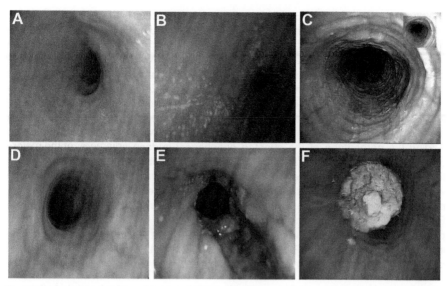

Fig. 1. Endoscopic aspects of eosinophilic esophagitis according to Endoscopic Reference System (EREFS) grading system. (*A*) Edema and furrows at 7 o' clock and 9 o' clock; (*B*) exudates covering greater than 10% of the esophageal surface area; (*C*) rings, edema, furrows, and exudates; (*D*) edema, rings, and stricture; (*E*) edema, exudates, rings, and a stricture at the gastroesophageal junction, leaving a mucosal tear after passage with the adult diagnostic endoscope (crepe paper esophagus); (*F*) edema, rings, furrows, and an impacted piece of chicken. (Image courtesy of Dr. Alain Schoepfer.)

have been influenced by the fact that less experienced endoscopists can miss endoscopic features. Several randomized controlled trials, in which endoscopic features were prospectively assessed, showed EREFS criteria to have sensitivities over 90% to diagnose EoE.[11,12]

Critical Appraisal of Distinct Endoscopic Features of Eosinophilic Esophagitis

The characteristic of edema (loss of vascularization) is explained by the mucosal inflammatory activity in the esophagus from EoE. Longitudinal furrows develop because of a folding of the edematous mucosa. Exudates represent mucosal areas characterized by a high eosinophil density.[8] In biopsies of exudates, eosinophilic microabscesses are typically observed. Circumferential rings and strictures are commonly a consequence of subepithelial fibrosis.[8,13] Of note, there exists an overlap between severe rings and strictures.[8] Strictures are typically diagnosed when the diagnostic adult endoscope (outer diameter between 8–9.5 mm) passes against a resistance or when passage is no longer possible. Given the fact that the normal esophageal caliber in an adult is around 25 mm, every reduction of esophageal caliber would formally qualify as stricture. Indeed, esophageal narrowing is frequently underappreciated at endoscopy in EoE.[8] As of yet, there is no widely accepted definition of which minimal esophageal caliber defines a stricture, which explains the heterogeneity of data reporting on esophageal strictures. Exudates, edema, and furrows represent *inflammatory features* whereas rings and strictures represent *fibrotic features*.[8] Hence, an anti-inflammatory therapy such as swallowed topical corticosteroids or dupilumab will have an effect particularly on inflammatory features but to a lesser degree on fibrotic features, whereas esophageal dilation will have an impact on rings and strictures but not on underlying inflammatory endoscopic features.[14–16]

A simple way to integrate EREFS into daily clinical practice is to annotate the letters of the acronym followed by the grading. As such, the grading E1R2Ex1F1S1 would be decoded as edema present, rings moderate, exudates mild, furrows present, and stricture present. While the assessment of edema, furrows, and rings is quite clear-cut, the authors propose to discuss some modifications that could be beneficial for standardizing the assessment of endoscopic activity of EoE. First, to avoid confusing the grading of exudates and edema, the authors propose to abbreviate edema by "E" and exudates by "Ex". Second, following the current grading system, exudates covering 11% to 100% of the esophageal surface area would all be graded as Ex2. Adding the percentage of the affected esophageal surface area can provide more granularity when judging the efficacy of a therapeutic intervention. For example, using the aforementioned example, E1R2Ex40%F1S1 would describe an esophagus in which 40% of the mucosal surface is affected by white exudates. Third, the authors propose the inclusion of the minimal esophageal caliber (measured in mm) into the EREFS grading system when strictures are encountered. In addition, the authors propose to describe the location of the stricture measured in cm from the dental line. Using the earlier example, Ex1R2Ex1F1S1(11 mm;30 cm/DL) would describe a stricture of 11 mm diameter at 30 cm from the dental line.

Use of Endoscopic Reference System Grading System to Assess Endoscopic Activity of Eosinophilic Esophagitis

In daily practice and in observational studies, global disease activity of EoE is measured using a combination of patient-reported outcomes (EoE-related symptoms and quality of life) and biologic disease activity, which encompasses histologic and endoscopic activity.[17–19] The American Society for Gastrointestinal Endoscopy recently published a consensus paper on the role of endoscopy in the diagnosis and monitoring of EoE patients.[20] Participating experts recommended to routinely use the EREFS grading system to assess endoscopic activity of EoE. There are several strong arguments to support this claim.

First, the correlation between EoE-related symptoms and histology is poor which advocates for the inclusion of endoscopic activity as a reliable physician-reported endpoint.[21,22] Symptom severity in adults is influenced by food avoidance and behavioral modification strategies which can lead to an underestimation of dysphagia.[21,22] Additionally, dysphagia is considered a symptom which occurs more commonly in adolescents and adults. Young patients may present with varied symptoms from food avoidance, malnutrition, abdominal pain, vomiting, and mealtime anxiety.[3] The variable symptoms of EoE in the pediatric population contribute even more to the difficulty in correlating symptoms to histology. This mandates additional measurements such as endoscopic assessments.

Second, currently accepted histopathologic assessments of peak eosinophil numbers in esophageal biopsies do not take into account the patchiness of histologic activity and furthermore lack acknowledgment of the contribution of inflammatory cell types other than eosinophils that are involved in EoE pathogenesis. Assessment of histologic inflammation by means of esophageal biopsies accounts for a very small fraction of the entire esophageal surface. Additionally, routine esophageal biopsies provide subepithelial tissue in only half of the cases.[23] Therefore, assessment of endoscopic disease activity provides a more global view of inflammatory and fibrotic esophageal alterations than the histopathologic assessment that is often limited to the assessment of inflammatory changes. Endoscopic rings and strictures are able to predict the future risk of food bolus impactions and need for esophageal dilation.[24] In summary, the assessment of endoscopic disease activity complements microscopic and symptom measures, providing thereby a holistic view of overall EoE symptom severity.[25]

Third, assessment of endoscopic activity using EREFS is easy to learn and to perform In dally clinical practice and does not require additional time compared to the standard of care procedures. The use of the acronym EREFS avoids lengthy descriptions in the endoscopy report. A Dutch group evaluated the interobserver agreement of EREFS features and showed it to be substantial for rings (κ 0.70), white exudates (κ 0.63), and crepe paper esophagus (κ 0.62), moderate for furrows (κ 0.49) and strictures (κ 0.54), and slight for edema (κ 0.12).[26] Intraobserver agreement was substantial for rings (median κ 0.64, interquartile range [IQR] 0.46–0.70), furrows (median κ 0.69, IQR 0.50–0.89), and crepe paper esophagus (median κ 0.69, IQR 0.62–0.83), moderate for white exudates (median κ 0.58, IQR 0.54–0.71) and strictures (median κ 0.54, IQR 0.33–0.70), and less than chance for edema (median κ 0.00, IQR 0.00–0.29). Furthermore, interobserver and intraobserver agreement was not substantially different between expert and trainee endoscopists.[26]

Fourth, the responsiveness of EREFS to a therapeutic intervention has been demonstrated in several randomized placebo-controlled clinical trials.[11,12,14,27] The usefulness of using EREFS as an objective therapeutic endpoint is highlighted by the low rate of change in EREFS score seen within placebo arms. Improvement of inflammatory endoscopic features several weeks after the introduction of an anti-eosinophil treatment provides the endoscopist with important information regarding the effectiveness of the treatment beyond that achieved by histology.[28] The EREFS grading system is formally validated as an endoscopy score.[27] In a randomized, placebo-controlled study evaluating fluticasone orodispersible tablets to treat clinically and histologically active EoE in adults, the EREFS scores, that assessed the proximal and distal esophagus separately, were no better at documenting the change in endoscopic findings of EoE than a simple EREFS score that was calculated from the worst feature (ie, most severe area of involvement) along the entire length of the esophagus.[27] Hence, for daily clinical practice and observational studies, the authors recommend a pan-esophageal scoring of the EREFS using the highest scored area (edema [absent or present], rings [absent, mild, moderate, or severe], exudates [absent, mild, or severe], furrows [absent or present], stricture [absent or present with estimation of diameter in mm and location of stricture measured in cm from the dental line]).

Fifth, some limitations of EREFS as therapeutic endpoint should be noted. Endoscopic features of EoE are not pathognomonic for EoE and can be found in other esophageal conditions.[29] While the EREFS grading system has been shown to identify the majority of patients with EoE, its performance in determining response to anti-inflammatory treatment is limited with an area under the curve ranging from 0.79 to 0.88 as compared to the gold standard of histologic remission defined as peak eosinophil count of ≤ 15/hpf. As such, 12% to 21% of patients would be misclassified regarding the therapeutic response.[30,31] Thus, the EREFS grading system should be used *together with, and not in place of* histologic findings to accurately assess physiologic disease activity in EoE. The role of endoscopy in the follow-up of EoE patients has also been highlighted in a recent consensus paper from an international expert group.[32]

CLINICS CARE POINTS

- Endoscopic features of EoE are edema, rings, exudates, furrows, and strictures (EREFS).
- Endoscopic activity of EoE should be graded using EREFS at every endoscopy.

- Endoscopic response to therapy should be graded using the EREFS score (total score range: 0–8 points).
- The EREFS applied to the highest scoring area should be used to assess the entire esophagus.
- Endoscopic activity should be assessed in conjunction with histologic activity to gain insights into biologic activity of EoE.

DISCLOSURE

A.M. Schoepfer received consulting fees and/or speaker fees and/or research grants from Avir Pharma, Inc., Adare/Ellodi Pharmaceuticals, Inc., AstraZeneca, AG, Switzerland, Receptos-Celgene-BMS Corp., Dr Falk Pharma, GmbH, Germany, Glaxo Smith Kline, AG, Nestlé S. A., Switzerland, Novartis, AG, Switzerland, and Regeneron-Sanofi Pharmaceuticals, Inc. E. Safroneeva reports (i) consulting fees from Avir Pharma, Inc., Aptalis Pharma, Inc., Celgene Corp., Novartis, AG, and Regeneron Pharmaceuticals Inc; (ii) being an employee of Tillotts Pharma AG. K. Peterson received (i) consulting fees and/or speaker fees from AGA, Alladapt, AstraZeneca, Allakos, Bristol Meyers Squibb, Ellodi, ITA group, Lecture LInx, Lucid, Nexstone (Ubiquity), WebMD, Peerview, PLatform Q health, Regeneron, Revolo, Sanofi, Takeda, WebMD; (ii) research support from AstraZeneca, Allakos, Regeneron-Sanofi, Revolo, Adare, Ellodi, Bristol Meyers Squibb, Celdex; and (iii) equity from Nexeos Bio.

REFERENCES

1. Furuta GT, Liacouras CA, Collins MH, et al. Eosinophilic esophagitis in children and adults: a systematic review and consensus recommendations for diagnosis and treatment. Gastroenterology 2007;133:1342–63.
2. Liacouras CA, Furuta GT, Hirano I, et al. Eosinophilic esophagitis: updated consensus recommendations for children and adults. J Allergy Clin Immunol 2011;128:3–20.
3. Lucendo AJ, Molina-Infante J, Arias A, et al. Guidelines on eosinophilic esophagitis: evidence-based statements and recommendations for diagnosis and management in children and adults. United European Gastroenterol J 2017;5:335–58.
4. Schoepfer AM, Safroneeva E, Bussmann C, et al. Delay in diagnosis of eosinophilic esophagitis increases risk for stricture formation in a time-dependent manner. Gastroenterology 2013;145:1230–6.
5. Dellon ES, Kim HP, Sperry SL, et al. A phenotypic analysis shows that eosinophilic esophagitis is a progressive fibrostenotic disease. Gastrointest Endosc 2014;79:577–85.
6. Lipka S, Kumar A, Richter JE. Impact of diagnostic delay and other risk factors on eosinophilic esophagitis phenotype and esophageal diameter. J Clin Gastroenterol 2016;50:134–40.
7. Arias-González L, Rey-Iborra E, Ruiz-Ponce M, et al. Esophageal perforation in eosinophilic esophagitis: A systematic review on clinical presentation, management and outcomes. Dig Liver Dis 2020;52:245–52.
8. Hirano I, Moy N, Heckman MG, et al. Endoscopic assessment of the oesophageal features of eosinophilic oesophagitis: validation of a noval classification and grading system. Gut 2013;62:498–595.
9. Mackenzie SH, Go M, Chadwick B, et al. , Kuwada S, et al. Eosinophilic oesophagitis in patients presenting with dysphagia–a prospective analysis. Aliment Pharmacol 2008;28:1140–6.

10. Liacouras CA, Spergel JM, Ruchelli E, et al. Eosinophilic esophagitis: a 10-year experience in 381 children. Clin Gastroenterol Hepatol 2005;3:1198–206.

11. Lucendo AJ, Miehlke S, Schlag C, et al. Efficacy of budesonide orodispersible tablets as induction therapy for eosinophilic esophagitis in a randomized placebo-controlled trial. Gastroenterology 2019;157:74–86.

12. Hirano I, Collins MH, Katzka DA, et al. Budesonide oral suspension improves outcomes in patients with eosinophilic esophagitis: results from a Phase 3 Trial. Clin Gastroenterol Hepatol 2022;20:525–34.

13. Hirano I, Furuta GT. Approaches and challenges to management of pediatric and adult patients with eosinophilic esophagitis. Gastroenterology 2020;158:840–51.

14. Straumann A, Lucendo AJ, Miehlke S, et al. Budesonide orodispersible tablets maintain remission in a randomized, placebo-controlled trial of patients with eosinophilic esophagitis. Gastroenterology 2020;159:1672–85.

15. Dellon ES, Rothenberg ME, Collins MH, et al. Dupilumab in adults and adolescents with eosinophilic esophagitis. N Engl J Med 2022;387:2317–30.

16. Schoepfer AM, Gonsalves N, Bussmann C, et al. Esophageal dilation in eosinophilic esophagitis: effectiveness, safety, and impact on the underlying inflammation. Am J Gastroenterol 2010;105:1062–70.

17. Schoepfer A, Safroneeva E, Straumann A. How to measure disease activity in eosinophilic esophagitis. Dis Esophagus 2016;29:959–66.

18. Schoepfer AM, Schürmann C, Trelle S, et al. Systematic review of outcome measures used in observational studies of adults with eosinophilic esophagitis. Int Arch Allergy Immunol 2021;182:1169–93.

19. COREOS Collaborators, Ma C, Schoepfer AM, Dellon ES, et al. Development of a core outcome set for therapeutic studies in eosinophilic esophagitis (COREOS). J Allergy Clin Immunol 2022;149:659–70.

20. Aceves SS, Alexander JA, Baron TH, et al. Endoscopic approach to eosinophilic esophagitis: American Society for Gastrointestinal Endoscopy Consensus Conference. Gastrointest Endosc 2022;96:576–92.

21. Safroneeva E, Straumann A, Coslovsky M, et al. Symptoms have modest accuracy in detecting endoscopic and histologic remission in adults with eosinophilic esophagitis. Gastroenterology 2016;150:581–659.

22. Safroneeva E, Straumann A, Schoepfer AM. Latest insights on the relationship between symptoms and biologic findings in adults with eosinophilic esophagitis. Gastrointest Endosc Clin N Am 2018;28:35–45.

23. Bussmann C, Schoepfer AM, Safroneeva E, et al. Comparison of different biopsy forceps models for tissue sampling in eosinophilic esophagitis. Endoscopy 2016; 48:1069–75.

24. Hirano I. How to approach a patient with eosinophilic esophagitis. Gastroenterology 2018;155:601–6.

25. Schoepfer AM, Panczak R, Zwahlen M, et al. How do gastroenterologists assess overall activity of eosinophilic esophagitis in adult patients? Am J Gastroenterol 2015;110:402–14.

26. van Rhijn B, Warners MJ, Curvers MJ, et al. Evaluating the endoscopic reference score for eosinophilic esophagitis: moderate to substantial intra- and interobserver reliability. Endoscopy 2014;46:1049–55.

27. Schoepfer AM, Hirano I, Coslovsky M, et al. Variation in endoscopic activity assessment and endoscopy score validation in adults with eosinophilic esophagitis. Clin Gastroenterol Hepatol 2019;17:1477–88.

28. Dellon ES, Gupta SK. A Conceptual Approach to understanding treatment response in eosinophilic esophagitis. Clin Gastroenterol Hepatol 2019;17: 2149–60.

29. Dellon ES, Gibbs WB, Fritchie KJ, et al. Clinical, endoscopic, and histologic findings distinguish eosinophilic esophagitis from gastroesophageal reflux disease. Clin Gastroenterol Hepatol 2009;7:1305–13.

30. Wechsler JB, Bolton SM, Amsden K, et al. Eosinophilic Esophagitis reference score accurately identifies disease activity and treatment effects in children. Clin Gastroenterol Hepatol 2018;16:1056–63.

31. Hori K, Watari J, Fukui H, et al. Do endoscopic features suggesting eosinophilic esophagitis represent histological eosinophilia? Dig Endosc 2014;26:156–63.

32. Von Arnim U, Biedermann L, Aceves SS, et al. Monitoring patients with eosinophilic esophagitis in routine clinical practice – International expert recommendations. Clin Gastroenterol Hepatol 2023;21:2526–33.

Histopathology of Eosinophilic Esophagitis

Margaret H. Collins, MD[a],*, Nicoleta C. Arva, MD, PhD[b],
Anas Bernieh, MD[c], Oscar Lopez-Nunez, MD[c],
Maria Pletneva, MD, PhD[d], Guang-Yu Yang, MD, PhD[e]

KEYWORDS

- Stricture • Smooth muscle • Remodeling • Fibrosis • Treatment • Esophagus
- Eosinophils

KEY POINTS

- Peak eosinophil count and additional abnormalities in esophageal biopsies should be included in eosinophilic esophagitis pathology reports.
- A web-based tool uses patient age and 3 epithelial abnormalities (basal zone hyperplasia, surface epithelial alteration, and dyskeratotic epithelial cells) to predict lamina propria fibrosis in biopsies lacking evaluable lamina propria.
- Samples of the deeper esophageal wall could aid clinical care by exposing pathology not represented in endoscopic samples.
- Smooth muscle, myofibroblasts, and extracellular matrix are significant components of pediatric esophageal strictures due to various causes.

BACKGROUND

Eosinophilic esophagitis (EoE), a chronic relapsing disease that afflicts both adults and children, is defined by clinical signs/symptoms and esophageal biopsy pathology.[1–3] The pathology portion of the diagnosis requires at least 15 intraepithelial eosinophils in at least 1 high power field (hpf) from any portion of the esophagus. Dysphagia is the most common symptom in adults and adolescents, and children have more protean manifestations including vomiting, failure to thrive, food aversion, etc. Although

[a] Department of Pathology and Laboratory Medicine, Cincinnati Children's Hospital Medical Center, University of Cincinnati College of Medicine, Pathology ML1035, 3333 Burnet Avenue, Cincinnati, OH 45229, USA; [b] Department of Pathology, Nationwide Children's Hospital, 700 Children's Drive, Columbus, OH 43205, USA; [c] Pathology ML1035, Cincinnati Children's Hospital Medical Center, 3333 Burnet Ave.nue Cincinnati, OH 45229, USA; [d] Department of Pathology, University of Utah School of Medicine, 50 North Medical Drive, Salt Lake City, UT 84132, USA; [e] Department of Pathology, Ward Building Ward 4-115, Northwestern University Feinberg School of Medicine, 303 East Chicago Avenue, Chicago, IL. 60611, USA
* Corresponding author.
E-mail address: margaret.collins@cchmc.org

Immunol Allergy Clin N Am 44 (2024) 205–221
https://doi.org/10.1016/j.iac.2023.12.008
0889-8561/24/© 2023 Elsevier Inc. All rights reserved.
immunology.theclinics.com

symptoms vary with age, esophageal biopsies from adults who have EoE resemble those from children,[4] except for very young ($\leq$12 months of age) children.[5]

Evaluation of Esophageal Biopsies for Eosinophilic Esophagitis

Microscopic examination of esophageal epithelium is the only means to confirm the presence of the diagnostic threshold value of eosinophil inflammation and therefore pathology is an essential component of clinical evaluation to diagnose EoE. A minimum of 6 biopsy pieces is recommended to ensure sufficient sampling because EoE has a patchy distribution.[6] Distal and proximal esophagus are most commonly sampled; however, biopsies from the mid esophagus may be the only biopsies that display abnormalities.[7]

The luminal surface of the normal human esophagus is lined by non-keratinized squamous epithelium. Biopsies obtained by conventional endoscopy often consist of squamous epithelium without underlying lamina propria, or lamina propria that shows crush artifact complicating the ability to adequately assess lamina propria pathology. In addition to conventional endoscopy, biopsies may be procured by transnasal endoscopy,[8] or cytosponge[9] which do not require anesthesia, an advantage especially attractive for pediatric patients. The esophageal string test yields data that correlate with disease activity.[10]

History of Eosinophilic Esophagitis Biopsy Evaluation

Distinguishing esophageal biopsies of gastroesophageal reflux disease (GERD) from EoE was an early goal. Numerous intraepithelial eosinophils in esophageal biopsies were emphasized as typical of EoE. In addition, other abnormalities, for example, basal zone hyperplasia,[11–14] were included in descriptions of EoE pathology; subsequently, eosinophil abscess[15,16] and surface layering[15] were added. The original histology scoring system consisted of acute inflammatory cells in addition to eosinophils, basal zone hyperplasia, and elongated papilla.[12] Early immunohistochemical studies demonstrated epithelial cell hyperplasia,[17] and the type 2 inflammatory nature of EoE.[18] Since the early studies, proposed markers to distinguish EoE from GERD include ALOX15,[19] or the number of T regulatory lymphocytes[20] or, of activated mast cells.[21]

Eosinophilic Esophagitis Histology Scoring System

A comprehensive histology scoring system was subsequently developed that evaluates 8 abnormalities for severity as a grade score and extent as a stage score (**Figs. 1–8, Table 1**).[22] Scoring is based on a 4-point scale: 0 = normal, or absence of an abnormality, and 3 = the most marked/extensive abnormality. The features may be reported in a dichotomous manner, as present or absent, but more detailed scoring helps determine improvement or deterioration over time, and response to therapy changes. Polytomous evaluation can be provided using numbers, or words such as mild, moderate, or marked. For example, "Numerous eosinophils are present along with basal zone hyperplasia (BZH) and dilated intercellular spaces" is less informative than "Peak intraepithelial eosinophil count is 57/hpf, most hpf appear to contain more than 15 eosinophils, and both marked BZH and markedly dilated intercellular spaces are seen diffusely." The latter narrative is even more meaningful if accompanied by, "The current biopsy appears significantly worse compared to the immediate previous biopsy."

Importance of Peak Eosinophil Count

All consensus statements/recommendations advise a peak count of $\geq$15 intraepithelial eosinophils/hpf from any region of the esophagus for diagnosis (see **Fig. 1**).[1–3]

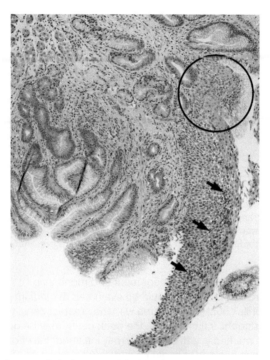

Fig. 1. Numerous intraepithelial eosinophils (grade 3, *arrows*) are found in esophageal squamous epithelium at the gastroesophageal junction (*circle*). 100 ×.

Therefore, a peak count should be generated, not estimates such as ≥ a number ≤, or a range of estimated numbers. Assuming that the endoscopist provides representative samples of esophageal pathology, and recognizing the limitations of patchy distribution, peak eosinophil count (PEC) provides the best opportunity for point-to-point comparisons among consecutive biopsies for this remitting/relapsing disease,

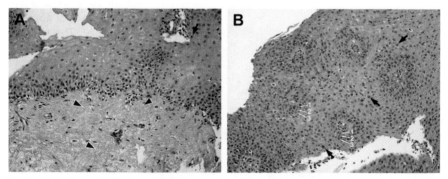

Fig. 2. (*A*) Delicate fibrils (*arrowheads*) populate this lamina propria. A single intraepithelial eosinophil is found (*arrow*). 200 ×. (*B*) A different piece from the same biopsy from the proximal esophagus as A shows numerous intraepithelial eosinophils (grade 3, *arrows*). The piece is not well-oriented but most papillae are surrounded by the normal number (3) of epithelial cell layers (numbers). 200 ×.

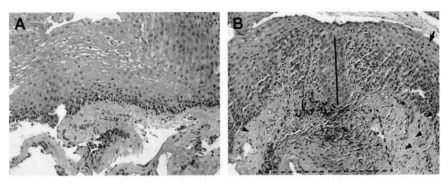

Fig. 3. (*A*) The epithelium and lamina propria appear normal in this mid esophageal biopsy. 200 ×. (*B*) This distal esophageal biopsy was obtained at the same endoscopy as A, and shows numerous intraepithelial eosinophils (*arrows*) (peak eosinophil count 148/hpt) and basal zone hyperplasia (BZH) (grade 3, bar). Lamina propria shows crush artifact inside the dashed lines, but adjacent to that area delicate fibrils are present (*arrowheads*). 200 ×.

and is recommended for disease management and monitoring.[23,24] To obtain a PEC, all pieces of all submitted biopsies should be evaluated at medium power (see **Figs. 2** and **3**), and eosinophils counted in the area with the greatest density. For biopsies with focal low-count eosinophil inflammation, the peak count may be quickly ascertained; for biopsies that are markedly, diffusely, uniformly inflamed, the effort is more arduous. Pathologists who have decided to evaluate additional abnormalities can assess the biopsy pieces for those abnormalities while surveying for the PEC.The slope of the learning curve to reproducibly evaluate multiple features simultaneously is not steep for experienced pathologists, but may be for less experienced pathologists,[25] suggesting that esophageal pathology is not well-taught in pathology training programs. After the peak eosinophil count is obtained, additional evaluations of numerous hpf(s) are unnecessary to generate word or numerical scores of other components of the Eosinophilic Esophagitis Histology Scoring System (EoEHSS) if those components were assessed during the search for a specific peak eosinophil count.

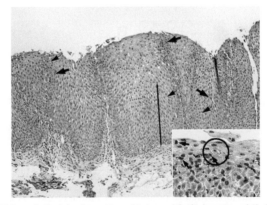

Fig. 4. Marked BZH (grade 2 at *bar*), scattered intraepithelial eosinophils (*black arrows*), and dilated intercellular spaces (*white-edge arrows*) are seen in this biopsy following therapy. 100 × The inset illustrates a dyskeratotic epithelial cell (*circle*) and intraepithelial eosinophils (*arrows*). 400 ×.

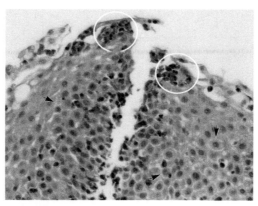

Fig. 5. Eosinophil abscesses (grade 2, *circles*) and dilated intercellular spaces (grade 1, *arrows*) are present in this biopsy. 400 ×.

Evaluating Additional Abnormalities

All EoE abnormalities may be patchy, including among pieces obtained at the same time from the same esophageal region (see **Figs. 2** and **3**). Some features are best evaluated in well-oriented pieces. BZH(see **Figs. 2–4, 6**) is most accurately evaluated in biopsies exhibiting the entire depth, but even in poorly-oriented biopsies there are usually a few areas sufficiently oriented to permit scoring. If not, counting the number

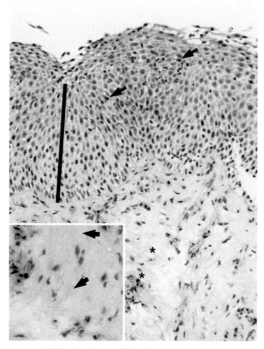

Fig. 6. Numerous intraepithelial eosinophils (*arrows*) populate markedly hyperplastic epithelium in this biopsy. Mildly coalescent fibrils form vague fibers (*asterisks*) in the lamina propria. 200 × Inset Higher power view of the lamina propria illustrates thin fibers (*arrows*). 400 ×.

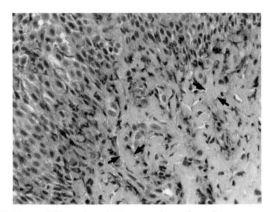

Fig. 7. Extremely thickened fibers (grade 3–*arrows*) are found in a non-compressed area of the lamina propria in this biopsy. 400 ×.

of layers (should not exceed 3 or 4) of basal zone surrounding papillae cut in cross section may be informative (see **Fig. 2**). Surface epithelial alteration (see **Fig. 8**) or eosinophil surface layering cannot be evaluated if surface epithelium is not present. Dilated intercellular spaces (see **Figs. 4, 5** and **8**) may not be evaluable in very superficial pieces. In contrast, eosinophil abscesses (see **Fig. 8**) and dyskeratotic epithelial cells

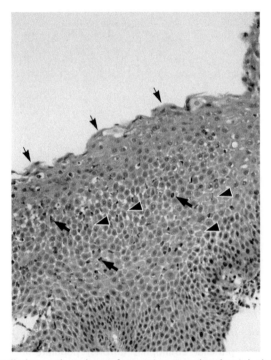

Fig. 8. Epithelial cells (*arrows*) at the surface stain more deeply pink than the underlying epithelium constituting surface epithelial alteration (grade 1). Dilated intercellular spaces (grade 2–*arrowheads*) are also present. 200 ×.

Table 1
Abnormalities evaluated in the eosinophilic esophagitis histology scoring system

Abnormality/ Component	Definition	Grade	Stage
Eosinophil inflammation (based on peak eosinophil count (PEC))	≥15 eosinophils in any hpf; intact cells are counted. Granules not associated with a nucleus are not counted unless forming a discrete aggregate surrounded by a cytoplasmic membrane.	0 - no eosinophils 1 - <15/hpf 2 - ≥15–44/hpf 3 - –45 - >60/hpf	0 - PEC ≤15/hpf PEC ≥15/hpf in 1 - <33% hpf 2%–33%–66% hpf 3 - >66% hpf
Basal zone hyperplasia	Cells in the basal zone have little cytoplasm, and are closely spaced separated by less than the diameter of their nucleus. Basal zone occupying 15% or more of total epithelial thickness is abnormal.	0 - no BZH 1 - BZH >15% < 33% total epithelial thickness 2%–33%–66% 3 - >66%	0 - no BZH 1 - any grade >0 in <33% of epithelium 2%–33%–66% 3 - >66%
Eosinophil abscess	Aggregates of eosinophils obscuring underlying architecture	0 - no EA 1 - 4–9 eosinophils in EA 2–10–20 3 - >30	0 - no EA 1 - any grade >0 in <33% of epithelium 2%–33%–66% 3 - >66%
Eosinophil surface layering	Eosinophils aligned parallel to the epithelial surface. One or more rows may comprise a focus of surface layering.	0 - no ESL 1 - 3–4 eosinophils 2 - 5–10 eosinophils 3 - >10 eosinophils	0 - no SL 1 - any grade >0 in <33% of epithelium 2%–33%–66% 3 - >66%
Dilated intercellular spaces	Spaces between epithelial cells exhibit tram-track-like portions of intercellular connections.	0 - no DIS 1 - DIS visible at 400x 2–200x 3–100x	0 - no DIS 1 - any grade >0 in <33% of epithelium 2%–33%–66% 3 - >66%
Surface epithelial alteration	Epithelial cells lining the esophageal lumen stain more deeply pink than underlying epithelial cells. Eosinophils may be admixed with the altered epithelial cells, which may become detached from the rest of the epithelium.	0 - no SEA 1 - no admixed eosinophils 2 - few eosinophils 3 - exudate	0 - no SEA 1 - any grade >0 in <33% epithelium 2%–33%–66% 3 - >66%

(continued on next page)

Table 1 (continued)			
Abnormality/ Component	**Definition**	**Grade**	**Stage**
Dyskeratotic epithelial cells	Individual epithelial cells anywhere in the epithelium exhibit small hyperchromatic nuclei and cytoplasm that is more pink than adjacent epithelial cells.	0 - no DEC 1 - cell/hpf 2 - 2–5 DEC/hpf 3 - >5/hpf	0 - no DEC 1 - any grade >0 in <33% of epithelium 2%–33%–66% 3 - >66%
Lamina propria fibrosis	Lamina propria fibrils are replaced by fibers that equal or exceed the diameter of basal cell nuclei.	0 - no LPF 1 - cohesive fibrils 2 - fiber diameter = basal cell nucleus diameter 3 - fiber diameter > cell nucleus diameter	0 - no LPF 1 - any grade >0 in <33% LP 2%–33%–66% 3 - >66%

(see **Fig. 4**) may be found in poorly-oriented epithelium and superficial epithelium. Lamina propria is often not present in biopsies or else may be compressed from prior handling. Areas of crush artifact must not be considered fibrotic, an error that may contribute to less than optimum interobserver agreement (see **Fig. 3**).[26–28] Nuclei that are exclusively elongated and hyperchromatic are indications of prior compression; in areas of true lamina propria fiber thickening, connective tissue and other nuclei are round and at least some are vesicular (see **Figs. 6** and **7**). The issues concerning lamina propria and the interpretation of its fibrosis may become irrelevant; a web-based tool (Available at: Model to Predict Lamina Propria Fibrosis [LPF] in Eosinophilic Esophagitis [shinyapps.io]) uses EoEHSS grade and stage scores for basal zone hyperplasia, surface epithelial alteration, and dyskeratotic epithelial cells plus patient age to predict lamina propria fibrosis.[29] The relationship between lamina propria remodeling and remodeling in deeper wall components is uncertain; a recent study of pediatric esophageal strictures suggests that lamina propria may not be necessary for stricture formation/maintenance (see esophageal remodeling below).

Additional Abnormalities Are Important

The EoEHSS is responsive[30–35] and reliable.[22,25,36] EoEHSS scores correlate with symptoms,[37,38] endoscopic features,[7,30,39] IgG4 levels,[40] eosinophil progenitor levels,[41] and endotypes.[42] EoEHSS scores distinguish active disease from remission, defined as fewer than 15 eosinophils/hpf, EoE and gastroesophageal reflux disease (GERD) that also has at most low eosinophil counts; however, the scores are higher in EoE remission biopsies compared to GERD biopsies.[43] EoEHSS scores do not distinguish active EoE biopsies from biopsies with ≥15 eosinophils/hpf from patients who do not have symptoms of esophageal dysfunction, although some of those patients subsequently exhibit characteristic EoE symptoms.[44] Individual EoEHSS components, specifically BZHin children and adults, and dilated intercellular spaces in children,[45–47] associate with persistent symptoms in biopsies considered inactive based on PEC of 0 to 14 eosinophils/hpf. Dilated intercellular spaces are good candidates to facilitate ongoing symptoms because they are associated with impaired barrier function.[48,49] Mast cells are increased in biopsies from patients who have persistent symptoms despite eosinophil reduction/deletion, and may contribute to those symptoms.[16] In fact, a suggested EoEHSS remission score correlates with reduced symptoms and reduced expression of mast cell genes, also suggesting a role for mast cells in EoE symptom generation.[38]

The EoEHSS correlates moderately but significantly and better than PEC with endoscopic scores in pediatric patients, and a combination of an endoscopic feature (furrows) and EoEHSS abnormalities (eosinophil inflammation, basal zone hyperplasia, eosinophil abscesses, and dilated intercellular spaces) predicts active EoE with high degrees of accuracy, sensitivity, and specificity.[39] A clinical activity index, the Index of Severity for Eosinophilic Esophagitis (I-SEE), intended for use in pediatric and adult patients, includes EoEHSS components (basal zone hyperplasia, and lamina propria fibrosis—or surface epithelial alteration and dyskeratotic epithelial cells if lamina propria is not present/evaluable).[50]

Esophageal Remodeling

The term "esophageal remodeling" is broad, including events in the epithelium and connective tissue, and activities in normal growth as well as pathologic alterations. Esophageal stricture represents the ultimately remodeled benign esophagus. The pathology of EoE-related esophageal strictures is not well-defined. Most esophagi with inflammation considered to represent EoE were resected because of food impaction-related perforation with,[51–53] or without stricture,[54] to rule out neoplasm that was shown following resection to be stricture,[55,56] or to resect a perforation associated with extensive mucosal dissection.[57] In addition to numerous eosinophils,[54,56,57] descriptions of resected esophagi include thickened esophageal wall due to fibrosis,[51,52] and/or muscularis propria hypertrophy.[53,55]

Strictured esophagi resected from pediatric patients, most (5/10) following caustic ingestion, others following surgery for congenital anomaly (3/10), or related to gastroesophageal reflux disease (2/10), were resected after repeated dilations and, for some, intralesional corticosteroid injections failed to relieve obstructive symptoms.[58] Compared to controls (studied at postmortem examinations of patients who did not have esophageal diseases), all strictures showed thickened muscularis propria, and submucosal obliterative muscularization resembling small bowel strictures due to Crohn disease (**Figs. 9–11**).[59] Distinct lamina propria, muscularis mucosa, or submucosa were not seen in the strictured areas, and unremarkable squamous epithelium covered spindled cells admixed with extracellular matrix. Some spindled cells expressed both alpha and gamma smooth muscle actin isoforms, possibly derived from persisting normal esophageal muscle layers, and others expressed alpha actin and vimentin, suggesting transformation to myofibroblasts (see **Fig. 10**). Periostin and fibronectin were both abundant in areas of submucosal obliterative muscularization documenting the presence of excessive extracellular matrix (see **Fig. 11**). Mast cells were also abundant in the abnormal strictured areas and were most likely the cells that expressed interleukin (IL)-13 and transforming growth factor beta (TGF-β).

The markedly altered esophageal strictures described earlier were not clinically reversible. Not all esophageal remodeling is irreversible. EoEHSS scores are reduced following swallowed topical corticosteroids, antibodies to IL-13, the shared IL-4/IL-13 receptor, and elimination diet.[30–33,60,61] Epithelial mesenchymal transition (EMT) that results in epithelial cells acquiring characteristics of mesenchymal cells was demonstrated in esophageal biopsies from children[62] and adults[63] with EoE, was correlated with fibrosis,[62] and was diminished by treatment that reduced intraepithelial

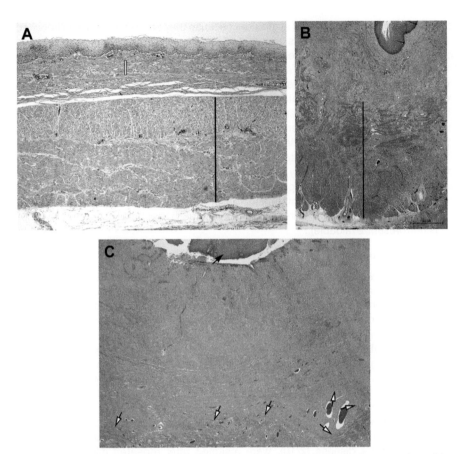

Fig. 9. (*A*) Control: squamous epithelium lines the surface (*top*), lamina propria resides beneath the epithelium, muscularis mucosa (*white bar*) and submucosa are beneath, and muscularis propria (*black bar*) is the outermost layer. 40 ×. (*B*) Stricture: In contrast, the exceedingly thick wall does not show distinct layers except for squamous epithelium and muscularis propria (*black bar*). Between the epithelium and the muscularis propria are fibers resembling smooth muscle. 20 ×. (*C*) Stricture: A closer view of another area shows squamous epithelium (*top–black arrow*), and the inner edge of the muscularis propria at the bottom of the photo (*black edge arrows*). The lamina propria, muscularis mucosa, and submucosa are not distinguishable, replaced by fibers that appear continuous with the muscularis propria (*black edge arrows at bottom right*). 40 ×. (Collins MH, Alexander ES, Martin LJ, et al. Acquired Esophageal Strictures in Children: Morphometric and Immunohistochemical Analyses. Pediatric and Developmental Pathology. 2022;25(2):124-133. https://doi.org/10.1177/10935266211041086).

eosinophil inflammation.[62,63] Non-transformed immortalized human esophageal epithelial cells treated with profibrotic cytokines acquired mesenchymal characteristics, and withdrawal of the stimulation incompletely rescued the treated cells[64] consistent with the in vivo data.

Symptoms in Eosinophilic Esophagitis

A predictable relationship between eosinophil inflammation and symptoms in EoE is not always demonstrable. Symptoms of esophageal dysfunction occur in patients

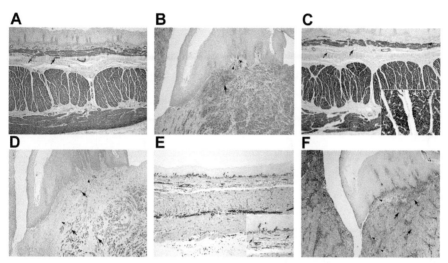

Fig. 10. (*A*) Control: Alpha actin antibody decorates the muscularis mucosa, muscularis propria, and blood vessel walls (*arrows*). 40 ×. (*B*) Stricture: Nodules of fibers replace the lamina propria, muscularis mucosa, and submucosa, and antibody to alpha actin stains them (*black arrow*) and blood vessels (*white edge arrows*). 40 ×. (*C*) Control: Gamma actin antibody decorates muscularis mucosa and muscularis propria, but not all blood vessels (*arrows*). The inset (100 ×) illustrates the characteristic globular staining pattern of gamma actin antibody. 40 ×. (*D*) Stricture: Some fibers stain with antibody to gamma actin (*black arrows*); vascular wall fibers do not (*white edge arrows*). 40 ×. (*E*) Control: Vimentin antibody does not stain smooth muscle fibers in muscularis mucosa or propria but stains thin fibers (*arrows*) (*inset*, 100 ×) representing fibroblasts. 40 ×. (*F*) Stricture: Vimentin antibody stains mainly thin fibers with variable intensity (*black arrows*) and blood vessel walls (*white edge arrows*). 40 ×. (Collins MH, Alexander ES, Martin LJ, et al. Acquired Esophageal Strictures in Children: Morphometric and Immunohistochemical Analyses. Pediatric and Developmental Pathology. 2022;25(2):124-133. https://doi.org/10.1177/10935266211041086).

whose esophageal biopsies have fewer than 15 eosinophils/hpf,[45–47] and eosinophil inflammation ≥15 eosinophils/hpf occurs in patients who do not have symptoms of esophageal dysfunction.[44] Early reports of discordance between eosinophil inflammation and symptoms[65–67] evoked explanations such as use of unvalidated symptoms instruments. Moderate but statistically significant correlations were demonstrated between symptom and EoEHSS scores, but not PEC, in children using the validated pediatric EoE symptom score (PEESS)v2.0 questionnaire.[37,38] Dysphagia is the predominant EoE symptom in adolescents and adults; budesonide oral suspension[33] and dupilumab, an antibody to the IL4-IL13 shared receptor,[31,60] significantly reduced peak eosinophil count, as well as dysphagia compared to placebo, measured by the validated Dysphagia Symptom Questionnaire (DSQ). However, an antibody to siglec-8, expressed on eosinophils (https://investor.allakos.com/news-releases 2021), an antibody to IL-5, the major promoter of eosinophil genesis,[65–67] or an antibody to the IL-5 receptor (Update on the MESSINA Phase III trial for Fasenra in eosinophilic esophagitis (astrazeneca.com). www.astrazeneca.com/media published 25Oct2022) did not result in convincing/significant symptom reductions despite eosinophil reduction/depletion. The inconstant discordance between symptoms and eosinophil inflammation in EoE may involve macro-anatomic and microanatomic factors. Esophageal dilation treats EoE symptoms, but not tissue eosinophil inflammation, and ablates symptoms/PEC association[68] suggesting that deeper aspects of the esophagus

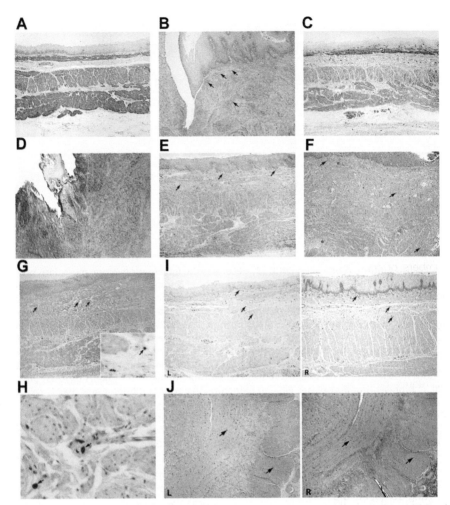

Fig. 11. (*A*) Control: Periostin antibody stains muscularis mucosa and propria and blood vessel walls. 40 ×. (*B*) Stricture: Periostin is present in this area of smooth muscle/myofibro-blast proliferation (*arrows*). 40 ×. (*C*) Control: Fibronectin antibody decorates the muscularis mucosa and propria. 40 ×. (*D*) Stricture: Fibronectin is present in the same area as periostin. 40 ×. (*E*) Control: Antibody to IL-13 decorates cells (*arrows*) mostly in inner layers. 40 ×. (*F*) Stricture: Cells stain with antibody to IL-13 (*arrows*). 40 ×. (*G*) Control: Antibody to TGFb shows a similar pattern in cells (*arrows*) with granular cytoplasm (*inset*, 400 ×). 40 ×. (*H*) Stricture: TGFb antibody stained similar cells (400 ×), suggestive of mast cells (*arrows*). (*I*) Control: Tryptase (L) and chymase (R) antibodies decorate mast cells (*arrows*) mainly in the inner layers. (L: 40 ×; R: 100 ×). (*J*) Stricture: Numerous mast cells are detected with tryp-tase antibody (L, *arrows*) and chymase antibody (R, *arrows*) in the residual muscularis prop-ria. (Collins MH, Alexander ES, Martin LJ, et al. Acquired Esophageal Strictures in Children: Morphometric and Immunohistochemical Analyses. Pediatric and Developmental Pathology. 2022;25(2):124-133. https://doi.org/10.1177/10935266211041086).

contribute to symptoms independent of intraepithelial eosinophils. On a microscopic level, epithelial cells that undergo EMT acquire the ability to move, secrete collagen and/or matrix, and become contractile, characteristics which may have consequences such as contributing to persistently dilated intercellular spaces that correlate with epithelial dysfunction.[48,49] The lack of symptom reduction compared to placebo in patients with significantly reduced eosinophils in multiple randomized, double-blind, placebo-controlled trials suggests that reconsideration of the recommended endpoints of trials testing drugs to treat EoE (download (fda.gov)) may be prudent. Changing the requirement for at least 15 eosinophils in at least 1 hpf for the pathology portion of the clinicopathologic diagnosis of EoE is not warranted currently, but inclusion of additional/other histopathologic changes such as BZHappears to be reasonable.

Future Directions

Artificial intelligence is increasingly impactful in medicine. The pathologic portion of the diagnosis of EoE rests on a specific focal metric, namely PEC. Artificial intelligence can accurately quantify intact and non-intact eosinophils in digitized images,[69] and accurately distinguish EoE biopsies from controls using PEC and global features, permitting correct classification with a small number of images.[70] As discussed earlier, pathologists simultaneously evaluate multiple features, as in EoE biopsies. This proficiency can be captured by artificial intelligence to generate meaningful models. Machine and deep learning can calculate peak eosinophil counts and the total numbers of eosinophils as well as create visual outputs that display their density and spatial distribution.[69,71] Similarly, additional features such as BZHcan be quantified and displayed spatially.[71] Models developed by machine learning have the potential to determine relationships between inflammatory cells and symptoms, develop additional predictive models using endoscopic biopsies that could predict pathology deeper in the wall, etc. Applying AI to preclinical models including organoids could shorten the time to the development and/or application of new drugs to treat EoE. Collaboration between AI and medical scientists to develop useful clinical models will reduce pathologist time required to produce comprehensive meaningful reports.

DISCLOSURES

M.H. Collins is a consultant for Allakos, Arena/Pfizer, AstraZeneca, Calypso Biotech, EsoCap Biotech, GlaxoSmithKline, Receptos/Celgene/BMS, Regeneron Pharmaceuticals, Robarts Clinical Trials Inc./Alimentiv, Inc. and Shire, a Takeda company. M. Pletneva is a consultant for Allakos. N.C. Arva, A. Bernieh, O. Lopez-Nunez and G.-Y. Yang do not have conflicts of interest.

REFERENCES

1. Furuta GT, Liacouras CA, Collins MH, et al. Eosinophilic esophagitis in children and adults: a systematic review and consensus recommendations for diagnosis and treatment. Gastroenterology 2007;133:1342–63.
2. Liacouras CA, Furuta GT, Hirano I, et al. Eosinophilic esophagitis: updated consensus recommendations for children and adults. J Allergy Clin Immunol 2011;128:3–20.
3. Lucendo AJ, Molina-Infante J, Arias A, et al. Guidelines on eosinophilic esophagitis: evidence-based statements and recommendations for diagnosis and management in children and adults. United European Gastroenterol J 2017;5:335–8.
4. Straumann A, Aceves SS, Blanchard C, et al. Pediatric and adult eosinophilic esophagitis: similarities and differences. Allergy 2012;67:477–90.
5. Lyles JL, Martin LJ, Shoda T, et al. Very early onset eosinophilic esophagitis is common, responds to standard therapy, and demonstrates enrichment of CAPN14 gene variants. J Allergy Clin Immunol 2012;147:244–54.

6. Gonsalves N, Policarpio-Nicolas M, Zhang Q, et al. Histopathology variability and endoscopic correlates in adults with eosinophilic esophagitis. Gastrointest Endosc 2006;64:313–9.

7. Chernetsova E, Agarwal A, Weir A, et al. Diagnostic value of mid-esophageal biopsies in pediatric patients with eosinophilic esophagitis. Pediatr Dev Pathol 2021;24:34–42.

8. Friedlander JA, DeBoer EM, Soden JS, et al. Unsedated transnasal esophagoscopy for monitoring therapy in pediatric eosinophilic esophagitis. Gastrointest Endosc 2016;83:299–306.

9. Katzka DA, Geno DM, Ravi A, et al. Accuracy, safety, and tolerability of tissue collection by cytosponge vs endoscopy for evaluation of eosinophilic esophagitis. Clin Gastroenterol Hepatol 2015;13:77–83.

10. Ackerman SJ, Kagalwalla AF, Hirano I, et al. One-hour esophageal string test: a nonendoscopic minimally invasive test that accurately detects disease activity in eosinophilic esophagitis. Am J Gastroenterol 2019;114:1614–25.

11. Attwood SE, Smyrk T, Demeester TR, et al. Esophageal eosinophilia with dysphagia. A distinct clinicopathologic syndrome. Dig Dis Sci 1993;38:109–16.

12. Kelly KJ, Lazenby AJ, Rowe PC, et al. Eosinophilic esophagitis attributed to gastroesophageal reflux: improvement with an amino acid-based formula. Gastroenterology 1995;109:1503–12.

13. Gupta SK, Fitzgerald JF, Chong SK, et al. Vertical lines in distal esophageal mucosa (VLEM): a true endoscopic manifestation of esophagitis in children? Gastrointest Endosc 1997;45:485–9.

14. Liacouras CA, Wenner WJ, Brown K, et al. Primary eosinophilic esophagitis in children: successful treatment with oral corticosteroids. J Pediatr Gastroenterol Nutr 1998;26:380–5.

15. Walsh SV, Antonioli DA, Goldman H, et al. Allergic esophagitis in children: a clinicopathologic entity. Am J Surg Pathol 1999;23:390–6.

16. Orenstein SR, Shalaby TM, Di Lorenzo C, et al. The spectrum of pediatric eosinophilic esophagitis beyond infancy: a clinical series of 30 children. Am J Gastroenterol 2000;95:1422–30.

17. Noel RJ, Putnam PE, Collins MH, et al. Clinical and immunopathologic effects of fluticasone for eosinophilic esophagitis. Clin Gastroenterol Hepatol 2004;2: 568–75.

18. Straumann A, Bauer M, Fischer B, et al. Idiopathic eosinophilic esophagitis is associated with T(H)2-type allergic inflammation. J Allergy Clin Immunol 2001; 108:954–61.

19. Matoso A, Allen D, Herzlinger M, et al. Correlation of ALOX15 expression with eosinophilic or reflux esophagitis in a cohort of pediatric patients with esophageal eosinophilia. Hum Pathol 2014;45:1205–12.

20. Fuentebella J, Patel A, Nguyen T, et al. Increased number of regulatory T cells in children with eosinophilic esophagitis. J Pediatr Gastroenterol Nutr 2010;51: 283–9.

21. Kirsch R, Bokhary R, Marcon MA, et al. Activated mucosal mast cells differentiate eosinophilic (allergic) esophagitis from gastroesophageal reflux disease. J Pediatr Gastroenterol Nutr 2007;44:20–6.

22. Collins MH, Martin LJ, Alexander ES, et al. Newly developed and validated eosinophilic esophagitis histology scoring system and evidence that it outperforms peak eosinophil count for disease diagnosis and monitoring. Dis Esophagus 2017;30:1–8.

23. Hirano I, Chan ES, Rank MA, et al. AGA Institute and the Joint Task Force on Allergy-Immunology Practice Parameters clinical guidelines for the management of eosinophilic esophagitis. Gastroenterology 2020;158:1776–86.

24. Arnim UV, Biedermann L, Aceves SS, et al. Monitoring patients with eosinophilic esophagitis in routine clinical practice – international expert recommendations. Clin Gastroenterol Hepatol 2022. https://doi.org/10.1016/j.cgh.2022.12.018.

25. Vieria MC, Gugelmin ES, Percicote AP, et al. Intra- and interobserver agreement of histopathological findings in pediatric patients with eosinophilic esophagitis. J Pediatr 2022;98:26–32.

26. Wang J, Park JY, Huang R, et al. Obtaining adequate lamina propria for subepithelial fibrosis evaluation in pediatric eosinophilic esophagitis. Gastrointest Endosc 2018;87:1207–14.

27. Thakker AI, Melo DM, Samandi LZ, et al. Esophageal fibrosis in eosinophilic gastrointestinal diseases. J Pediatr Gastroenterol Nutr 2021;72:392–7.

28. Thakker AI, Smith J, Pathak M, et al. Challenges in inter-rater agreement on lamina propria fibrosis in eosinophilic esophagitis. Pediatr Dev Pathol 2023;26:106–14.

29. Hiremath G, Sun L, Correa H, et al. Development and validation of web-based tool to predict lamina propria fibrosis in eosinophilic esophagitis. Am J Gastroenterol 2022;117:272–9.

30. Collins MH, Dellon ES, Katzka DA, et al. Budesonide oral suspension significantly improves eosinophilic esophagitis histology scoring system results: analysis from a 12-week, phase 2, randomized, placebo-controlled clinical trial. Am J Surg Pathol 2019;43:1501–9.

31. Hirano I, Dellon ES, Hamilton JD, et al. Efficacy of dupilumab in a phase 2 randomized trial of adults with active eosinophilic esophagitis. Gastroenterology 2020;158:111–22.

32. Dellon ES, Collins MH, Rothenberg ME, et al. Long-term efficacy and tolerability of RPC4046 in an open-label extension trial of patients with eosinophilic esophagitis. Clin Gastroenterol Hepatol 2021;19:473–83.

33. Hirano I, Collins MH, Katzka DA, et al. Budesonide oral suspension improves outcomes in patients with eosinophilic esophagitis: results from a phase 3 trial. Clin Gastroenterol Hepatol 2022;20:525–34.

34. Ma C, Jairath V, Feagan BG, et al. Responsiveness of a histologic scoring system compared with peak eosinophil count in eosinophilic esophagitis. Am J Gastroenterol 2022;117:264–71.

35. Cruz J, Irvine MA, Avinashi V, et al. Application of the eosinophilic esophagitis histology scoring system grade scores in patients at British Columbia Children's Hospital. Fetal Pediatr Pathol 2022;41:962–76.

36. Warners MJ, Ambarus CA, Bredenoord AJ, et al. Reliability of histologic assessment in patients with eosinophilic esophagitis. Aliment Parmacol Ther 2018;47:940–50.

37. Aceves SS, King E, Collins MH, et al. Alignment of parent- and child-reported outcomes and histology in eosinophilic esophagitis across multiple CEGIR sites. J Allergy Clin Immunol 2018;142:130–8.

38. Collins MH, Martin LJ, Wen T, et al. Eosinophilic esophagitis histology remission score: significant relations to measures of disease activity and symptoms. J Pediatr Gastroenterol Nutr 2020;70:598–603.

39. Hiremath G, Correa H, Acra S, et al. Correlation of endoscopic signs and mucosal alterations in children with eosinophilic esophagitis. Gastrointest Endosc 2020;91:785–94.

40. Rosenberg CE, Mingler MK, Caldwell JM, et al. Esophageal IgG4 levels correlate with histopathologic and transcriptomic features in eosinophilic esophagitis. Allergy 2018;73:1892–901.

41. Schwartz JT, Morris DW, Collins MH, et al. Eosinophil progenitor levels correlate with tissue pathology in eosinophilic esophagitis. J Allergy Clin Immunol 2019; 143:1221–4.

42. Shoda T, Wen T, Aceves SS, et al. Eosinophilic esophagitis endotype classification by molecular, clinical and histopathologcal analyses: a cross-sectional study. Lancet Gastroenterol Hepatol 2018;3:477–88.

43. Lin B, Rabinowitz S, Haseeb MA, et al. Usefulness of the eosinophilic esophagitis histology scoring system in distinguishing active eosinophilic esophagitis from remission and gastroesophageal reflux disease. Gastroenterol Res 2021;14: 220–6.

44. Suzuki Y, Iizuka T, Hosoi A, et al. Clinicopathological differences between eosinophilic esophagitis and asymptomatic esophageal eosinophilia. Intern Med 2022; 61:1319–27.

45. Bolton SM, Kagalwalla AF, Arva NC, et al. Mast cell infiltration is associated with persistent symptoms and endoscopic abnormalities despite resolution of eosinophilia in eosinophilic esophagitis. Am J Gastroenterol 2020;115:224–33.

46. Whelan KA, Godwin BC, Wilkins B, et al. Persistent basal cell hyperplasia is associated with clinical and endoscopic findings in patients with histologically inactive eosinophilic esophagitis. Clin Gastroenterol Hepatol 2020;18:1475–82.

47. Wenzel AA, Wadhwani N, Wechsler JB. Continued basal zone expansion after resolution of eosinophilia in a child with eosinophilic esophagitis on benralizumab. J Pediatr Gastroenterol Nutr 2022;74:e31–4.

48. Katzka DA, Ravi K, Geno DM, et al. Endoscopic mucosal impedance measurements correlate with eosinophilia and dilated intercellular spaces in patients with eosinophilic esophagitis. Clin Gastroenterol Hepatol 2015;13:1242–8.

49. Marietta EV, Geno DM, Smyrk TC, et al. Presence of intraepithelial food antigen in patients with active eosinophilic oesophagitis. Aliment Pharmacol Ther 2017;45: 427–33.

50. Dellon ES, Khoury P, Muir AB, et al. A clinical severity index for eosinophilic esophagitis: development, consensus, and future directions. Gastroenterology 2022;163:59–76.

51. Riou PJ, Nicholson AG, Pastorino U. Esophageal rupture in a patient with idiopathic eosinophilic esophagitis. Ann Thorac Surg 1996;62:1854–6.

52. Nicholson AG, Li D, Pastorino U, et al. Full thickness eosinophilia in oesophageal leiomyomatosis and idiopathic eosinophilic oesophagitis. A common allergic inflammatory profile? J Pathol 1997;183:233–6.

53. Fontillon M, Lucendo AJ. Transmural eosinophil infiltration and fibrosis in a patient with non-traumatic Boerhaave's syndrome due to eosinophilic esophagitis. Am J Gastroenterol 2012;107:1762.

54. Shim LSE, Grehan M. Oesophageal perforation during endoscopy for food impaction in eosinophilic esophagitis. J Gastroenterol Hepatol 2010;25:428.

55. Stevoff C, Rao S, Parsons W, et al. EUS and histopathologic correlates in eosinophilic esophagitis. Gastrointest Endosc 2001;54:373–7.

56. Evrard S, Louis H, Kahaleh M, et al. Idiopathic eosinophilic oesophagitis: atypical presentation. Acta Gastroenterol Belg 2004;67:232–5.

57. Ligouri G, Cortale M, Cimino F, et al. Circumferential mucosal dissection and esophageal perforation in a patient with eosinophilic esophagitis. World J Gastroenterol 2008;14:803–4.

58. Collins MH, Alexander ES, Martin LJ, et al. Acquired esophageal strictures in children: morphometric and immunohistochemical analyses. Pediatr Dev Pathol 2022;25:124–33.
59. Koukoulis G, Ke Y, Henley JD, et al. Obliterative muscularization of the small bowel submucosa in Crohn disease: a possible mechanism of small bowel obstruction. Arch Pathol Lab Med 2001;125:1331–4.
60. Dellon ES, Rothenberg ME, Collins MH, et al. Dupilumab in adults and adolescents with eosinophilic esophagitis. N Engl J Med 2022;387:2317–30.
61. Kliewer KL, Gonsalves N, Dellon ES, et al. One-food versus six-food elimination diet therapy for the treatment of eosinophilic oesophaitis: a multicentre, randomized, open-label trial. Lancet Gastroenterol Hepatol 2023;8:408–21.
62. Kagalwalla AF, Akhtar N, Woodruff SA, et al. Eosinophilic esophagitis: epithelial mesenchymal transition contributes to esophageal remodeling and reverses with treatment. J Allergy Clin Immunol 2012;129:1387–96.
63. Gann PH, Deaton RJ, McMahon N, et al. An anti-IL13 antibody reverses epithelial-mesenchymal transition biomarkers in eosinophilic esophagitis: Phase 2 trial results. J Allergy Clin Immunol 2020;146:367–76.
64. Muir A, Dods K, Noah Y, et al. Esophageal epithelial cells acquire functional characteristics of activated myofibroblasts after undergoing an epithelial to mesenchymal transition. Exp Cell Res 2015;330:102–10.
65. Pentiuk S, Putnam PE, Collins MH, et al. Dissociation between symptoms and histological severity in pediatric eosinophilic esophagitis. J Pediatr Gastroenterol Nutr 2009;48:152–60.
66. Assa'ad AH, Gupta SK, Collins MH, et al. An antibody against IL-5 reduces numbers of esophageal intraepithelial eosinophils in children with eosinophilic esophagitis. Gastroenterology 2011;141:1593–604.
67. Spergel JM, Rothenberg ME, Collins MH, et al. Reslizumab in children and adolescents with eosinophilic esophagitis: results of a double-blind, randomized, placebo-controlled trial. J Allergy Clin Immunol 2012;129:456–63.
68. Safroneeva E, Pan Z, King E, et al. Long-last dissociation of esophageal eosinophilia and symptoms after dilation in adults with eosinophilic esophagitis. Clin Gastroenterol Hepatol 2022;20:766–75.
69. Daniel N, Larey A, Aknin E, et al. A Deep Multi-Label Segmentation Network For Eosinophilic Esophagitis Whole Slide Biopsy Diagnostics. Annu Int Conf IEEE Eng Med Biol Soc 2022;3211–7.
70. Czyzewski T, Daniel N, Rochman M, et al. Machine Learning Approach for Biopsy-based Identification of Eosinophilic Esophagitis Reveals Importance of Global Features. IEEE Open Journal of Engineering in Medicine and Biology 2021;2:218–23.
71. Larey A, Aknin E, Daniel N. Harnessing Artificial Intelligence to Infer Novel Spatial Biomarkers for the Diagnosis of Eosinophilic Esophagitis. Front Med Pathology 2022. https://doi.org/10.3389/fmed.2022.950728.

Dietary Management of Eosinophilic Esophagitis

Alfredo Lucendo, MD, PhD[a,b,c], Marion Groetch, MS, RDN[d],
Nirmala Gonsalves, MD, AGAF[e],*

KEYWORDS

- Eosinophil • Food allergy • Diet • Eosinophilic esophagitis • Dysphagia
- Dietary therapy • Elimination diet

KEY POINTS

- Eosinophilic esophagitis is a chronic immune-mediated food allergy–driven disease characterized by eosinophilic inflammation of the esophagus leading to symptoms of esophageal dysfunction.
- The etiopathogenesis of eosinophilic infiltration in the esophagus is multifactorial including genetic predisposition, epithelial barrier dysfunction, exposure to food and aeroallergens, and Th-2 immune dysregulation.
- Prior studies have supported the key role of food allergen exposure as the main driver behind the etiopathogenesis showing that removal of food antigens can result in disease remission.

INTRODUCTION

Eosinophilic esophagitis (EoE) is a chronic immune-mediated food allergy–driven disease characterized by eosinophilic inflammation of the esophagus leading to symptoms of esophageal dysfunction. The etiopathogenesis of eosinophilic infiltration in the esophagus is multifactorial. Prior studies have supported the key role of food allergen exposure as the main driver behind the etiopathogenesis showing that removal of food antigens can result in disease remission. These landmark studies serve as the basis for the rising interest and evolution of dietary therapy in EoE. This

[a] Department of Gastroenterology, Hospital General de Tomelloso, Tomelloso, Spain; [b] Centro de Investigación Biomédica en Red de Enfermedades Hepáticas y Digestivas (CIBERehd); [c] Instituto de Investigación Sanitaria de Castilla-La Mancha (IDISCAM), Tomelloso, Ciudad Real 13700, Spain; [d] Department of Pediatric Allergy & Immunology, Icahn School of Medicine at Mount Sinai, 1 Gustave L. Levy Place, New York, NY 10029, USA; [e] Division of Gastroenterology and Hepatology, Northwestern University-Feinberg School of Medicine, 676 North St. Claire, Suite 1400, Chicago, IL 60611, USA
* Corresponding author.
E-mail address: n-gonsalves@northwestern.edu

Immunol Allergy Clin N Am 44 (2024) 223–244
https://doi.org/10.1016/j.iac.2023.12.009
0889-8561/24/© 2024 Elsevier Inc. All rights reserved.

immunology.theclinics.com

article will focus on the rationale for dietary therapy in EoE and provide helpful tools for the implementation of dietary therapy in practice.

BACKGROUND

The role of dietary therapy for EoE was first described in the pediatric literature in a pivotal study by Kelley and colleagues in the late 1990s. In their case series of 10 children with esophageal eosinophilia who failed to respond to anti-reflux therapy, they showed that esophageal inflammation was triggered by sensitivity to dietary proteins.[1] Larger retrospective pediatric studies showed similar results after treatment with elemental diet with an amino acid–based formula (AAF).[2–4] Subsequent studies in both the pediatric and adult population also showed improvement in EoE after a partial elimination diet with the empiric 6-food elimination diet (6FED).[4,5] These and other pioneering studies supported the concept that EoE is an antigen-mediated inflammatory disorder triggered by food antigens, and thus manageable by food elimination diets.

ELEMENTAL DIET: THE MOST EFFECTIVE MODALITY

Exclusively feeding patients with an AAF[6] was crucial in demonstrating the role of food allergy in the origin of EoE[1] and was impactful in defining the first effective therapy for achieving disease remission. A meta-analysis published in 2014 summarizing the results of 13 studies over 429 patients (including 411 children but only 18 adults) exclusively fed with an elemental diet provided an extremely homogenous overall effectiveness of 91%,[7] making this one of the most effective therapies for EoE, superior to almost any pharmacologic alternative.

Although adherence to the diet by adults can be challenging, elemental diet has been also successful in inducing remission in adults.[8,9] In the first study by Peterson and colleagues, 29 adults with active disease were advised to avoid any kind of food except an elemental formula for 4 weeks: 11 patients abandoned the study but the 17 of 18 patients who adhered to the diet achieved complete disease remission, providing a per-protocol effectiveness of 94.4%, which went down to 58.8% when intention-to treat data were analyzed. During the study, participants lost between 3 and 7 kg of weight.[8] In a study[9] of 21 adult participants, 4 participants were not adherent with the recommended volume of daily formula intake and in the 17 who adhered to elemental diet, 88% became completely asymptomatic and 12 patients (71%) achieved histologic remission (defined as $\leq$15 eosinophils per high-power field [eos/hpf]). Weight loss in 4 weeks was only 1.4 kg, but patients experienced a decline in social functioning during the study period.[9]

The American Gastroenterological Association and the Joint Task Force recommended, with moderate certainty of evidence, an elemental diet over no therapy as it was the treatment alternative with the least probability of failure compared to placebo.[10]

Limitations of Elemental Diets Threaten Their Effectiveness

Despite its high effectiveness, the use of the elemental diet is limited in clinical practice due to its numerous drawbacks. First, the palatability of elemental formulas is poor and diet adherence is consequently low. Due to poor volume adherence, patients are at risk of receiving fewer daily calories than necessary. Most young patients required administration through a nasogastric or gastrostomy tube[2,3] to reduce the possibility of weight loss.[8] Second, elemental formulas are costly and not universally reimbursed by insurances.[8,9] Third, long-term avoidance of solid food in children under 2 year old or with known feeding dysfunction may lead to delayed oral-motor skill development.[11] The most important deterrent for elemental diets is the negative impact on social activities, psychological well-being, and health-related quality of life (HRQoL) since this involves complete avoidance of any kind of table food.[12] The prolonged time required for food reintroduction after an elemental diet is also quite challenging. Thus the elemental diet has a limited role in treating EoE.[10,13,14] Despite these limitations, elemental formulas are an allergen-free supplement capable of supporting adequate intake of nutrients and calories,[15] which may improve adherence to other diet restrictions and contribute to maintaining HRQoL of patients.[16] An elemental diet may be useful for a short period of time to (a.) treat infants and toddlers who were highly to selective removal of foods, as a bridge therapy while waiting for investigational drugs, (b.) for patients who wish to remain in remission while investigating the casual role of unusual foods and aeroallergens in their disease,[17] or (c.) for those not responding to an extended exclusion diet or not eating solids.[18] These very selected circumstances have not been investigated in real-world clinical practice.[19]

ALLERGY TESTING–BASED DIET

Given the limitations of elemental diet, the prospect of individualized and directed dietary therapy through allergy testing became an attractive option. Over a decade, different researchers used various allergy tests, including skin prick testing (SPT), atopy patch testing (APT), and serum food-specific immunoglobulin (Ig) E (sIgE) testing, to search for the dietary trigger for EoE.[20]

Initial results of testing a combination of SPT and APT to target potential foods triggering EoE were promising but studies over the last 2 decades have not identified a key role for this testing to identify EoE-related food triggers. In 2002, a retrospective series of 26 children[21] found that 19 had a positive SPT, most commonly for milk and eggs (36% each), and 21 also had a positive APT, with wheat and rye being the most common. Following avoidance of foods for 4 to 6 weeks, histologic and symptomatic remission was achieved by 49% patients. In a follow-up study in 2012, 53% of patients normalized esophageal biopsies after the SPT/APT approach and when milk was also removed, the remission rate increased to 77%.[22]

A major challenge in all treatment studies has been the lack of correlation between symptoms and histologic inflammation in patients of all ages.[23–25] This factor has confounded subsequent results that indicated improvement in symptoms but recurrence of inflammation with food reintroduction. The accuracy of allergy skin tests in identifying milk, the most common culprit food involved in triggering EoE. has been lacking with a negative predictive value (NPV) of APT for milk as low as 31.4%; the NPV of SPT for milk was even worse (29.3%). Therefore, a negative test for milk on SPT or APT does not rule out milk as a trigger food.[22,26] The NPV of the combination of both methods for milk is only 44%.[22] Another small study in adult patients who were sensitized to wheat and rye found no changes in endoscopy and histopathologic examination of the esophagus after an elimination diet of wheat, rye, and barley for 6 weeks, with only symptomatic improvement in 1 patient.[27]

Food triggers of EoE identified by reintroduction challenge results also provide further evidence of the limited accuracy of allergy testing with SPT accurately predicting only 13% of causal agents, and 67% of patients who had a food trigger identified by the reintroduction process had a negative SPT for all foods.[5] Sensitivity values for sIgE and SPT were only 32.5% and 22.8%, respectively, in another study.[15]

A meta-analysis published in 2014 summarized the effectiveness of allergy testing–based diets in 14 studies involving 594 children and 32 adults.[7] Overall efficacy was 45.5%, with better results in children compared to adults (47.9% vs. 32.2%, respectively). The European Academy of Allergy, Asthma, and Immunology stated in 2016 that measuring specific immunoglobulin (Ig) E levels and/or SPT was not sufficient to identify foods that cause EoE and recommended against dietary advice exclusively based on IgE-mediated sensitization to foods, because it does not improve EoE in a significant number of patients.[28] New systematic reviews updated the effectiveness of food allergy testing–directed diets in EoE by compiling most recent evidence, but a very similar efficacy of 45.7% was provided.[29]

Other allergy test modalities were also evaluated further in EoE. Philpott and colleagues assessed 5 different modalities (SPT, APT, allergen-specific IgE, basophil activation test, and sIgG) in 56 adults with EoE and found no test was accurate to predict culprit food triggers.[30]

Thus, no clinical practice guidelines recommend allergy tests to inform food restriction in EoE.[13,14,31]

Future Directions in Allergy Testing for Eosinophilic Esophagitis

Despite the fact that IgG4 concentrations in esophageal tissues are increased compared to controls in adults and children with EoE, these reduce after effective treatment,[32–37] and tissue IgG4 levels correlate with esophageal peak eosinophil count, severity of histologic features, and Th2 cytokine gene expression levels[36] the ability of tissue IgG4 testing to guide dietary elimination therapy in EoE has provided poor results.[38] One recent randomized clinical trial showed a potential role for serum concentrations of cow's milk-specific IgG4 against α-lactalbumin, β-lactoglobulin, and casein in the pathogenesis of EoE but further studies investigating the role of this modality as a reliable predictor of dietary therapy in EoE are needed.

EMPIRIC ELIMINATION DIETS

Due to the limitations with the use of elemental diets and allergy testing–directed diets, empiric elimination strategies consisting of excluding common food allergens from a patient's diet have evolved and shown promising clinical success.

The 6-Food Elimination Diet: Effective and Highly Reproducible

In 2006, a 6FED, excludingcow's milk protein, soy, egg, wheat, peanut/tree nut, and seafood,[21,39] was compared with an elemental diet in 35 and 25 children with EoE, respectively.[4] After 6 weeks, peak esophageal eosinophil counts decreased in 74% of patients treated with a 6FED and in 88% of those treated with an elemental diet.[4] To identify EoE food triggers sequential single-food reintroductions were performed in those patients in remission followed by endoscopic assessments (average 5.6 per patient).[40] As with the initial food restrictions, dietetic supervision was provided during the reintroduction process. Results demonstrated that the most common triggers were cow's milk (74%), followed by wheat (26%) and eggs (17%).[40]

Similar treatments with follow-up endoscopic assessments during reintroductions were subsequently investigated in adults in 2 studies carried out in the United States and Spain.[5,15] In the first one investigating 6FED in adults, Gonsalves and colleagues[5] found that 95% had decreased dysphagia scores and 74% achieved histologic remission after 6 weeks. Reintroduction of 1 food group every 2 weeks was offered to patients, followed by an endoscopy after 2 foods were introduced. When present, symptom recurrence occurred with a median time of 3 days after exposure to trigger foods, with the most common being wheat (60%) and milk (50%); 15% of patients had more than 1 trigger identified. No patient had seafood as an EoE trigger.[5]

In Spain, Lucendo and colleagues reported a 73.1% histologic remission with a 6-week treatment with an extended and modified 6FED (excluding cereals, milk, eggs, fish/seafood, legumes/soy, and peanuts).[15] This trial used a longer introduction of 6 weeks of regular intake and found the triggers as follows: cow's milk (61.9%), wheat (28.6%), eggs (26.2%), and legumes (23.8%).[15] Adherence to the diet resulted in maintenance of EoE remission for up to 3 years.

A first meta-analysis that summarized 7 studies comprising 197 patients (75 children and 122 adults) who underwent a 6FED provided a homogenous effectiveness of 72% (95% confidence interval [CI]: 66%–78%) histologic remission rate.[29,41] In this sense, a technical review of 10 single-arm observation studies over 633 patients overall showed that 32.1% of patients failed to achieve histologic remission (defined as<15 eos/hpf) compared with 86.7% in a placebo comparison group.[10]

Limitations of the 6-food elimination diet

The difficulties in implementing a 6FED and its complexity, diet effectiveness at reducing symptoms, navigating social situations, and diet-related anxiety, together with the costs related to the higher costs of allergen-free and unprocessed foods,[42] limit the implementation and acceptance of this treatment option in some patients, supporting the long-term adherence to 6FED of 57%. Despite these limitations, the majority of diet users recommended diet therapy to other EoE patients.[43]

FOUR-FOOD ELIMINATION DIET AND STEP-UP APPROACHES

To simplify the dietary approach, a 4-food elimination diet (4FED) has been studied consisting of excluding dairy products (cow's, goat's or sheep's milk), gluten-containing grains, eggs, soy and all legumes (comprising lentil, chickpeas, peas, beans, and peanuts).

The 4-Food Elimination Diet

This was first studied in a prospective multicenter Spanish study involving adult EoE patients.[44] After 6 weeks, 54% achieved histologic remission. In children, a similar 4FED (that excluded cow's milk, wheat, egg, and soy) induced histologic remission in 64% of patients after 8 weeks[45]; 1 single food trigger was identified in 62% of patients, most commonly cow's milk. A meta-analysis of 8 studies summarized the effectiveness of a 4FED in 302 patients of all ages with active EoE, estimating that 49.4% (95% CI, 32.5%–66.3%) of patients could achieve remission with this approach.[29]

Reversing Restriction Approach: the 2-4-6 Elimination Diet Study

In 2018, to simplify the diet approach further, adult and pediatric patients reversed the order of food elimination diets, so that the most extensive avoidance diet was reserved for patients not responding to less restrictive diets. . In this multicenter study of adult and pediatric patients on a 2-food elimination diet (2FED) consisting of a 6-week avoidance of gluten-containing cereals and mammalian milk, results showed that 43% of patients achieved clinical and histologic remission, irrespective of age. Non-responders were offered a 4FED, with a 6FED reserved as the final rescue therapy only for motivated patients who failed both prior alternatives.[46] Milk was the culprit food in 81%, and most responders to either a 2FED or 4FED presented 1 or 2 triggers for EoE.

A computer-based simulation model has shown step-up approaches are the most efficient empiric elimination strategies for EoE.[47] All simulations started with the elimination of dairy products and were based on reported prevalence values for foods that trigger EoE. In all simulations, the 1,4,8-food and 1,3-food strategies appeared to be the most efficient in identifying EoE food triggers, providing the highest rate of correct identification of food triggers balanced by the number of endoscopies required.

The 1-Food Elimination Diet

Since milk and dairy products are the most common triggers for EoE in patients of all ages[48]; a 1-food elimination diet (1FED) or a milk-free diet has been the next advancement. A recent systematic review has shown that avoiding cow's milk induced clinical and histologic remission in 51.4% of patients, with most research on a 1FED having been carried out in children.[49–54] Despite the ubiquity of milk in processed foods, this approach may be more acceptable for some patients who wish to avoid more extensive restrictions.

RANDOMIZED TRIALS WITH DIET THERAPIES IN EOSINOPHILIC ESOPHAGITIS

Recently, 2 multicenter randomized trials have provided comparative evidence on different dietary approaches for EoE. In the first trial, children and adolescents were randomized to 1FED (n = 38) versus 4FED (n = 25); after 12 weeks of diet therapy, symptoms improved significantly in both groups and histologic remission rates were similar between the 1FED (44.1%) and 4FED (41.2%). Not surprisingly, improvements in psychosocial and emotional well-being scores were better with the 1FED.[54]

The second randomized trial compared a 1FED (animal milk including cow, sheep, and goat milk products) to a 6FED (animal milk, egg, wheat, soy, fish and shellfish, and peanut and tree nut elimination) in adults with EoE for 6 weeks with 34% reaching histologic remission after the 1FED and 40% after the 6FED.[55] Some patients without histologic response after the 1FED underwent a 6FED, but only 43% achieved remission.

The unexpected low effectiveness of the 4FED and 6FED in this study could be caused by inadequate selection of candidates (enrolling not sufficiently motivated patients), poor control of proper elimination diet adherence, or the greater presence of novel allergens (legume, mycoproteins, seeds, and so forth) in the US food supply in particular in common substitute foods. These results prompt the need to continue carrying out new trials that identify and minimize these risks.

HOW TO DISCUSS DIET THERAPY WITH PATIENTS

Dietary therapy offers the potential for long-term remission without medication, and the proven efficacy of less restrictive diets in children[46,56] and adults[44,46] makes dietary therapy a more attractive option. Despite the desire to use diet treatment, a recent survey of EoE providers found the greatest barrier to offering dietary therapy was the belief that patients are disinterested and unlikely to adhere to elimination diets (58%).[43,57] Still, implementing dietary therapy can be a challenge and requires knowledge on the part of the provider and motivation and significant effort on the part of the patient/caregiver. The choice of EoE therapy should be individualized based on patient preference and also feasibility from a medical, nutritional, and lifestyle standpoint. Using a shared decision-making approach will help families choose the most appropriate therapy option.

Nutritional Considerations/Assessments with Implementing Diet Therapy

Dieticians are vital members of any team using diet therapy to treat EoE for several reasons. First, pediatric patients may initially present with macronutrient or micronutrient deficiencies,[58] feeding difficulties,[59–62] and poor growth.[58,60,63] In these cases, nutritional deficiency is not necessarily a contraindication to dietary therapy but a full assessment, including anthropometrics and dietary history, to address nutritional needs and correct malnutrition or nutrient deficiency is indicated. Second, dietitians are well versed in the resources to access food allergy educational materials available through organizations such as Food Allergy Research and Education (FARE; www. foodallergy.org/), using the *Meet FARE Trained Registered Dietitians* link, and the American Partnership for Eosinophilic Disorders (APFED www.apfed.org/), and the *Specialist Finder* tool. Dietitians will be knowledgeable about the availability of tele-health medical nutrition therapy in regions with a limited access to food allergy–trained/EoE-trained experts as well as licensure laws that vary by state in the United States. Food allergy[64] and EoE[3,65,66] guidelines strongly recommend involvement of a registered dietitian (RD) who is well versed in food allergy when available. These RDs with food allergy training can provide dietary guidance including plans to meet nutritional needs within the context of the elimination diet, assess elimination diet adherence, and monitor weight and dietary intake for nutritional risk (**Fig. 1**).

NUTRITION ASSESSMENT
Anthropometrics

Length-for-age/height-for-age, weight-for-length, or body mass index are important factors to assess malnutrition[67] (eg, wasting, stunting, overweight/obesity (**Table 1**).

In children, reductions in growth velocity as well as involuntary weight loss may provide additional indicators of poor growth; these patients may need additional nutrition (energy, macronutrients, and micronutrients) and a dietary plan to account for these needs.

Diet History

The diet history may expose decreased intake of calories, macronutrients (in particular protein and fat), micronutrients, or missing food groups. One important cause of this is feeding difficulties, a concern examined by Mukkada and colleagues[59] in 200 children (median age 34 months) with EoE. They found 16.5% of children had significant feeding disorders (food refusal, low volume/variety of intake, poor acceptance of new foods) and 93.9% of parents had learned maladaptive feeding behaviors (lack of mealtime structure, prompting child to eat). Other causes of decreased intake include reduction in ingestion of IgE-mediated food allergens,[7] difficulty in managing food textures, religious dietary restrictions, harmful dietary beliefs (fasting, skipping meals, fad diets), diets that heavily rely on a food that is targeted for elimination, and personal dietary preferences (eg, vegetarian/vegan diets). Therefore, the involvement of a dietitian is

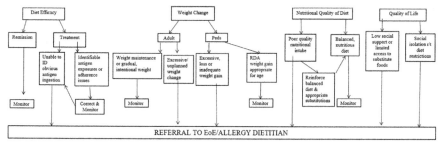

Fig. 1. When to refer to a registered dietitian. (With permission from: Groetch M, Venter C, Skypala I, Vlieg-Boerstra B, Grimshaw K, Durban R, Cassin A, Henry M, Kliewer K, Kabbash L, Atkins D, Nowak-Węgrzyn A, Holbreich M, Chehade M; Eosinophilic Gastrointestinal Disorders Committee of the American Academy of Allergy, Asthma and Immunology. Dietary Therapy and Nutrition Management of Eosinophilic Esophagitis: A Work Group Report of the American Academy of Allergy, Asthma, and Immunology. J Allergy Clin Immunol Pract. 2017 Mar-Apr;5(2):312-324.e29.)

Table 1
Malnutrition and nutrition risk assessment criteria

Pediatric[a]: Primary Indicator with 1 Data Point

Growth parameters[e]	Moderate (z-score)	Severe (z-score)
Underweight (weight-for-age)	Below −2 to −3	Below −3
Wasting (weight-for-length or BMI)	Below −2 to −3	Below −3
Stunting (length-for-age/height-for-age)	Below −2 to −3	Below −3
Overweight (weight-for-length or BMI)	Above +2 to +3	Above +3 (obese)

Pediatric: Primary Indicator With Multiple Data Points

<2 y of age Weight gain velocity (weight-for-age)	<50% of the norm for expected weight gain	<25% of the norm for expected weight gain
2–20 y Decreasing growth velocity (weight-for-length)	Decline of 2 z-scores	Decline of 2 z-scores
2–20 y Weight loss	7.5% usual body weight	10% usual body weight
Inadequate energy/protein intake	25%–50% estimated needs	<25% estimated needs

Adult[b]

Underweight (BMI)	<18.5 kg/m²	
Overweight (BMI)	>25 kg/m²	
Involuntary weight loss (chronic)	Moderate[c] 5% in 1 mo 7.5% in 3 mo 10% in 6 mo 20% in 1 y	Severe[d] 5% in 1 mo 7.5% in 3 mo 10% in 6 mo 20% in 1 y

Abbreviation: BMI, body mass index.
   [a] Pediatric malnutrition classification.
   [b] Criteria to diagnose adult chronic malnutrition.
   [c] Criteria to diagnose adult moderate chronic malnutrition require at least 2 signs (weight loss, mild to moderate body fat depletion, mild to moderate muscle mass depletion, or mild to moderate fluid accumulation).
   [d] Criteria to diagnose adult severe chronic malnutrition require at least 2 signs and 1 must be severe (weight loss, severe body fat depletion, severe muscle mass depletion, or severe fluid accumulation).
   [e] For children, standing height (>2 y)/recumbent length (<24 mo), weight, and head circumference (<36 mo) should be measured and plotted on the appropriate growth chart based on country-specific guidelines. In the United States, it is recommended to use the World Health Organization growth charts for 0 to less than 2 years of age and the Centers for Disease Control and Prevention growth charts for 2 to 20 years of age.

critical to assess the foods being eaten and tolerated, the foods avoided and why they are being avoided, and the ability and willingness to accept substitute foods to replace important nutrition.

In patients unable to meet nutritional needs in the context of the elimination diet, a nutritionally complete AAF or plant-based formula (PBF) if available, feasible, and accepted can help fill nutritional gaps. PBFs may include food proteins such as soy, pea, almond, rice, and other grains, are less expensive than AAFs, and are useful if they align with the patient's elimination diet.

If a nutritionally sound diet is not possible based on the patient's medical and nutrition assessments, then pursuing an alternative therapy and deferring dietary elimination until such time that nutritional needs can be met within the context of the elimination diet would be advisable (**Table 2**).

IMPLEMENTING DIET THERAPY

Education needs to teach how to eliminate the target food(s) and plan for a nutritionally balanced diet (See supplement for patient education handouts: *Reading a Product Label*).

Avoidance Skills

Avoidance requires understanding how to read product labels to identify the eliminated food and also how to avoid cross-contact risk. Since the threshold level for triggering EoE is unknown, strict avoidance during the initial diagnostic phase of dietary elimination is commonly recommended so trigger foods can be clearly identified.[6,7,68–70]

Label Reading

Priority allergens are identified by food allergen labeling laws, which mandate full disclosure of the priority allergen on food product labels. In the United States, milk, egg, wheat, soy, peanut, tree nut, fish, crustacean shellfish, and sesame must be identified in the ingredient list or in the *Contains* statement on food product labels using their common name, for example, "milk" or "wheat." Priority allergens vary by country or region, but the 6FED allergens associated with EoE are also priority allergens in Canada, the United Kingdom, the European Union, Australia, and New Zealand. Patients must read product labels every time and avoid the target food(s) if listed in the ingredient list or *Contains* statement.

Table 2 Screening for factors associated with increased nutritional risk	
Physical	Assess for underweight, overweight, involuntary weight loss, wasting, stunting, or decreasing growth velocity; signs or symptoms of nutritional or nutrient deficiency; chest pain, abdominal pain, heartburn, or food impaction associated with eating.
Dietary	Assess for low volume intake, low variety intake, the ability to meet energy and protein needs, or micronutrient adequacy.
Feeding and eating barriers	Assess for texture modification needs, increased time required to eat, early satiety, picky eating, food avoidance or refusal, or the ability to accept alternative nutrition sources.
Other potential dietary restrictions	Immunoglobulin E-mediated food allergy, religious dietary laws, fad diets, dietary goals and values, financial, or food access or food preparation barriers
Consider referral to a registered dietitian if increased nutritional risk.	

Precautionary allergen labels (PALs) indicate the potential for allergen presence due to unintentional cross-contact. PALs are voluntary and are not regulated in most countries; therefore, the lack of a PAL does not necessarily mean the product is without risk of cross-contact.[2,3,9,10] Overall, the risk is low (around 10%), but higher for certain allergens, such as milk.[8] The type of statement used (eg, "may contain" vs "manufactured in a shared facility") does not reflect more or less risk of cross-contact.[10] Therefore, patients should assume that any PAL statement carries the same risk of cross-contact and avoid PAL products during the initial phases of dietary therapy.

EMPIRIC ELIMINATION DIETS

(Supplement to this article contains patient handouts for 1FED, 2FED, 4FED, and 6FED)

1-Food Elimination Diet: Milk

Cow's milk versus other animals' milk
Although cow's milk is the common form of milk consumed in the Western diet, it should be noted that other mammalian milks such as goat's milk and sheep's milk must also be eliminated due to shared homologous proteins.[11] Other mammalian milks (for example, mare, donkey) have less reported risk of cross-reactivity but have not been used extensively to treat cow's milk allergy. Hence, when treating EoE, all mammalian milks should be avoided.

Baked milk
Eliminating milk results in the elimination of all dairy foods (milk, cheese, yogurt, butter, ice cream, pudding, and so forth) and products with any milk ingredients, including baked goods containing milk. A small retrospective study[71] reported on the tolerance of baked milk. Eleven patients (73%) maintained histologic remission and 4 patients had disease recurrence after baked milk ingestion. Another small prospective study enrolled 18 patients with confirmed milk-triggered EoE and advised them to drink 200 mL of sterilized milk (boiled for 20 minutes) twice daily for 8 weeks, and 12 maintained EoE remission.[72]

Nutrition impact and risk of milk elimination
Infants, toddlers, and young children. Eliminating milk from a child's diet can have significant nutritional impact, as milk and milk products such as yogurt and cheese provide key nutrients for growth and development[73] (**Table 3**). It is inappropriate to

Table 3
Nutrients in foods commonly eliminated during eosinophilic esophagitis elimination diet therapy

Foods	Main Nutrients
Milk	Protein, calcium, magnesium, phosphorus, vitamins A, B_6, B_{12}, D, riboflavin, pantothenic acid, iodine
Wheat	Carbohydrate, thiamine, niacin, riboflavin, folic acid, iron, fiber
Soy	Protein, calcium, phosphorus, magnesium, iron, zinc, thiamine, riboflavin, Vitamin B_6. (folate)
Eggs	Protein, iron, choline, selenium, biotin, vitamins A, B_{12}, pantothenic acid, folate, riboflavin
Peanut/tree nuts	Protein, selenium, zinc, manganese, magnesium, niacin, phosphorus, vitamins E and B_6, alpha linolenic acid, and linoleic acid
Fish/shellfish	Protein, iodine, zinc, phosphorus, selenium, niacin Fatty fish oil: vitamins A and D, omega-3 fatty acids.

use plant-based beverages (PBBs) in very young toddlers (<2 years) without a complete nutrition assessment. For infants and young toddlers, breast milk or an infant or toddler substitute formula (AAF or PBF) may be recommended.[74] The World Allergy Organization suggests breast milk or substitute formulas for children under 2 years of age on milk elimination.[75] (**Table 4**).

Milk avoidance in older children and adults. Milk and milk products continue to support vital nutritional needs in older children (>2 years) and adults and are recommended as an essential food group for daily consumption throughout the life cycle. For older children and adults, PBFs may be appropriate but this should be individualized based on the specific patient's nutritional status. If the older child or adult patient has sufficient intake of solid foods to meet energy and macronutrient needs, then the addition of a PBB is not necessary but micronutrient supplementation, particularly calcium, vitamin D, and magnesium, should be considered to meet but not exceed needs.

   At all ages, exceeding the recommended daily intake of milk substitute is also an inappropriate use of PBBs as they are not nutritionally complete and a large volume can displace other important nutritional components (**Table 5**). Inappropriate use of a PBB can lead to poor growth and in rare cases kwashiorkor/marasmus, electrolyte disorders, kidney stones, and severe nutrient deficiencies including iron deficiency, anemia, rickets, and scurvy.[76–81]

2-Food Elimination Diet: Milk and Wheat or Gluten

In a 2FED, milk and wheat or gluten are eliminated. It is unclear if wheat (inclusive of all wheat derivatives) or all gluten-containing grains (wheat and their derivatives, barley, and rye) should be eliminated,[82] as multiple empiric elimination clinical research trials report differing approaches.[4,44,46,56] In a post hoc analysis of the 1FED versus 6FED, Kliewer and colleagues[55] reported on histologic remission rates in 59 patients who consumed and who did not consume other gluten-containing grains when randomized to a 6FED. Patients who consumed barley grains (5/17, 29%) had a nonsignificantly lower remission rate (29%) than patients who did not (48%). Further studies are required to determine if clinical and histologic outcomes would improve if wheat avoidance was expanded to gluten avoidance.

   In general, barley and rye are often combined with wheat in our food supply and thus should be avoided, and[82] oats should be certified gluten free.[66] Handouts available in the supplement to this article offer options of both wheat elimination and gluten elimination.

Nutritional impact of wheat elimination
Wheat and wheat-base foods are important sources of iron, folate, niacin, riboflavin, thiamin, and dietary fiber, and thus the micronutrients (iron and B vitamins) fortification should be considered. Reading product labels to choose fortified grains or choosing nutritionally dense gluten-free whole-grain substitutes such as amaranth, millet, quinoa, buckwheat, oat, and sorghum will help replace the nutrients lost to the elimination diet.

4-Food Elimination Diet: Including Milk, Wheat, Eggs, and Soy; and 6-Food Elimination Diet: Including Milk, Egg, Wheat, Soy, Seafood (Fish and Shellfish), and Nuts (Peanut and Tree Nuts)

As more foods are eliminated, AAFs or substituted foods are needed to replace lost calories and protein. Some replacements, such as meats, may be difficult textures to swallow with active EoE (see **Table 5**). Nutrients in foods are commonly eliminated during EoE elimination diet therapy.

Table 4
Comparison of cow's milk and plant-based beverages[a]

Nutrient	Whole Cow's Milk	Soy	Pea Protein Kids Version	Pea Protein	Oat	Hemp	Cashew	Coconut	Flax[b]	Almond	Rice
Calories	150	110	140	100	140	70	80	70	25	60	120
Protein (g)	8	✓✓	✓✓	✓✓	✓	✓	–	–	✓	–	–
Fat (g)	8	✓✓	✓✓	✓✓	✓✓	✓✓	✓	✓✓	✓	–	–

Good source ✓✓ 7–8g protein, >4–8g fat.
Moderate source ✓ ≥ 3g protein, 4g fat.
Poor source – <3g protein, <4g fat.

[a] All plant-based beverages are original versions (typically sweetened) when available. Nutritional content may vary based on the brand. Other formulations may be available with "protein" versions (for instance, flax protein beverage) typically with added soy or pea protein. The product nutrition facts and ingredient label are the best sources for ingredient and nutrition information.

[b] Unsweetened version.

Table 5
Recommended food group goals to meet nutritional needs

Food Group	Daily Servings	Child Age			Adult Daily Energy Requirement			
		1–3 y	4–8 y	>8 y	2000 kcal	2400 kcal	2600 kcal	3000 kcal
		Recommended serving size per age			Recommended Daily Amount			
Grains	6	$^{1}/_{4}$–1/3 cup $^{1}/_{4}$–$^{1}/_{2}$ slice	1/2 cup $^{3}/_{4}$ slice	1/2 cup 1 slice	6 ounces	8 ounces	9 ounces	10 ounces
Rice, corn, potato, gluten-free oats, Alternative grains (quinoa, millet, amaranth, teff, sorghum, buckwheat) Breads, cereals, crackers, baked goods made from alternative whole grains								
Fruits/vegetables	5	$^{1}/_{4}$ cup	1/2 cup	1/2 cup	Veg 2 ½ cups Fruit 2 cups	Veg 3 cups Fruit 2 cups	Veg 3 ½ cups Fruit 2 cups	Veg 4 cups Fruit 2 ½ cups
Fresh or frozen, prepared without allergenic ingredients								
Dairy or milk substitute or amino acid-based formula		12–16 fluid ounces	18–24 fluid ounces	24–32 fluid ounces	3 cups	3 cups	3 cups	3 cups
Fortified milk alternatives (drinks based on rice, coconut, hemp, flax) Amino acid-based formulas								
Proteins	2–3	1 ounce 2–4 Tbsp	2 ounces $^{1}/_{4}$ – 1/3 cup	3 ounces 1/2 cup	5 ½ ounces	6 ½ ounces	6 ½ ounces	7 ounces
Fresh or frozen meats (poultry, beef, pork, lamb) Dried legumes (peanut and soy may be excluded)		Recommended serving size						

(continued on next page)

Table 5
(continued)

Food Group	Daily Servings	Child Age			Adult Daily Energy Requirement			
		1–3 y	4–8 y	>8 y	2000 kcal	2400 kcal	2600 kcal	3000 kcal
		Serving size			Recommended Daily Amount			
Fats and oils	Milk-free and soy-free margarine				Total fat intake from all sources (30%–35% total energy intake)			
	Vegetable oils (olive, canola, heat-pressed soybean oil)	1 tsp	1 tsp	1 tsp	67–78 g	80–93g	87–101g	100–117g
	3, depending on energy needs							

All portion sizes are for US foods and measures. A US cup is equivalent to 237 mLs, 1 fluid ounce to 29.5 mLs, 1 tablespoon (tbsp.) to 15 mL, and 1 teaspoon (tsp) to 5 mL. 1 ounce is equivalent to 28.3 g. 1 cup of fruit is equivalent to 1 large banana, 8 strawberries, and 2 large plums. 1 cup of vegetables is equivalent to 10 broccoli florets, 12 baby carrots, 1 large sweet potato. 1 cup of rice weighs approximately 200g, and 1 cup of oats approximately 100g.

Table 6 Avoidance pearls	
Allergen	**Risks**
Cow's milk	• Other mammalian milks such as goat and sheep milk should be avoided due to shared homologous proteins. • The risk of cross-contact with milk in certain food products such as dark chocolate and nutrition meal bars is high. • Animal-free bioidentical milk proteins made by precision fermentation should be avoided. These must be labeled as "milk" in the United States and in the European Union. • Strict milk elimination is required for some, but not all, patients, and therefore it is prudent to recommend a strict milk elimination diet for the initial empiric diet prescription. Baked or boiled milk should be avoided with initial empiric elimination diets.
Wheat	• Further studies are required to determine if clinical and histologic outcomes would improve if wheat avoidance was expanded to gluten avoidance. • The risk of cross-contact with wheat in barley and rye is high; therefore, a gluten-free diet may be prudent. • It is important to consider the risk of cross-contact with wheat in other grains, particularly oats; therefore, we recommend choosing oats that are certified gluten free.
Soy	• Soy oil and soy lecithin do not contain significant soy protein and are allowed on a soy elimination diet.
Eggs	• Animal-free bioidentical egg proteins made by precision fermentation should be avoided. These must be labeled as "milk" in the United States and in the European Union.
Novel allergens	• Pea and other legume proteins, seeds, insects, and other novel allergens are added to many substitute foods and may play an antigenic role. The diet should be evaluated for novel food allergens when dietary elimination fails.

Novel Foods and Ingredients

Novel foods and ingredients are increasingly used in food formulations as manufacturers respond to evolving consumer health trends, concern for the environment and animal welfare, and a growing demand for sustainable foods.[83] Dietary elimination, even when just 1 food or food group is eliminated, results in the use of substitute foods that may introduce novel ingredients in the diet such as legumes (lentil, chickpea, green, and yellow pea), alternative and ancient grains (buckwheat, millet, quinoa), or seed proteins (sunflower, chia, and flax), which may be potential EoE triggers. Patients/caregivers and health care practitioners should not only focus on the eliminated food(s), but also the foods and ingredients in the diet at the time of remission to assist in documenting tolerated foods moving forward (**Table 6**).

When dietary elimination fails, it is important to first evaluate adherence to the diet to avoid misinterpreting poor adherence for refractory disease. Dietary intake should be carefully assessed, and if noncompliance or accidental allergen ingestion is found, consider providing re-education and additional 6 weeks of dietary elimination therapy. Treatment of comorbid gastroesophageal reflux disease may also be needed.[84,85] For patients who have been compliant, the removal of additional foods is an option to consider with motivated patients.[84] Lastly, medication management is another alternative therapy that can be discussed with patients/caregivers in a shared decision-making approach.

MAKING DIETARY THERAPY WORK FOR LONG-TERM MAINTENANCE

Dietary therapy can maintain remission.[84,86–88] Patients who choose dietary therapy have additional restrictions including traveling for vacation, special holidays, work, or school schedules and may benefit from treatment with medical therapy and taking a break from the diet for a while and then resuming. Additional ways to promote success are to avoid times when patients are traveling a lot for work, starting diets before winter holidays, or starting right before a young adult is leaving for college.[84]

SUMMARY

Dietary therapy has been found to be an effective first-line treatment for both children and adults with EoE and has advantages of finding a patient's food triggers while avoiding the need for concomitant medical therapy. Given these multiple choices, it is important to discuss these approaches with patients to formulate the best diet plan that aligns with their goals of care. Consultation with a trained dietitian is important to assist with a patient's baseline nutritional status, provide patient-facing education about dietary elimination, and help to monitor for adherence and contamination. Careful monitoring of patients' nutritional status, quality of life, and continued assessment of patients' goals of care should be pursued after diet implementation. If at any point dietary therapy is no longer aligning with patient goals, a transition to medical therapy is advised.

CLINICS CARE POINTS

- Dietary elimination is an effective therapy for treating adults and children with EoE.
- Empiric elimination diets are favored over elemental and allergy testing directed diets in the treatment of EoE.
- Multiple options for empiric elimination diets exist and the right approach should be pursued in a shared decision approach with patients.
- Dietary elimination should be pursued for a period of 6-8 weeks and repeat endoscopy should be used to assess response to treatment prior to food reintroduction.
- Food reintroduction is a critical part of dietary elimination to identify culprit foods triggering the disease.
- Working with a registered dietitan to assist with patient education and implementation of dietary elimination is essential.
- Timing of diet initiation is essential to success of dietary therapy (ie when patients have the time dedicated to pursue this treatment).

DISCLOSURE

N. Gonsalves: Consultant for AstraZeneca, Allakos, BMS, Sanofi-Regeneron; Speaking: Sanofi-Regeneron. M. Groetch: Received royalties from UpToDate and the Academy of Nutrition and Dietetics and consulting fees from FARE; Serves on the Medical Advisory Board of the International Food Protein-Induced Enterocolitis Syndrome Association as a Senior Advisor to FARE, as a Health Sciences Advisor for APFED, and is on the editorial board of the Journal of Food Allergy; and has no commercial interests to disclose. A. Lucendo: Consultant for Dr Falk Pharma and EsoCap.

REFERENCES

1. Kelly KJ, Lazenby AJ, Rowe PC, et al. Eosinophilic esophagitis attributed to gastroesophageal reflux: improvement with an amino acid based formula. Gastroenterology 1995;109(5):1503–12.
2. Markowitz JE, Spergel JM, Ruchelli E, et al. Elemental diet is an effective treatment for eosinophilic esophagitis in children and adolescents. Am J Gastroenterol 2003;98(4):777–82.
3. Liacouras CA, Spergel JM, Ruchelli E, et al. Eosinophilic esophagitis: A 10-year experience in 381 children. Clin Gastroenterol Hepatol 2005;3(12):1198–206.
4. Kagalwalla AF, Sentongo TA, Ritz S, et al. Effect of Six-Food Elimination Diet on Clinical and Histologic Outcomes in Eosinophilic Esophagitis. Clin Gastroenterol Hepatol 2006;4(9):1097–102.
5. Gonsalves N, Yang G-Y, Doerfler B, et al. Elimination diet effectively treats eosinophilic esophagitis in adults; food reintroduction identifies causative factors. Gastroenterology 2012;142(7):1451–9.e1 [quiz: e14-15].
6. Molina-Infante J, Lucendo AJ. Dietary therapy for eosinophilic esophagitis. J Allergy Clin Immunol 2018. https://doi.org/10.1016/j.jaci.2018.02.028.
7. Arias A, Gonzalez-Cervera J, Tenias JM, et al. Efficacy of dietary interventions for inducing histologic remission in patients with eosinophilic esophagitis: a systematic review and meta-analysis. Gastroenterology 2014;146(7):1639–48.
8. Peterson KA, Byrne KR, Vinson LA, et al. Elemental diet induces histologic response in adult eosinophilic esophagitis. Am J Gastroenterol 2013;108(5): 759–66.
9. Warners MJ, Vlieg-Boerstra BJ, Verheij J, et al. Elemental diet decreases inflammation and improves symptoms in adult eosinophilic oesophagitis patients. Aliment Pharmacol Therapeut 2017;45(6):777–87.
10. Rank MA, Sharaf RN, Furuta GT, et al. Technical Review on the Management of Eosinophilic Esophagitis: A Report From the AGA Institute and the Joint Task Force on Allergy-Immunology Practice Parameters. Gastroenterology 2020; 158(6):1789–810.e15.
11. Delaney AL, Arvedson JC. Development of swallowing and feeding: prenatal through first year of life. Dev Disabil Res Rev 2008;14(2):105–17.
12. Lucendo AJ, Arias-González L, Molina-Infante J, et al. Systematic review: health-related quality of life in children and adults with eosinophilic oesophagitis-instruments for measurement and determinant factors. Aliment Pharmacol Ther 2017;46(4):401–9.
13. Lucendo AJ, Molina-Infante J, Arias Á, et al. Guidelines on eosinophilic esophagitis: evidence-based statements and recommendations for diagnosis and management in children and adults. United European Gastroenterol J 2017;5(3): 335–58.
14. Dhar A, Haboubi HN, Attwood SE, et al. British Society of Gastroenterology (BSG) and British Society of Paediatric Gastroenterology, Hepatology and Nutrition (BSPGHAN) joint consensus guidelines on the diagnosis and management of eosinophilic oesophagitis in children and adults. Gut 2022. https://doi.org/10.1136/gutjnl-2022-327326. gutjnl-2022-327326.
15. Lucendo AJ, Arias Á, González-Cervera J, et al. Empiric 6-food elimination diet induced and maintained prolonged remission in patients with adult eosinophilic esophagitis: A prospective study on the food cause of the disease. J Allergy Clin Immunol 2013;131(3):797–804.

16. de Rooij WE, Vlieg-Boerstra B, Warners MJ, et al. Effect of amino acid-based formula added to four-food elimination in adult eosinophilic esophagitis patients: A randomized clinical trial. Neuro Gastroenterol Motil 2022;34(7):e14291.

17. Peterson KA, Boynton KK. Which patients with eosinophilic esophagitis (EoE) should receive elemental diets versus other therapies? Curr Gastroenterol Rep 2014;16(1):364.

18. Ribes-Koninckx C, Amil-Dias J, Espin B, et al. The use of amino acid formulas in pediatric patients with allergy to cow's milk proteins: Recommendations from a group of experts. Front Pediatr 2023;11:1110380.

19. Cianferoni A, Shuker M, Brown-Whitehorn T, et al. Food avoidance strategies in eosinophilic oesophagitis. Clin Exp Allergy 2019;49(3):269–84.

20. Anyane-Yeboa A, Wang W, Kavitt RT. The Role of Allergy Testing in Eosinophilic Esophagitis. Gastroenterol Hepatol 2018;14(8):463–9.

21. Spergel JM, Beausoleil JL, Mascarenhas M, et al. The use of skin prick tests and patch tests to identify causative foods in eosinophilic esophagitis. J Allergy Clin Immunol 2002;109(2):363–8.

22. Spergel JM, Brown-Whitehorn TF, Cianferoni A, et al. Identification of causative foods in children with eosinophilic esophagitis treated with an elimination diet. J Allergy Clin Immunol 2012;130(2):461–7.e5.

23. Pentiuk S, Putnam PE, Collins MH, et al. Dissociation between symptoms and histological severity in pediatric eosinophilic esophagitis. J Pediatr Gastroenterol Nutr 2009;48(2):152–60.

24. Alexander JA, Jung KW, Arora AS, et al. Swallowed fluticasone improves histologic but not symptomatic response of adults with eosinophilic esophagitis. Clin Gastroenterol Hepatol 2012;10(7):742–9.e1.

25. Safroneeva E, Straumann A, Coslovsky M, et al. Symptoms Have Modest Accuracy in Detecting Endoscopic and Histologic Remission in Adults With Eosinophilic Esophagitis. Gastroenterology 2016;150(3):581–90.e4.

26. Ballmer-Weber BK. Value of allergy tests for the diagnosis of food allergy. Dig Dis 2014;32(1–2):84–8.

27. Simon D, Straumann A, Wenk A, et al. Eosinophilic esophagitis in adults – no clinical relevance of wheat and rye sensitizations. Allergy 2006;61(12):1480–3.

28. Simon D, Cianferoni A, Spergel JM, et al. Eosinophilic esophagitis is characterized by a non-IgE-mediated food hypersensitivity. Allergy 2016;71(5):611–20.

29. Mayerhofer C, Kavallar AM, Aldrian D, et al. Efficacy of Elimination Diets in Eosinophilic Esophagitis: A Systematic Review and Meta-analysis. Clin Gastroenterol Hepatol 2023;21(9):2197–210.e3.

30. Philpott H, Nandurkar S, Royce SG, et al. Allergy tests do not predict food triggers in adult patients with eosinophilic oesophagitis. A comprehensive prospective study using five modalities. Aliment Pharmacol Ther 2016;44(3):223–33.

31. Pitsios C, Vassilopoulou E, Pantavou K, et al. Allergy-Test-Based Elimination Diets for the Treatment of Eosinophilic Esophagitis: A Systematic Review of Their Efficacy. JCM 2022;11(19):5631.

32. Clayton F, Fang JC, Gleich GJ, et al. Eosinophilic esophagitis in adults is associated with IgG4 and not mediated by IgE. Gastroenterology 2014;147(3):602–9.

33. Quinn L, Nguyen B, Menard-Katcher C, et al. IgG4+ cells are increased in the gastrointestinal tissue of pediatric patients with active eosinophilic gastritis and duodenitis and decrease in remission. Dig Liver Dis 2023;55(1):53–60.

34. Mohammad N, Avinashi V, Chan E, et al. Pediatric Eosinophilic Esophagitis Is Associated With Increased Lamina Propria Immunoglobulin G4-Positive Plasma Cells. J Pediatr Gastroenterol Nutr 2018;67(2):204–9.

35. Schuyler AJ, Wilson JM, Tripathi A, et al. Specific IgG4 antibodies to cow's milk proteins in pediatric patients with eosinophilic esophagitis. J Allergy Clin Immunol 2018,142(1):139 48.o12.

36. Rosenberg CE, Mingler MK, Caldwell JM, et al. Esophageal IgG4 levels correlate with histopathologic and transcriptomic features in eosinophilic esophagitis. Allergy 2018. https://doi.org/10.1111/all.13486.

37. Wright BL, Kulis M, Guo R, et al. Food-specific IgG4 is associated with eosinophilic esophagitis. J Allergy Clin Immunol 2016;138(4):1190–2.e3.

38. Dellon ES, Guo R, McGee SJ, et al. A Novel Allergen-Specific Immune Signature-Directed Approach to Dietary Elimination in Eosinophilic Esophagitis. Clin Transl Gastroenterol 2019;10(12):e00099.

39. Sampson HA. Update on food allergy. J Allergy Clin Immunol 2004;113(5): 805–19.

40. Kagalwalla AF, Shah A, Li BUK, et al. Identification of specific foods responsible for inflammation in children with eosinophilic esophagitis successfully treated with empiric elimination diet. J Pediatr Gastroenterol Nutr 2011;53(2):145–9.

41. Cotton CC, Erim D, Eluri S, et al. Cost Utility Analysis of Topical Steroids Compared to Dietary Elimination for Treatment of Eosinophilic Esophagitis. Clin Gastroenterol Hepatol 2017;15(6):841–9.e1.

42. Asher Wolf W, Huang KZ, Durban R, et al. The Six-Food Elimination Diet for Eosinophilic Esophagitis Increases Grocery Shopping Cost and Complexity. Dysphagia 2016;31(6):765–70.

43. Wang R, Hirano I, Doerfler B, et al. Assessing Adherence and Barriers to Long-Term Elimination Diet Therapy in Adults with Eosinophilic Esophagitis. Dig Dis Sci 2018. https://doi.org/10.1007/s10620-018-5045-0.

44. Molina-Infante J, Arias A, Barrio J, et al. Four-food group elimination diet for adult eosinophilic esophagitis: A prospective multicenter study. J Allergy Clin Immunol 2014;134(5):1093–9.e1.

45. Kagalwalla AF, Wechsler JB, Amsden K, et al. Efficacy of a 4-Food Elimination Diet for Children With Eosinophilic Esophagitis. Clin Gastroenterol Hepatol 2017;15(11):1698–707.e7.

46. Molina-Infante J, Arias Á, Alcedo J, et al. Step-up empiric elimination diet for pediatric and adult eosinophilic esophagitis: The 2-4-6 study. J Allergy Clin Immunol 2018;141(4):1365–72.

47. Zhan T, Ali A, Choi JG, et al. Model to Determine the Optimal Dietary Elimination Strategy for Treatment of Eosinophilic Esophagitis. Clin Gastroenterol Hepatol 2018;16(11):1730–7.e2.

48. Lucendo AJ. Nutritional approach to eosinophilic esophagitis: which diet and when. Minerva Gastroenterol Dietol 2020. https://doi.org/10.23736/S1121-421X.20.02797-X.

49. Kagalwalla AF, Amsden K, Shah A, et al. Cow's milk elimination: a novel dietary approach to treat eosinophilic esophagitis. J Pediatr Gastroenterol Nutr 2012; 55(6):711–6.

50. Wechsler JB, Schwartz S, Arva NC, et al. A Single-Food Milk Elimination Diet Is Effective for Treatment of Eosinophilic Esophagitis in Children. Clin Gastroenterol Hepatol 2022;20(8):1748–56.e11.

51. Teoh T, Mill C, Chan E, et al. Liberalized Versus Strict Cow's Milk Elimination for the Treatment of Children with Eosinophilic Esophagitis. J Can Assoc Gastroenterol 2019;2(2):81–5.

52. Wong J, Goodine S, Samela K, et al. Efficacy of Dairy Free Diet and 6-Food Elimination Diet as Initial Therapy for Pediatric Eosinophilic Esophagitis: A Retrospective Single-Center Study. Pediatr Gastroenterol Hepatol Nutr 2020;23(1):79–88.

53. Kruszewski PG, Russo JM, Franciosi JP, et al. Prospective, comparative effectiveness trial of cow's milk elimination and swallowed fluticasone for pediatric eosinophilic esophagitis. Dis Esophagus 2016;29(4):377–84.

54. Kliewer K, Aceves SS, Atkins D, et al. 817 – Efficacy of 1-Food and 4-Food Elimination Diets for Pediatric Eosinophilic Esophagitis in a Randomized Multi-Site Study. Gastroenterology 2019;156(6). S-173.

55. Kliewer KL, Gonsalves N, Dellon ES, et al. One-food versus six-food elimination diet therapy for the treatment of eosinophilic oesophagitis: a multicentre, randomised, open-label trial. The Lancet Gastroenterology & Hepatology 2023;8(5): 408–21.

56. Kliewer K, Aceves SS, Atkins D, et al. Efficacy of 1-Food and 4-food elimination diets for peditric eosinophilic esophagitis in a randomized multisite study. Gastroenterology 2019;156(Suppl 1). S-172-S-173.

57. Chang JW, Kliewer K, Katzka DA, et al. Provider Beliefs, Practices, and Perceived Barriers to Dietary Elimination Therapy in Eosinophilic Esophagitis. Am J Gastroenterol 2022;117(12):2071–4.

58. Votto M, De Filippo M, Olivero F, et al. Malnutrition in Eosinophilic Gastrointestinal Disorders. Nutrients 2020;13(1):E128.

59. Mukkada VA, Haas A, Maune NC, et al. Feeding dysfunction in children with eosinophilic gastrointestinal diseases. Pediatrics 2010;126(3):e672–7.

60. Jensen ET, Huang KZ, Chen HX, et al. Longitudinal Growth Outcomes Following First-line Treatment for Pediatric Patients With Eosinophilic Esophagitis. J Pediatr Gastroenterol Nutr 2019;68(1):50–5.

61. Haas AM, Maune NC. Clinical Presentation of Feeding Dysfunction in Children with Eosinophilic Gastrointestinal Disease. Immunol Allergy Clin 2009;29(1): 65–75.

62. Menard-Katcher C, Henry M, Furuta GT, et al. Significance of feeding dysfunction in eosinophilic esophagitis. World J Gastroenterol 2014;20(31):11019–22.

63. Pelz BJ, Wechsler JB, Amsden K, et al. IgE-associated food allergy alters the presentation of paediatric eosinophilic esophagitis. Clin Exp Allergy 2016;46(11): 1431–40.

64. Boyce JA, Assa'ad A, Burks AW, et al. Guidelines for the Diagnosis and Management of Food Allergy in the United States: Summary of the NIAID-Sponsored Expert Panel Report. J Allergy Clin Immunol 2010;126(6):1105–18.

65. Dellon ES, Gonsalves N, Hirano I, et al. ACG clinical guideline: Evidenced based approach to the diagnosis and management of esophageal eosinophilia and eosinophilic esophagitis (EoE). Am J Gastroenterol 2013;108(5):679–92.

66. Groetch M, Venter C, Skypala I, et al. Dietary Therapy and Nutrition Management of Eosinophilic Esophagitis: A Work Group Report of the American Academy of Allergy, Asthma, and Immunology. J Allergy Clin Immunol Pract 2017;5(2): 312–24.e29.

67. Becker P, Carney LN, Corkins MR, et al. Consensus Statement of the Academy of Nutrition and Dietetics/American Society for Parenteral and Enteral Nutrition: Indicators Recommended for the Identification and Documentation of Pediatric Malnutrition (Undernutrition). Nut in Clin Prac 2015;30(1):147–61.

68. Katzka DA, Smyrk TC, Alexander JA, et al. Accuracy and Safety of the Cytosponge for Assessing Histologic Activity in Eosinophilic Esophagitis: A Two-Center Study. Am J Gastroenterol 2017;112(10):1538–44.

69. Friedlander JA, Deboer EM, Soden JS, et al. Unsedated transnasal esophagoscopy for monitoring therapy in pediatric eosinophilic esophagitis. Gastrointest Endosc 2016;83(2):299–306.e1.

70. Friedlander JA, Fleischer DM, Black JO, et al. Unsedated transnasal esophagoscopy with virtual reality distraction enables earlier monitoring of dietary therapy in eosinophilic esophagitis. J Allergy Clin Immunol Pract 2021;9(9):3494–6.

71. Leung J, Hundal NV, Katz AJ, et al. Tolerance of baked milk in patients with cow's milk–mediated eosinophilic esophagitis. J Allergy Clin Immunol 2013;132(5): 1215–6.e1.

72. González-Cervera J, Arias Á, Navarro P, et al. Tolerance to sterilised cow's milk in patients with eosinophilic oesophagitis triggered by milk. Aliment Pharmacol Ther 2022;56(6):957–67.

73. U.S. Department of Agriculture and U.S. Department of Health and Human Services. Dietary Guidelines for Americans, 2020-2025. 9th Edition. 2020. Available at: DietaryGuidelines.gov. Accessed February 8, 2024.

74. Merritt RJ, Fleet SE, Fifi A, et al. North American Society for Pediatric Gastroenterology, Hepatology, and Nutrition Position Paper: Plant-based Milks. J Pediatr Gastroenterol Nutr 2020;71(2):276–81.

75. World Allergy Organization (WAO). Diagnosis and Rationale for Action against Cow's Milk Allergy (DRACMA) Guidelines. Pediatr Allergy Immunol 2010;21(s21): 1–125.

76. Agostoni C, Terracciano L, Varin E, et al. The Nutritional Value of Protein-hydrolyzed Formulae. Crit Rev Food Sci Nutr 2016;56(1):65–9.

77. Meyer R, De Koker C, Dziubak R, et al. The impact of the elimination diet on growth and nutrient intake in children with food protein induced gastrointestinal allergies. Clin Transl Allergy 2016;6(1):25.

78. Maslin K, Oliver EM, Scally KS, et al. Nutritional adequacy of a cows' milk exclusion diet in infancy. Clin Transl Allergy 2016;6(1):20.

79. Nachshon L, Goldberg MR, Schwartz N, et al. Decreased bone mineral density in young adult IgE-mediated cow's milk–allergic patients. J Allergy Clin Immunol 2014;134(5):1108–13.e3.

80. Vitoria Miñana I. The nutritional limitations of plant-based beverages in infancy and childhood. Nutr Hosp 2017. https://doi.org/10.20960/nh.931.

81. Verduci E, D'Elios S, Cerrato L, et al. Cow's Milk Substitutes for Children: Nutritional Aspects of Milk from Different Mammalian Species, Special Formula and Plant-Based Beverages. Nutrients 2019;11(8):1739.

82. Kliewer KL, Venter C, Cassin AM, et al. Should wheat, barley, rye, and/or gluten be avoided in a 6-food elimination diet? J Allergy Clin Immunol 2016;137(4): 1011–4.

83. Calabrese C, Bortolotti M, Fabbri A, et al. Reversibility of GERD Ultrastructural Alterations and Relief of Symptoms After Omeprazole Treatment. Am J Gastroenterol 2005;100(3):537–42.

84. Zalewski A, Doerfler B, Krause A, et al. Long-Term Outcomes of the Six-Food Elimination Diet and Food Reintroduction in a Large Cohort of Adults With Eosinophilic Esophagitis. Am J Gastroenterol 2022;117(12):1963–70.

85. van Rhijn BD, Weijenborg PW, Verheij J, et al. Proton pump inhibitors partially restore mucosal integrity in patients with proton pump inhibitor-responsive esophageal eosinophilia but not eosinophilic esophagitis. Clin Gastroenterol Hepatol 2014;12(11):1815–23.e2.

86. Hirano I, Chan ES, Rank MA, et al. AGA Institute and the Joint Task Force on Allergy-Immunology Practice Parameters Clinical Guidelines for the Management of Eosinophilic Esophagitis. Gastroenterology 2020;158(6):1776–86.

87. Lucendo A, Molina-Infante. Current treatment options and long-term outcomes in patients with eosinophilic esophagitis. Expet Rev Clin Immunol 2022;18(8): 859–72.

88. Aceves SS, Alexander JA, Baron TH, et al. Endoscopic approach to eosinophilic esophagitis: American Society for Gastrointestinal Endoscopy Consensus Conference. Gastrointest Endosc 2022;96(4):576–92.e1.

Pharmacologic Management of Eosinophilic Esophagitis

Gary W. Falk, MD, MS[a], Robbie Pesek, MD[b],*

KEYWORDS

- Eosinophilic esophagitis • Corticosteroids • Proton pump inhibitors
- Potassium-competitive acid blockers • Biologic therapy • Dupilumab

KEY POINTS

- Medications, including proton pump inhibitors (PPIs), swallowed topical corticosteroids (STSs), and biologics, are a mainstay in the treatment of eosinophilic esophagitis (EoE). Only one medication, dupilumab, is Food and Drug Administration (FDA) approved.
- PPIs function as anti-inflammatories in EoE and are effective for both short-term and long-term treatment. Response to PPIs is no longer required to diagnose EoE.
- Potassium-competitive acid blockers demonstrate similar efficacy as PPIs and may be an alternative therapy for EoE in the future.
- STSs have broad anti-inflammatory activity and are effective for both short-term and long-term use in EoE. However, loss of response may develop over time.
- Biologics provide a more targeted mechanism of action than PPIs or STSs. Dupilumab is the only FDA-approved therapy for EoE but other agents are under development.

INTRODUCTION

Medications, in addition to food elimination diets, are the mainstay of treatment for eosinophilic esophagitis (EoE). The ultimate choice of therapy depends on shared decision-making, accounting for factors such as efficacy, ease of use, safety, and cost. Until recently, there have been 2 classes of medications used: proton pump inhibitors (PPIs) and swallowed topical corticosteroids (STSs). More recently, 2 new classes of medication have emerged including potassium-competitive acid blockers (P-CABs) and biologics. Each of these medication classes is effective in improving the clinical symptoms, endoscopic findings, and histologic abnormalities in some but not all patients with EoE. Until recently, response to PPI was considered a key step in diagnosing

[a] Division of Gastroenterology & Hepatology, Department of Medicine, Hospital of the University of Pennsylvania, University of Pennsylvania Perelman School of Medicine, 7th Floor South Pavilion PCAM, 3400 Civic Center Boulevard, Philadelphia, PA 19104, USA; [b] Division of Allergy and Immunology, Department of Pediatrics, Arkansas Children's Hospital, University of Arkansas for Medical Sciences, 13 Children's Way, Slot 512-13, Little Rock, AR 72202, USA
* Corresponding author.
E-mail address: rdpesek@uams.edu

Immunol Allergy Clin N Am 44 (2024) 245–264
https://doi.org/10.1016/j.iac.2023.12.010
0889-8561/24/© 2023 Elsevier Inc. All rights reserved.

EoE, and STSs or dietary therapy was initiated in patients who did not improve. PPIs and STSs are both excellent initial treatment options and both classes are typically well tolerated, safe, and effective for long-term use. Targeted biologic therapy has undergone considerable investigation and holds tremendous promise for the treatment of EoE. Dupilumab, a monoclonal antibody that blocks interleukin (IL)-4 and IL-13 signaling, is currently the only Food and Drug Administration (FDA)–approved treatment for EoE. In this articler, each class of medication utilized to treat EoE will be reviewed with an in depth discussion of efficacy, safety, and guidelines for use.

PROTON PUMP INHIBITORS

The role of PPIs in the treatment of EoE has evolved dramatically over the last 3 decades as our understanding of the disease has changed. In 2006, a case series of 3 patients with esophageal eosinophilia, endoscopic, and clinical findings suggestive of EoE demonstrated normalization of endoscopic findings, elimination of symptoms, and near normalization of histology after treatment with PPIs.[1] Early clinical guidelines suggested that the best way to distinguish esophageal eosinophilia related to gastroesophageal reflux disease (GERD) from EoE was an initial trial of a PPI for 8 weeks.[2] Subsequent guideline iterations described an entity known as PPI-REE (PPI-responsive esophageal eosinophilia) in which patients had esophageal symptoms and histologic findings of esophageal eosinophilia but demonstrated a symptomatic and histologic response to a PPI trial. This entity was viewed as separate from "traditional" allergic EoE.[3] This all changed in 2018 with the publication of the AGREE consensus conference that removed the PPI trial requirement for the diagnosis of EoE and instead classified PPIs as a bona fide treatment option for EoE.[4]

Mechanism of Action

PPIs bind irreversibly to the hydrogen potassium ATPase (H^+/K^+ ATPase) proton pump in gastric parietal cells, thereby decreasing gastric acid production. This has led to the well-described efficacy of this class of drugs in acid peptic disorders such as GERD and peptic ulcer disease. In addition to these antisecretory effects, PPIs have a variety of anti-inflammatory effects independent of gastric acid secretion in EoE. These include antioxidant properties, inhibition of immune cell function, reduction of inflammatory cytokine production by esophageal squamous cells, and a decrease in adhesion molecule expression by endothelial cells.[5] Recently, a non-gastric H^+/K^+ ATPase has been identified in esophageal squamous cells from patients with EoE.[6] Blockade of this non-gastric proton pump with a PPI decreases Th2 cytokine–induced secretion of the eosinophil chemokine eotaxin-3. PPI therapy can also reverse nearly all of the allergic inflammatory gene expression profile characteristics of EoE.[7] All of these effects lead to the improvement of impaired mucosal integrity and permeability characteristic of EoE.[8]

Efficacy

Two large systematic reviews have examined the efficacy of PPIs in EoE. The first, by Lucendo and colleagues in 2016, examined 33 studies, including 2 randomized controlled trials, comprising 619 pediatric and adult patients.[9] Symptomatic improvement was seen in 60.8% (95% confidence interval [CI], 48.3%–72.2%) and histologic remission (<15 eosinophils/high power field [eos/hpf]) in 50.5% (95% CI, 42.2%–58.7%), albeit with moderate to high heterogeneity. Furthermore, no differences in response were observed between pediatric and adult populations. A second systematic review, conducted by the American Gastroenterological Association (AGA) and

Joint Task Force for Allergy-Immunology Practice Parameters (JTF), examined 23 observational studies and found a histologic response (<15 eos/hpf) in 42%.[10] Thus, a subset of patients will respond histologically and clinically to PPI therapy.

Predictors of Response

A number of studies have examined predictors of response to PPI therapy. The largest of these was a cross-sectional study of 650 patients in the European EoE CONNECT registry that reflects real-world practice in Europe.[11] In this study, 630 patients had induction therapy with PPIs; symptomatic improvement occurred in 71% and histologic remission (<15 eos/hpf) in 48.8%. Importantly, the histologic response rate was higher for double-dose therapy than for standard-dose therapy (50.7% vs 36.7%), as was symptom improvement (73.9% vs 54.6%). The presence of inflammatory endoscopic features led to a higher clinicohistologic response than did fibrotic features (odds ratio [OR] 3.7; 95%, CI 1.4–9.5) as did prolonging length of therapy from 8 to 12 weeks (OR 2.7; 95% CI, 1.3–5.3). No differences were observed among the various different PPIs, and PPIs appeared to be less effective in individuals who failed STSs or dietary therapy. Thus, dose, duration of therapy, and inflammatory features on endoscopy are all features that may predict a positive response to PPIs. Other studies also suggest that fibrotic endoscopic features predict nonresponse to PPIs.[12–14]

Maintenance Therapy

There are limited data on the efficacy of long-term PPI therapy in the maintenance of remission. A multicenter international study of 75 patients in remission on high-dose PPIs subsequently had low-dose maintenance therapy (omeprazole equivalent of 20 mg once daily), which resulted in the maintenance of histologic remission in 73% over a mean follow-up of 26 months.[15] Interestingly, loss of response was associated with the CYP2C19 rapid metabolizer genotype that leads to lower PPI plasma levels. Other evidence for step-down PPI therapy comes from Spain, in a study of 40 patients who achieved histologic remission on high-dose PPI therapy (omeprazole 40 mg twice daily).[16] Histologic remission (<15 eos/hpf) was maintained in 81% after a dose reduction to omeprazole 40 mg daily for 8 weeks and was still maintained in 83% after a further reduction in dose to 20 mg once daily. Similar results for maintenance therapy have been described in other adult and pediatric studies as well.[17,18] Thus, maintenance therapy is effective in most but not all patients responding to a PPI, and an effort should be made to titrate down to the lowest PPI dose that maintains remission. Once the optimal maintenance therapy dose is achieved, the issue of loss of response to treatment over time remains unclear.

Safety Concerns

A wide variety of potential adverse events have been associated with chronic PPI use in observational studies. These include kidney disease, Clostridioides difficile infection, pneumonia, dementia, bone fracture, myocardial infarction, small intestinal bacterial overgrowth, spontaneous bacterial peritonitis, and micronutrient deficiencies, among others.[19] However, the magnitude of these purported risks is low, they fall within a zone of potential bias uncertainty, and criteria for causality are generally not met.[20] In the only randomized controlled trial to examine this issue, patients with underlying cardiovascular disease were administered pantoprazole 40 mg daily or placebo for a median of 3 years.[21] No difference in safety outcomes was found between the 2 groups with the exception of a slight increase in enteric infections in the PPI group (OR 1.33; 95% CI, 1.01–1.75). Thus, evidence to date suggests that when PPIs are appropriately used, treatment benefits clearly outweigh the risks of therapy.

Guideline Recommendations

The most recent clinical practice guideline published in 2022 by the British Society of Gastroenterology (BSG) and the British Society of Pediatric Gastroenterology, Hepatology, and Nutrition strongly recommends PPI therapy to induce remission in EoE based on a moderate GRADE (Grading of Recommendations, Assessment, Development and Evaluation) level of evidence.[22] The recommendation also suggests twice-daily therapy (omeprazole equivalent of 20 mg twice daily) for 8 to 12 weeks prior to the assessment of response. Finally, the guideline strongly recommends considering long-term maintenance therapy after induction of a remission with a low GRADE of evidence. The AGA/JTF guideline conditionally recommends PPI therapy based on very low GRADE quality of evidence.[23]

Summary

PPIs have the advantages of low cost, easy availability, excellent tolerability, and safety profile, making this class of drugs a reasonable option for many, but perhaps not all, patients with EoE for both induction of remission and maintenance therapy. Predictors of initial response include inflammatory features at the time of endoscopy, initial use of high dose therapy, and prolonged initial therapy for at least 12 weeks. If a response is achieved, efforts should be made to titrate down to the lowest PPI dose that maintains clinical, histologic, and endoscopic remission. Patients should be reassured as to the excellent safety profile of this class of drugs based on best available evidence.

POTASSIUM-COMPETITIVE ACID BLOCKERS

P-CABs are a new class of antisecretory drugs that act by blocking the potassium channel of the H^+/K^+ ATPase proton pump through reversible binding of both active and inactive proton pumps. Compared to PPIs, P-CABs have a more rapid onset and longer duration of antisecretory effect.[24] Given the similarity in mechanism of action, P-CABs are now being investigated in EoE as well, although limited data are available to date. A case series of 4 EoE patients not responding to 12 weeks of esomeprazole 20 mg daily found that switching to the P-CAB vonoprazan led to resolution of all symptoms and histologic response (<15 eos/hpf) in 3 of the 4 patients.[25] Since then, 2 additional case series from Japan showed no difference in symptomatic, histologic, or endoscopic responses between vonoprazan and 2 different PPIs.[26,27] P-CABs have been widely used in Asia but are only approved by the FDA for *Helicobacter pylori* therapy. The eventual role of PCABs in the treatment of EoE remains to be determined.

CORTICOSTEROIDS

Successful treatment of EoE with both topical and systemic corticosteroids was first described in 1998.[28,29] A subsequent randomized clinical trial comparison of oral prednisone and topical fluticasone in 80 children found no difference in clinical and histologic efficacy between the systemic and topical steroids, but, not surprisingly, far greater adverse events in the prednisone group.[30] Since these publications, topical corticosteroids have emerged as a mainstay of therapy for EoE. However, the evidence supporting the use of topical corticosteroids comes primarily from studies using off-label steroid preparations designed for the treatment of asthma and not from esophageal specific preparations.[31] Both budesonide liquid respules, mixed in a wide variety of delivery vehicles to make a viscous slurry, and fluticasone propionate, administered via a metered dose inhaler that is swallowed rather than inhaled, have emerged as the 2 most common topical steroids in use today.[32] Both of these steroids may also be prepared by compounding pharmacies, but considerable variation in compounding practices has been noted as well.[33,34] Other small case series have described other steroids including mometasone and ciclesonide.[35,36]

Regardless of the steroid preparation chosen, a number of barriers exist that present challenges for the use of these compounds in clinical practice. These include cost, issues with insurance coverage for off-label use, compliance, and the practical hurdle of administering compounds developed for asthma instead of EoE. Furthermore, while no topical steroid preparation has been approved by FDA in the United States, budesonide orally disintegrating tablets were first approved by the European Medicines Agency (EMA) in 2018 and then subsequently by regulatory agencies in Canada and Australia. Other novel new compounds to enhance esophageal delivery are being developed as outlined in the following sections.

Mechanism of Action

Topical corticosteroids have broad anti-inflammatory activities in EoE. These include reduction of eosinophils, mast cells, T lymphocytes, and genes encoding for inflammatory cytokines such as IL-5, IL-13, eotaxin-3, periostin, and TSLP.[37–40] Successful treatment with fluticasone leads to reversal of 98% of the unique transcriptome of 574 differentially expressed genes seen in EoE.[41] Topical steroid therapy also results in enhanced mucosal integrity, decreased mucosal permeability, and a decrease in basal cell hyperplasia while also increasing gene expression of the barrier integrity proteins filaggrin and desmoglein.[37]

The impact of topical corticosteroids on fibrosis is somewhat more challenging to sort out. Seminal work by Aceves and colleagues in 2010 in 16 pediatric EoE patients found that successful treatment with topical corticosteroids led to a decrease in fibrosis and remodeling, as well as mediators of fibrosis including TGF-β and pSMAD2/3, along with a decrease in vascular activation.[42] On the other hand, 1 year of fluticasone therapy in 10 adults resulted in no decrease in subepithelial fibrosis despite a downregulation of profibrogenic cytokine gene expression.[43]

Efficacy

The systematic review conducted by the AGA/JTF examined 8 randomized clinical trials of 437 patients and found a histologic response rate (<15 eos/hpf) of 65%.[10] A more recent meta-analysis of 9 randomized controlled trials of topical steroids found a complete histologic response (using variable definitions) in 62% along with improved symptoms (OR 2.53; 95% CI, 1.14–5.60) and endoscopic appearance (OR 3.51; 95% CI, 1.47–8.36), when compared to placebo.[44] The aforementioned systematic reviews aggregated all the different topical steroid preparations but did not offer a direct comparison of the different steroids. A randomized clinical trial that compared 8 weeks of oral viscous budesonide (1 mg twice daily) to fluticasone (880 mcg twice daily) found no difference in the trial endpoints of eosinophil counts, dysphagia symptoms, and endoscopic scores (EREFS) between the 2 preparations.[45] Histologic remission defined as less than 15 eos/hpf was comparable as well: 71% in the budesonide group and 64% in the fluticasone group.

Predictors of Response

Considerable efforts have been made to identify predictors of response to topical corticosteroids. Predictors of nonresponse to steroids include need for dilation at baseline examination, presence of a hiatal hernia, obesity (body mass index≥ 30), younger age, and edema on endoscopy.[46–48] Predictors of a positive response to therapy include older age and the presence of food allergies. More sophisticated biomarkers have also been investigated but baseline whole transcriptome gene expression could not predict response.[49] A more recent study identified 3 epigenetic DNA methylation sites that were associated with treatment response but further validation is still needed.[50]

Maintenance Therapy

Clinical, histologic, and endoscopic relapse is the norm after cessation of successful induction therapy with corticosteroids. This was shown nicely by Dellon and colleagues when 58 patients from the randomized controlled trial of budesonide viscous suspension versus fluticasone described earlier were observed off therapy after completion of the trial.[51] Symptomatic recurrence prior to 1 year was seen in 33/58 responders (57%) and 78% had histologic relapse at the time of symptom recurrence.

Long-term maintenance therapy with topical corticosteroids has been described in a number of observational studies. The work by Andreae and colleagues described maintenance therapy in 54 children who were administered chronic fluticasone over a mean follow-up of 20 months with dose adjusted by patient age.[52] Maintenance therapy was continued at the same dose as induction therapy and led to a sustained decrease in eosinophils, accompanied by improvement in endoscopic findings and symptoms as well. However, 30% of patients did have a histologic relapse while maintained on the same dose of fluticasone. An observational study of 229 patients from the Swiss EoE database examined the long-term effectiveness of topical steroids in patients initially given 1 mg of topical steroids twice daily and then maintained on 0.25 mg twice daily indefinitely.[53] At a median follow-up of 5 years, a higher proportion of patients on topical steroids were in clinical, histologic, and endoscopic remission compared to individuals who were not on maintenance therapy: 31% versus 4.5%; 44.8% versus 10.1%, and 48.8% versus 17.8%, respectively. Complete remission, which was defined as a combined clinical, histologic, and endoscopic response, was seen in 16.1% versus 1.3%, respectively. Higher cumulative doses of corticosteroids and longer duration of therapy were both associated with clinical and complete remission. Other studies have confirmed the effectiveness of chronic corticosteroid therapy in some, but not all, patients who achieve histologic remission on induction therapy.[54]

There are a number of questions to consider when using chronic topical corticosteroid maintenance therapy in EoE:

- What is the relapse rate while on chronic therapy, that is, loss of response?
- Can remission be maintained on a lower dose than induction therapy?
- Is chronic therapy safe?
- How adherent is the patient?

Loss of histologic response to induction doses is clearly seen in a subset of patients on chronic therapy. In a case series of 55 patients from Chapel Hill, 61% of patients with an initial response to therapy had loss of histologic response at a median follow-up of 11.7 months.[55] Of note, loss of response was lower in patients who were maintained on their original dose of steroids. A larger study of 82 patients in histologic remission who were administered chronic steroids at varying doses for a median of 2.2 years found histologic relapse in 67% with no difference between those on low-dose (≤0.5 mg/day) or high-dose steroids (>0.5 mg/day).[56] However, histologic relapse occurred earlier in the low-dose group than in the high=dose group. Finally, a small pediatric study of 26 patients examined the common clinical practice of inducing remission on a given dose of topical corticosteroids and then decreasing the dose to the lowest effective dose to maintain remission by progressively cutting the dose of therapy in half and, if histologic or clinical relapse occurred, resuming the previously effective dose.[57] While 54% of patients reached the lowest effective dose, 27% relapsed during dose reduction and required resumption of the higher dose of therapy. Overall 81% remained in remission. Maintenance therapy may be associated with other beneficial effects including a decrease in the need for subsequent dilations and decreased risk of food bolus impaction.[58,59]

Regardless of the aforementioned issues, adherence to any mode of maintenance therapy presents challenges in a chronic disease such as EoE, especially in younger patients.[60]

Taken together, the following can be said about chronic topical steroid therapy:

- Chronic therapy is effective in some, but not all, patients after successful initial response
- Loss of response is encountered in a subset of patients
- Dose reduction is effective in a subset of patients
- Chronic therapy may decrease complications of EoE
- Long-term compliance is problematic

Safety Concerns

Several studies have examined the safety profile of topical corticosteroid therapy for EoE. The most recent is an integrated safety analysis of 6 phase 1 to 3 clinical trials of the investigational formulation of budesonide oral suspension.[61] Esophageal candidiasis was found in 5.8% of patients given budesonide 2 mg twice daily and 5.4% given any dose, compared to 1.2% of the placebo group. Oral candidiasis was encountered in 4.1% compared to 0% in the placebo group. A decrease in serum cortisol was seen in 6.2% in the budesonide 2 mg twice-daily group compared to 1.2% in the placebo group, and an abnormal adrenocorticotropic hormone stimulation test was found in 4.8% and 1.8%, respectively.

An earlier systemic review of 17 studies encompassing 596 EoE patients administered topical corticosteroids found abnormal adrenal testing in 15.8% but not in any of the 7 randomized controlled clinical trials analyzed.[62] However, in this analysis it was noted that adrenal insufficiency was defined heterogeneously, often without baseline adrenal function testing and concomitant steroid use for asthma, rhinitis, or dermatitis was not considered. There have been other scattered reports of adrenal insufficiency in children treated with chronic STSs.[63–65] Currently, there are no guideline recommendations for screening of adrenal insufficiency in children or adults to inform optimal clinical care. Taken together, topical corticosteroid use appears to be safe, but patients and physicians should be aware of the underlying low rates of both candidiasis and abnormalities in adrenal function. Until more data become available, it seems reasonable to check a fasting cortisol annually in patients on chronic corticosteroid therapy.

New Agents

Three different novel steroid preparations optimized for esophageal delivery have been studied to date. Budesonide orodispersible tablets are placed on the tongue, pressed against the hard palate, and subsequently dissolved in saliva, allowing for drug delivery into the esophagus. This compound has been studied for both induction and maintenance of remission. In the 6-week induction study of 86 patients, clinicohistologic remission (<5 eos/hpf and symptom severity $\leq$ 2 on a numerical rating scale) was seen in 58% given budesonide orodispersible 1 mg twice daily compared to 0%

given placebo.[66] Importantly, the response rate increased to 85% if treatment was extended out to 12 weeks. Furthermore, histologic remission alone at week 6 was 93% in the active treatment group compared to 0% in the placebo group. A subsequent 48 week maintenance study of patients in clinical remission compared 0.5 mg twice daily, 1 mg twice daily, and placebo and found maintenance of clinical remission in 74%, 75%, and 4%, respectively.[67] Median time to relapse was 87 days in the placebo group compared to greater than 350 days in the active treatment arms. Budesonide orodispersible tablets were approved by the EMA in 2018 and subsequently by regulatory authorities in Canada and Europe, but this compound has not been approved by the FDA.

A large phase 3 study of a second esophageal-specific steroid preparation, budesonide oral suspension, found that budesonide oral suspension 2mg twice daily for 12 weeks was superior to placebo for improvement of histologic, symptomatic, and endoscopic endpoints.[68] The FDA has just approved this compound for a 12 week course of therapy at a dose of 2 mg twice daily in February of 2024.

Fluticasone propionate orally disintegrating tablets are a new esophageal-specific formulation of fluticasone that disintegrates on the tongue and then swallowed to coat the esophagus with minimal systemic absorption. A small phase 1 b/2s proof of principle study established safety and tolerability as well as potential efficacy for endoscopic, clinical, and histologic endpoints.[69] A subsequent 12-week phase 2b induction therapy dose finding study found histologic response (<6 eosinophils/hpf) in 80%, 67%, 86%, and 48% of subjects given 3 mg twice daily, 3 mg at bedtime, 1.5 mg twice daily, and 1.5 mg at bedtime, respectively, all of which were superior to placebo which had a 0% histologic response.[70] Histologic response was maintained in 30% to 84% depending on the dose administered at 52 weeks and no safety signals were noted. A 24-week induction study of fluticasone propionate 3 mg administered at bedtime versus placebo followed by an open label extension phase is currently ongoing (ClinicalTrials.gov, Number NCT05634746).

Guideline Recommendations

Both the AGA/JTF and the BSG guidelines give a strong recommendation for the use of topical corticosteroids for induction therapy in EoE with GRADE of evidence moderate and high, respectively.[22,23] However, as outlined earlier, the relapse rate after cessation of therapy is high, making maintenance therapy an important consideration. The AGA/JTF guideline suggests continuation of topical corticosteroids with a conditional recommendation based on very low GRADE quality of evidence and the BSG guideline strongly recommends maintenance therapy with moderate GRADE evidence. Not surprisingly, both guidelines recommend against the use of systemic steroids in EoE.

BIOLOGICS

Over the past decade, no class of medication has received more attention for the treatment of EoE than biologics. The most successful of the biologics have targeted cytokines including IL-4, IL-5, and IL-13, but other targets, including several novel pathways and molecules, have also been evaluated (**Fig. 1**). Multiple studies, including several phase 3 clinical trials, have evaluated the effectiveness of these molecules in the treatment of EoE. Unfortunately, many of these trials fell short in achieving improvement across all outcome measures including symptoms, endoscopic, and histologic endpoints. It was not until 2022 that one of these medications, dupilumab, finally broke through and became the first FDA-approved therapy for EoE.

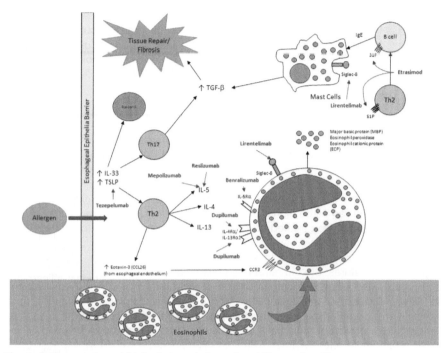

Fig. 1. Pathogenesis and biologic targets in eosinophilic esophagitis.

Dupilumab

Dupilumab is a humanized monoclonal antibody that binds to the IL-4 receptor alpha-subunit and inhibits signaling through both the IL-4 and IL-13 receptors. Dupilumab is approved for the treatment of multiple other atopic conditions including atopic dermatitis, asthma, and chronic rhinosinusitis with nasal polyposis. Its effectiveness for the treatment of EoE was evaluated in 2 phase 3 studies of adolescents, 12 years and older, and adults.[71] Both studies utilized the same primary endpoints of histologic remission ($\leq$6 eos/hpf) and changes in dysphagia, as defined by the absolute change from baseline in the Dysphagia Symptom Questionnaire (DSQ). The first study (Part A) enrolled 81 participants who were randomized to either placebo or dupilumab 300 mg weekly. The second trial (Part B) enrolled 159 participants who were randomized to placebo, dupilumab 300 mg weekly, or dupilumab 300 mg every 2 weeks. At the end of 24 weeks, 59% to 60% of participants who received weekly dupilumab in Part A and B achieved the primary histologic endpoint, compared to 5% to 6% of the placebo group. Weekly dupilumab was also associated with significant reductions in dysphagia, compared to placebo, although there was no difference between treated participants and placebo with dosing every 2 weeks. In a 28-week extension study (Part C), placebo-treated participants from the initial trial rolled over to dupilumab weekly or every 2 weeks. Those participants who were treated with dupilumab in Part A were eligible to continue treatment, for a total of 52 weeks. In this group, 56% maintained histologic remission while in those who rolled over from placebo to weekly dupilumab, 18/30 (60%) achieved histologic remission. During the trials, adverse events were reported by 60% to 86% of participants, although only 7 patients discontinued therapy due to a treatment-emergent adverse event. The most commonly reported adverse events were injection site reactions/erythema, nasopharyngitis, and headache. Conjunctivitis, which has been reported as a side effect in trials of dupilumab for atopic dermatitis, was only a rare occurrence. In May 2022, dupilumab was approved by the FDA for adolescents and adults with EoE. A similar phase 3 trial in children of ages 1 to less than 12 years is ongoing with results expected in late 2023 (ClinicalTrials.gov, Number NCT04394351).

Cendakimab

Cendakimab, a monoclonal antibody that prevents bindings to the IL-13 receptor, has also been evaluated in EoE. In a phase 2, randomized, double-blind trial of 90 adults with EoE, treatment with cendakimab was associated with significant reductions in esophageal eosinophils compared to placebo.[72] Nearly 50% of treated participants had less than 15 eos/hpf, and 20% to 25% had less than 6 eos/hpf, compared to none in the placebo group. Treated participants demonstrated a significant reduction in patient and clinician perceptions of disease severity; however, there were no significant differences between treated participants and the placebo group in changes in DSQ scores. Subgroup analysis of 47 steroid-refractory participants also demonstrated significant improvements in esophageal eosinophils as well as improvements in endoscopic features. Steroid refractory patients also had a more significant reduction in dysphagia symptoms compared to the overall study group. In a 52-week extension trial, cendakimab was associated with continued histologic and endoscopic improvement in treated participants. Those who received placebo in the initial trial demonstrated significant reductions in tissue eosinophils and improvement in endoscopic appearance after treatment with cendakimab and obtained similar eosinophil levels as those who were treated throughout both trials.[73] In the initial phase 2 trial, the safety profile of cendakimab was similar to that of dupilumab with 64.5% to 85.3% of participants reporting an adverse event. The most common reported adverse events included headache, upper respiratory tract infection, arthralgia, nasopharyngitis, diarrhea, and nausea. A phase 3 clinical trial is currently underway (ClinicalTrials.gov, Numbers NCT04753697, NCT04991935).

Compounds Targeting Interleukin 5

Several monoclonal antibodies against IL-5 or the IL-5 receptor have been evaluated in EoE. Mepolizumab and reslizumab bind directly to the IL-5 molecule, while benralizumab binds to the alpha-subunit of the IL-5 receptor, preventing signaling. Mepolizumab was the first biologic molecule evaluated for the treatment of EoE. In an early study, mepolizumab led to significant reductions in tissue eosinophils, mast cells, and peripheral eosinophils, and an improvement in hyperplasia of esophageal epithelium.[74] In 2 subsequent clinical trials, treatment with mepolizumab did not consistently lead to histologic remission (<5 eos/hpf) or significant improvement in clinical symptoms or endoscopic findings, compared to placebo.[75,76] The most recent study of mepolizumab evaluated its efficacy in 66 adolescents and adults with EoE, half of whom were steroid refractory.[77] In this study, participants were randomized to mepolizumab 300 mg monthly for 3 months (and were eligible to continue for an additional 3 months) or placebo. Those who initially received placebo were subsequently rolled over to mepolizumab 100 mg monthly for 3 months. At the end of 3 months, 34% of mepolizumab-treated participants achieved histologic remission (<6 eos/hpf) compared to 3% of the placebo group. Treated participants also demonstrated significant improvements in endoscopic findings. There were also reductions in symptoms, although not statistically significant, compared to placebo. Participants who were initially treated with placebo also demonstrated improvements in symptoms, and endoscopic and histologic outcomes after treatment with mepolizumab, although only 3 participants (11%) achieved histologic remission.

Reslizumab has demonstrated similar efficacy in reducing tissue eosinophils but is not associated with significant changes in clinical symptoms or quality of life measures, compared to placebo.[78] Benralizumab is currently under investigation for EoE as well as eosinophilic gastritis (EoG). In a trial of 24 participants with hypereosinophilic syndrome , 7 of which had coexisting eosinophilic gastrointestinal disease, benralizumab was associated with complete depletion of gastrointestinal eosinophils.[79] A phase 3, randomized, placebo-controlled trial of benralizumab in adolescents and adults with EoE has also been performed with results pending (ClinicalTrials.gov Number: NCT04543409).

Novel Pathways/Molecules

Siglec-8
Siglec-8 is a cell surface protein expressed on eosinophils, mast cells, and basophils. Binding to this molecule leads to inhibition of cell activity and promotion of eosinophil apoptosis, leading to eosinophil depletion.[80] A siglec-8 monoclonal antibody, lirentelimab, has been evaluated in the treatment of EoG and eosinophilic enteritis.[81] In a phase 2 study of 64 patients, lirentelimab led to a 95% reduction in gastrointestinal eosinophil (per-protocol analysis) with 95% of treated subjects achieving less than 30 eos/hpf, compared to 15% of the placebo group. Of the enrolled participants, 23 (14 treatment group, 9 placebo group) also experienced esophageal eosinophilia. Following treatment with lirentelimab, 13 of the 14 demonstrated histologic remission (<5 eos/hpf) compared to only 1 participant in the placebo group. Following these results, a phase 2/3 study was completed in adolescents and adults with EoE.[82] Key outcome measures included the number of participants who achieved histologic remission (≤6 eos/hpf) and changes in DSQ after 24 weeks of treatment. A total of 276 participants were enrolled and randomized to lirentelimab 1 mg/kg for 1 dose then 3 mg/kg monthly for 5 doses, 1 mg/kg monthly for 6 doses, or placebo. At the end of the study period, 88% to 92% of the treated group achieved histologic remission compared to 11% of the placebo group. There was a reduction in DSQ but this change was not significantly different than that in placebo-treated participants. However, in a supplementary analysis, participants who had a higher tissue eosinophil burden (>24 eos/hpf) were more likely to achieve remission and have significant reductions in DSQ compared to placebo, suggesting that the severity of disease may impact response to treatment.[83]

Thymic stromal lymphopoietin
Thymic stromal lymphopoietin (TSLP) has become an increasingly common target for therapy across multiple atopic conditions. TSLP is an alarmin that plays a role in disrupting the epithelium/endothelium. It can bind to receptors on type 2 innate lymphoid cells, produce IL-5 and IL-13, and activate other cells such as mast cells.[84] In addition, there is increased gene expression of TSLP in active EoE which decreases during disease remission.[85] In mouse models of EoE, TSLP also plays a role in the development of esophageal fibrosis.[86] Currently, tezepelumab, an anti-TSLP monoclonal antibody, is approved for the treatment of severe asthma. In contrast to other biologics such as dupilumab, mepolizumab, or benralizumab, it appears to be effective regardless of eosinophil levels.[87] A phase 3 clinical trial of tezepelumab for adolescents and adults with EoE is underway (ClinicalTrials.gov, Number NCT05583227).

Other novel pathways and molecules
Several other molecules/pathways have received attention for their potential role in the treatment of EoE (**Table 1**). While eosinophils have received much of the focus as mediators of disease activity, other cells, including mast cells, likely play a role.

Table 1
Current status of biologics and novel molecules in eosinophilic esophagitis

Drug	Mechanism of Action	Current Status
Dupilumab	Binds the α-subunit of IL-4 receptor (inhibits signaling through IL-4 and IL-13)	• FDA-approved for EoE in adolescents (≥12 y) and adults who weight at least 40 kg • Ongoing clinical trial in children 1–11 y with EoE
Mepolizumab	Binds directly to IL-5	• No ongoing trials
Reslizumab	Binds directly to IL-5	• No ongoing trials
Benralizumab	Binds to the α-subunit of the IL-5 receptor	• Phase 3 clinical trial stopped— did not meet primary clinical outcome
Cendakimab	Inhibits binding at the IL-13 receptor	• Phase 3 clinical trial ongoing
Lirentelimab	Anti-Siglec-8 monoclonal antibody	• Phase 2/3 clinical trial completed
Tezepelumab	Anti-TSLP monoclonal antibody	• Phase 3 clinical trial ongoing
Barzolvolimab	Binds to tyrosine kinase KIT	• Phase 2 clinical trial ongoing
IRL201104	Peptide fragment of chaperonin 60.1	• Phase 2 recently completed
Etrasimod	Selective S1P receptor blocker	• Phase 2 clinical trial ongoing

Abbreviations: EoE, eosinophilic esophagitis; FDA, Food and Drug Administration; IL, interleukin; S1P, sphingosine 1-phosphate; TSLP, thymic stromal lymphopoietin.

Barzolvolimab, a monoclonal antibody that inhibits phosphorylation of the tyrosine kinase KIT, resulting in decreased mast cell degranulation and decreased mast cell numbers, is currently under investigation (ClinicalTrials.gov, Number NCT05774184). Etrasimod (APD-334), a selective sphingosine 1-phosphate (S1P) receptor blocker that partially and reversibly reduces lymphocyte levels at sites of inflammation, is also being evaluated in a phase 2 EoE clinical trial (ClinicalTrials.gov, Number NCT04682639). S1P plays a role in the regulation of endothelial barrier function and lymphocyte trafficking. S1P also plays a role in eosinophil migration through increased expression of CCR3, the primary eosinophil chemokine. A peptide fragment (IRL201104) of chaperonin 60.1, a protein derived from *Mycobacterium tuberculosis*, is also under investigation (ClinicalTrials.gov, Number NCT05084963). IRL201104 increases the production of A20, an ubiquitin that inhibits NF-kappa B, and also increases activity of regulatory T and B cells. All of these actions serve to prevent the proinflammatory immune response and provide a protective effect against allergic disease.[88]

Lastly, the JAK-STAT pathway has been identified as important to the development of fibrosis in EoE. Through STAT6 phosphorylation, production of eotaxin-3 and activation of esophageal fibroblasts is increased. Early work in fibroblast cultures suggests that blockage of this pathway through use of JAK-STAT6 inhibitors can reverse these changes and potentially modify the risk of esophageal fibrosis.[89] A case report of a 34-year old with EoE and arthritis demonstrated clinical, endoscopic, and histologic improvement after 3 months of treatment with the JAK-STAT inhibitor tofacitinib.[90]

Safety Concerns—Could You Speculate on Long-Term Use Concerns Please

Overall, biologics utilized for EoE appear to have a good safety profile. As previously discussed, in clinical trials of dupilumab for EoE, the most common adverse event was injection-site reactions, followed by nasopharyngitis, and headache.[71] Conjunctivitis, which has been associated with use of dupilumab for atopic dermatitis, was rarely seen. Safety of dupilumab has been evaluated for up to 3 years in patients with atopic dermatitis. In an open-label extension study of 347 participants treated for a total of 148 weeks, only 9.6% of participants reported a serious treatment-emergent adverse event. No significant increase in the rate of adverse events was seen with long-term use. The most common of these were nasopharyngitis, worsening atopic dermatitis, upper respiratory tract infection, conjunctivitis, oral herpes, and injection site reactions.[91] Discontinuation of biologics due to serious adverse events or hypersensitivity reactions is rare. Given the long-term safety data from the use of dupilumab for atopic dermatitis, it is reasonable to expect a similar safety profile when utilized for EoE. Other biologics such as mepolizumab, benralizumab, cendakimab, and tezepelumab all have similar short-term safety profiles as dupilumab but long-term data are lacking. One additional concern is the potential development of antidrug antibodies (ADAs) to the biologics. Development of these antibodies is associated with reduced efficacy and increased risk of adverse events. Although this has not been studied to date in EoE, a meta-analysis of biologics utilized for asthma suggested an overall ADA incidence of 2.91% and 7.61% for dupilumab.[92]

Guideline Recommendations

While multiple biologics have been or are currently under investigation in EoE, currently dupilumab is the only biologic (and medication) that is FDA approved. However, it can be challenging to determine the best point in a patient's course to initiate dupilumab. Dupilumab is expensive and may not be covered by all insurance carriers. It also requires weekly injections and many patients experience "needle phobia." As summarized in a recent review by Aceves and colleagues,[93] there are several scenarios where dupilumab should be considered as first-line or step-up therapy:

- Multiple atopic conditions (atopic dermatitis, asthma, chronic rhinosinusitis with nasal polyposis)
- Failure of other EoE therapies including PPIs and/or STSs
- More severe clinical symptoms (failure to thrive, poor growth) or frequent use of rescue therapies
- Adverse effects or inability to tolerate other therapies

SUMMARY

Medications, including PPIs, STSs, and dupilumab, are highly effective therapies for the treatment of EoE. Choice of therapy is dependent on shared decision-making, and factors such as ease of use, safety, cost, and efficacy all should be discussed with patients and/or families prior to embarking on therapy. Response to PPI is no longer required to diagnose EoE. However, given the safety profile and ease of use, PPIs are the most common medication utilized early in the disease course. For those who do not respond to PPIs, topical corticosteroids are an excellent alternative and can be effective for both short-term and long-term use. Neither class of medication is disease modifying, and both require consistent dosing to be effective. P-CABs are a novel class of medication that could serve as an alternative to PPIs in the future, although more work is needed to understand their efficacy in EoE. Biologics provide a more targeted mechanism of action with similar efficacy for dupilumab as for topical corticosteroids. While early trials of biologics were disappointing, recent investigation has seen more success including the first FDA-approved medication for EoE. Dupilumab is not likely to replace PPIs or topical corticosteroids as first-line therapy except in highly specific circumstances, such as in patients with multiple atopic conditions. Identification of novel biologic pathways and the development of small molecules may lead to a wider diversity of treatment options in the future.

CLINICS CARE POINTS

- If EoE is suspected, endoscopy should be performed prior to the initiation of any therapy, including PPIs.
- Response to PPIs is no longer a requirement to diagnose EoE. Patients that demonstrate clinical, endoscopic, and/or histologic response to PPIs are also likely to respond to topical corticosteroids or even food elimination. Initial dosing of PPIs for EoE is typically higher than what is utilized in GERD.
- PPI safety is a common concern for many patients. Overall, PPIs are safe with limited potential side effects for most patients.
- Topical corticosteroids are highly effective in the treatment of EoE. The starting dose is typically 0.5 to 1 mg twice daily of budesonide or 880 mcg twice daily of fluticasone propionate. Topical corticosteroids are not disease modifying and require long-term use to prevent recurrence of the disease.
- Dupilumab is the only FDA-approved biologic for EoE. For many patients, dupilumab is not recommended as first-line therapy, given the cost of use. However, for patients with multiple atopic diseases (asthma, atopic dermatitis, and so forth), dupilumab may be appropriate for early use to control several disorders with 1 medication.
- Shared decision-making, including a discussion of safety and efficacy, with patients and families should be utilized to determine the most effective therapy for a specific patient.

DISCLOSURES

Dr G.W. Falk: Research funding: Adare/Ellodi, Allakos, ARENA, Australia/Pfizer, Bristol-Myers Squibb, United States/Celgene, Celldex, United States, Lucid, Nexteos, Regeneron, United States/Sanofi, Shire/Takeda; consulting: Adare/Ellodi, Bristol Myers Squibb/Celgene, Nexstone, Regeneron/Sanofi, Shire/Takeda. Dr R. Pesek: Research funding: Astra Zeneca AB, Regeneron; consulting: Regeneron.

REFERENCES

1. Ngo P, Furuta GT, Antonioli DA, et al. Eosinophils in the esophagus – peptic or allergic eosinophilic esophagitis? Case series of three patients with esophageal eosinophilia. Am J Gastroenterol 2006;101:1666–70.
2. Furuta GT, Liacouras CA, Collins MH, et al. Eosinophilic esophagitis in children and adults: systematic review and consensus recommendations for diagnosis and management. Gastroenterology 2007;133:1342–63.
3. Dellon ES, Gonsalves N, Hirano I, et al. ACG clinical guideline: Evidence based approach to the diagnosis and management of esophageal eosinophilia and eosinophilic esophagitis (EoE). Am J Gastroenterol 2013;108:679–92.
4. Dellon ES, Liacouras CA, Molina-Infante J, et al. Updated international consensus diagnostic criteria for eosinophilic esophagitis: proceedings of the AGREE conference. Gastroenterology 2018;155:1022–33.
5. Molina-Infante J, Bredenoord AJ, Cheng E, et al. Proton pump inhibitor-responsive oesophageal eosinophilia: an entity challenging current diagnostic criteria for eosinophilic oesophagitis. Gut 2016;65:524–31.

6. Odiase E, Zhang X, Chang Y, et al. In esophageal squamous cells from eosinophilic esophagitis patients, Th2 cytokines increase eotaxin-3 secretion through effects on intracellular calcium and a non-gastric proton pump. Gastroenterology 2021;160:2072–88.

7. Wen T, Dellon ES, Moawad FJ, et al. Transcriptome analysis of proton pump inhibitor responsive esophageal eosinophilia reveals proton pump inhibitor reversible allergic inflammation. J Allergy Clin Immunol 2015;135:187–97.

8. van Rhijn BD, Weijenborg PW, Verheij J, et al. Proton pump inhibitors partially restore mucosal integrity in patients with proton pump inhibitor responsive esophageal eosinophilia but not eosinophilic esophagitis. Clin Gastroenterol Hepatol 2014;12:1815–23.

9. Lucendo AJ, Arias A, Molina-Infante J. Efficacy of proton pump inhibitor drugs for inducing clinical and histologic remission in patients with symptomatic esophageal eosinophilia: a systematic review and meta-analysis. Clin Gastroenterol Hepatol 2016;14:13–22.

10. Rank MA, Sharaf RN, Furuta GT, et al. Technical review on the management of eosinophilic esophagitis: a report from the AGA Institute and the Joint Task Force on Allergy-Immunology Practice Parameters. Gastroenterology 2020;158:1789–810.

11. Laserna-Mendieta EJ, Casabona S, Guagnozzi D, et al. Efficacy of proton pump inhibitor therapy for eosinophilic oesophagitis in 630 patients: results from the EoE connect registry. Aliment Pharmacol Ther 2020;52:798–807.

12. Gutierrez-Junquera C, Fernandez-Fernandez S, Dominguez-Ortega G, et al. Proton pump inhibitor therapy in pediatric eosinophilic esophagitis: predictive factors and long-term step-down efficacy. J Pediatr Gastroenterol Nutr 2023;76:191–8.

13. Alexander R, Alexander JA, Akambase J, et al. Proton pump inhibitor therapy in eosinophilic esophagitis: predictors of nonresponse. Dig Dis Sci 2021;66:3096–104.

14. Golden AH, Muftah M, Mangla S, et al. Assessment of the clinical and allergy profiles of PPI responsive and non-responsive eosinophilic esophagitis. Dis Esophagus 2023;36:1–7.

15. Molina-Infante J, Rodriguez-Sanchez J, Martinek J, et al. Long-term loss of response in proton pump inhibitor responsive esophageal eosinophilia is uncommon and influenced by CYP2C19 genotype and rhinoconjunctivitis. Am J Gastroenterol 2015;110:1567–75.

16. Gomez-Torrijos E, Garica-Rodriguez R, Castro-Jimenez A, et al. The efficacy of step down therapy in adult patients with proton pump inhibitor responsive oesophageal eosinophilia. Aliment Pharmacol Ther 2016;43:534–40.

17. Thakkar KP, Folwer M, Keene S, et al. Long-term efficacy of proton pump inhibitors as a treatment modality for eosinophilic esophagitis. Dig Liver Dis 2022;54:1179–85.

18. Gutierrez-Junquera C, Fernandez-Fernandez S, Cilleruelo ML, et al. Long-term treatment with proton pump inhibitors is effective in children with eosinophilic esophagits. J Pediatr Gastroenterol Nutr 2018;67:210–6.

19. Freedberg DE, Kim LS, Yang YX. The risks and benefits of long-term use of proton pump inhibitors: expert review and best practice advice from the American Gastroenterological Association. Gastroenterology 2017;152:706–15.

20. Vaezi MF, Yang YX, Howden CW. Complications of proton pump inhibitor therapy. Gastroenterology 2017;153:35–48.

21. Moayyedi P, Eikelboom JW, Bosch J, et al. Safety of proton pump inhibitors based on a large, multi-year, randomized trial of patients receiving rivaroxaban or aspirin. Gastroenterology 2019;157:682–91.

22. Dhar A, Haboubi HN, Attwood SE, et al. British Society of Gastroenterology (BSG) and British Society of Paediatric Gastroenterology, Hepatology and Nutrition (BSPGHAN) joint consensus guidelines on the diagnosis and management of eosinophilic oesophagitis in children and adults. Gut 2022;71:1459–87.

23. Hirano I, Chan ES, Rank MA, et al. AGA Institute and the Joint Task Force on Allergy-Immunology Practice Parameters Clinical Guidelines for the management of eosinophilic esophagitis. Gastroenterology 2020;158:1776–86.

24. Katzka DA, Kahrilas PJ. Potassium competitive acid blocker suppression of gastric acid in erosive esophagitis: Is stronger and longer better? Gastroenterology 2023;164:14–5.

25. Ishimura N, Ishihara S, Kinoshita Y. Sustained acid suppression by potassium-competitive acid blocker (P-CAB) may be an attractive treatment candidate for patients with eosinophilic esophagitis. Am J Gastroenterol 2016;111:1203–4.

26. Kuzumoto T, Tanaka F, Sawada A, et al. Vonoprazan shows efficacy similar to that of proton pump inhibitors with respect to symptomatic, endoscopic, and histological response in patients with eosinophilic esophagitis. Esophagus 2021;18:372–9.

27. Fujiwara Y, Sawada A, Ominami M, et al. Responses of proton pump inhibitors and potassium-competitive acid blockers according to outcomes of symptom, endoscopy, and histology in patients with eosinophilic esophagitis. J Clin Gastroenterol 2023, in press.

28. Faubion WA Jr, Perrault J, Burgart LJ, et al. Treatment of eosinophilic esophagitis with inhaled corticosteroids. J Pediatr Gastroenterol Nutr 1998;27:90–3.

29. Liacouras CA, Wenner WJ, Brown K, et al. Primary eosinophilic esophagitis in children: successful treatment with oral corticosteroids. J Pediatr Gastroenterol Nutr 1998;26:380–5.

30. Schaefer ET, Fitzgerald JF, Molleston JP, et al. Comparison of oral prednisone and topical fluticasone in the treatment of eosinophilic esophagitis: a randomized trial in children. Clin Gastroenterol Hepatol 2008;6:165–73.

31. Visaggi P, Barberio B, Del Corso G, et al. Comparison of drugs for active eosinophilic oesophagitis: systematic review and network meta-analysis. Gut 2023;72(11):2019–30.

32. Syverson EP, Tobin M, Patton T, et al. Variability in swallowed topical corticosteroid practice patterns for treatment of pediatric eosinophilic esophagitis. J Pediatr Gastroenterol Nutr 2023;77:256–9.

33. Joshi S, Rubenstein JH, Dellon ES, et al. Variability in practices of compounding budesonide for eosinophilic esophagitis. Am J Gastroenterol 2021;116:1336–8.

34. Ketchem CJ, Reed CC, Stefanadis Z, et al. Treatment with compounded fluticasone suspension improves the clinical, endoscopic, and histologic features of eosinophilic esophagitis. Dis Esophagus 2021;34:1–8.

35. Syverson EP, Hait E, McDonald DR, et al. Oral viscous mometasone is an effective treatment for eosinophilic esophagitis. J Allergy Clin Immunol Pract 2020;8:1107–9.

36. Nistel M, Nguyen N, Atkins D, et al. Ciclesonide impacts clinicopathological features of eosinophilic esophagitis. J Allergy Clin Immunol Pract 2021;9:4069–74.

37. van Rhijn BD, Verheij J, van den Bergh Weerman MA, et al. Histological response to fluticasone proprionate in patients with eosinophilic esophagitis is associated

with improved functional esophageal mucosal integrity. Am J Gastroenterol 2015; 110:1289–97.

38. Lucendo AJ, De Rezende L, Comas C, et al. Treatment with topical steroids downregulates IL-5, eotaxin-1/CCL11, and eotaxin-3/CCL26 gene expression in eosinophilic esophagitis. Am J Gastroenterol 2008;103:2184–93.

39. Konikoff MR, Noel RJ, Blanchard C, et al. A randomized, double-blind, placebo-controlled trial of fluticasone propionate for pediatric eosinophilic esophagitis. Gastroenterology 2006;131:1381–91.

40. Noel RJ, Putnam PE, Collins MH, et al. Clinical and immunopathologic effects of swallowed fluticasone for eosinophilic esophagitis. Clin Gastroenterol Hepatol 2004;2:568–75.

41. Blanchard C, Mingler MK, Vicario M, et al. IL-13 involvement in eosinophilic esophagitis: transcriptome analysis and reversibility with glucocorticoids. J Allergy Clin Immunol 2007;120:1292–300.

42. Aceves SS, Newbury RO, Chen D, et al. Resolution of remodeling in eosinophilic esophagitis correlates with epithelial response to topical corticosteroids. Allergy 2010;65:109–16.

43. Lucendo AJ, Arias A, De Rezende LC, et al. Subepithelial collagen deposition, profibrogenic cytokine gene expression, and changes after prolonged fluticasone propionate treatment in adult eosinophilic esophagitis: a prospective study. J Allergy Clin Immunol 2011;128:1037–46.

44. Hao LX, Lu Y, Li T, et al. A meta-analysis of efficacy of topical steroids in eosinophilic esophagitis: From the perspective of histologic, clinical, and endoscopic outcome. Gastroenterol Hepatol 2021;44:251–60.

45. Dellon ES, Woosley JT, Arrington A, et al. Efficacy of budesonide vs fluticasone for initial treatment of eosinophilic esophagitis in a randomized controlled trial. Gastroenterology 2019;157:65–73.

46. Eluri S, Selitsky SR, Perjar I, et al. Clinical and molecular factors associated with histologic response to topical steroid treatment in patients with eosinophilic esophagitis. Clin Gastroenterol Hepatol 2019;17:1081–8.

47. Wolf WA, Cotton CC, Green DJ, et al. Predictors of response to steroid therapy for eosinophilic esophagitis and treatment of steroid-refractory patients. Clin Gastroenterol Hepatol 2015;13:452–8.

48. Ketchem CJ, Ocampo AA, Xue Z, et al. Higher body mass index Is associated with decreased treatment response to topical steroids in eosinophilic esophagitis. Clin Gastroenterol Hepatol 2023;21:2252–9.

49. Dellon ES, Tsai YS, Coffey AR, et al. Pre-treatment differential correlation of gene expression and response to topical steroids in eosinophilic esophagitis. Dis Esophagus 2023;36:1–7.

50. Jensen ET, Langefeld CD, Howard TD, Dellon ES. Validation of Epigenetic Markers for the Prediction of Response to Topical Corticosteroid Treatment in Eosinophilic Esophagitis. Clin Transl Gastroenterol 2023;14(9):e00622.

51. Dellon ES, Woosley JT, Arrington A, et al. Recurrence of eosinophilic esophagitis activity after successful treatment in the observation phase of a randomized, double-blind, double-dummy trial. Clin Gastroenterol Hepatol 2020;18:1483–92.

52. Andreae DA, Hanna MG, Magid MS, et al. Swallowed fluticasone propionate is an effective long-term maintenance therapy for children with eosinophilic esophagitis. Am J Gastroenterol 2016;111:1187–97.

53. Greuter T, Safroneeva E, Bussmann C, et al. Maintenance treatment of eosinophilic esophagitis with swallowed topical steroids alters disease course over a

5-year follow-up period in adult patients. Clin Gastroenterol Hepatol 2019;17: 419–28.

54. Dellon ES, Katzka, Collins MH, et al. Safety and efficacy of budesonide oral suspension maintenance therapy in patients with eosinophilic esophagitis. Clin Gastroenterol Hepatol 2019;17:555–73.

55. Eluri S, Runge TM, Hansen J, et al. Diminishing effectiveness of long-term maintenance topical steroid therapy in PPI non-responsive eosinophilic esophagitis. Clin Transl Gastroenterol 2017;15:e97.

56. Greuter T, Godat A, Ringel A, et al. Effectiveness and safety of high vs low dose swallowed topical steroids for maintenance treatment of eosinophilic esophagitis: a multicenter observational study. Clin Gastroenterol Hepatol 2021;19:2514–23.

57. Oliva S, Volpe D, Russo G, et al. Maintenance therapy with the lowest effective dose of oral viscous budesonide in children with eosinophilic esophagitis. Clin Gastroenterol Hepatol 2022;20:2005 7.

58. Runge TM, Eluri S, Woosley JT, et al. Control of inflammation decreases the need for subsequent esophageal dilation in patients with eosinophilic esophagitis. Dis Esophagus 2017;30:1–7.

59. Kuchen T, Straumann A, Safroneeva E, et al. Swallowed topical corticosteroids reduce the risk for long-lasting bolus impactions in eosinophilic esophagitis. Allergy 2014;69:1248–54.

60. Haasnoot ML, Safi S, Bredenoord AJ. Poor Adherence to Medical and Dietary Treatments in Adult Patients With Eosinophilic Esophagitis. Am J Gastroenterol 2022;117:1412–8.

61. Hirano I, Dellon ES, Gupta SK, et al. Safety of an investigational formulation of budesonide (budesonide oral suspension) for eosinophilic oesophagitis: an integrated safety analysis of six phase 1-3 clinical trials encompassing 514 patients. Aliment Pharmacol Ther 2023;57:1117–30.

62. Philpott H, Dougherty MK, Reed CC, et al. Systematic review: adrenal insufficiency secondary to swallowed topical corticosteroids in eosinophilic oesophagitis. Aliment Pharmacol Ther 2018;47:1071–8.

63. Harel S, Hursh BE, Chan ES, et al. Adrenal suppression in children treated with oral viscous budesonide for eosinophilic esophagitis. J Pediatr Gastroenterol Nutr 2015;61:190–3.

64. Golekoh MC, Hornung LN, Mukkada VA, et al. Adrenal insufficiency after chronic swallowed glucocorticoid therapy for eosinophilic esophagitis. J Pediatr 2016; 170:240–5.

65. Bose P, Kumar S, Nebesio TD, et al. Adrenal insufficiency in children with eosinophilic esophagitis treated with topical corticosteroids. J Pediatr Gastroenterol Nutr 2020;70:324–9.

66. Lucendo AJ, Miehlke S, Schlag C, et al. Efficacy of budesonide orodispersible tablets as induction therapy for eosinophilic esophagitis in a randomized placebo-controlled trial. Gastroenterology 2019;157:74–86.

67. Straumann A, Lucendo AJ, Miehlke S, et al. Budesonide orodispersible tablets maintain remission in a randomized, placebo-controlled trial of patients with eosinophilic esophagitis. Gastroenterology 2020;159:1672–85.

68. Hirano I, Collins MH, Katzka DA, et al. Budesonide oral suspension improves outcomes in patients with eosinophilic esophagitis: results from a phase 3 trial. Clin Gastroenterol Hepatol 2022;20:525–34.

69. Hirano I, Safroneeva E, Roumet MC, et al. Randomised clinical trial: the safety and tolerability of fluticasone propionate orally disintegrating tablets versus placebo for eosinophilic oesophagitis. Alimemt Pharmacol Ther 2020;51:750–9.

70. Dellon ES, Lucendo AJ, Schlag C, et al. Fluticasone propionate orally disintegrating tablet (APT 1011) for eosinophilic esophagitis: randomized controlled trial. Clin Gastroenterol Hepatol 2022;20:2485–94.

71. Es Dellon, Rothenberg ME, Collins I, et al. Dupilumab in adults and adolescents with eosinophilic esophagitis. N Engl J Med 2022;387:2317–30.

72. Hirano I, Collins MH, Assouline-Dayan Y, et al. RCP4046, a monoclonal antibody against IL13, reduced histologic and endoscopic activity in patients with eosinophilic esophagitis. Gastroenterology 2019;156:592–603.

73. Dellon ES, Collins MH, Rothenberg ME, et al. Long-term efficacy and tolerability of RPC4046 in an open-label extension trial of patients with eosinophilic esophagitis. Clin Gastroenterol Hepatol 2021;19:473–83.

74. Stein ML, Collins MH, Villanueva JM, et al. Anti-IL-5 (mepolizumab) therapy for eosinophilic esophagitis. J Allergy Clin Immunol 2006;118:1312–9.

75. Straumann A, Conus S, Grzonka P, et al. Anti-interleukin-5 antibody treatment (mepolizumab) in active eosinophilic oesophagitis: a randomized, placebo-controlled, double-blind trial. Gut 2010;59:21–30.

76. Assa'ad AH, Gupta SK, Collins MH, et al. An antibody against IL-5 reduces numbers of esophageal eosinophils in children with eosinophilic esophagitis. Gastroenterology 2011;141:1593–604.

77. Dellon ES, Peterson KA, Mitlyng BL, et al. Mepolizumab for treatment of adolescents and adults with eosinophilic oesophagitis: a multicentre, randomised, double-blind, placebo-controlled clinical trial. Gut 2023;72(10):1828–37.

78. Spergel JM, Rothenberg ME, Collins MH, et al. Reslizumab in children and adolescents with eosinophilic esophagitis: results of a double-blind, randomized, placebo-controlled trial. J Allergy Clin Immunol 2012;129:456–63.

79. Kuang FL, De Melo MS, Makiya M, et al. Benralizuamb completely depletes gastrointestinal tissue eosinophils and improves symptoms in eosinophilic gastrointestinal disease. J Allergy Clin Immunol Pract 2022;10:1598–605.

80. Kiwamoto T, Nawasaki N, Paulson JC, et al. Siglec-8 as a drugable target to treat eosinophil and mast cell-associated conditions. Pharmacol Ther 2012;135:327–36.

81. Dellon ES, Peterson KA, Murray JA, et al. Anti-Siglec-8 antibody for eosinophilic gastritis and duodenitis. N Engl J Med 2020;383:1624–34.

82. Dellon ES, Chehade M, Genta RM, et al. Results from KRYPTOS, a phase 2/3 study of lirentelimab (AK002) in adults and adolescents with EoE. Am J Gastroenterol 2022;117:S446.

83. Dellon ES, Chehade M, Genta RM, et al. Lirentelimab (AK002) safety and efficacy in patients with higher eosinophil thresholds: supplementary analysis of phase 2/3 EoE KRYPTOS trial. Am J Gastroenterol 2022;117:S449.

84. Rizzi A, Presti EL, Chini R, et al. Emerging role of alarmins in food allergy: an update on pathophysiologica insights, potential use as disease biomarkers, and therapeutic implications. J Clin Med 2023;12:2699.

85. Kottyan LC, Davis BP, Sherill JD, et al. Genome-wide association analysis of eosinophilic esophagitis provides insight into tissue specificity of this allergic disease. Nat Genet 2014;46:895–900.

86. Collinson AM, Sokulsky LA, Sherrill JD, et al. TNF-related apoptosis-inducing ligand (TRAIL) regulates midline-1, thymic stromal lymphopoietin, inflammation, and remodeling in experimental eosinophilic esophagitis. J Allergy Clin Immunol 2015;136:971–82.

87. Corren J, Menzies-Gow A, Chupp G, et al. Efficacy of tezepelumab in severe, uncontrolled asthma: pooled analysis of the PATHWAY and NAVIGATOR clinical trials. Am J Respir Crit Care Med 2023;208:13–24.

88. Riffo-Vasquez Y, Kanabar V, Keir SD, et al. Modulation of allergic inflammation in the lung by a peptide derived from Mycobacteria tuberculosis chaperonin 60.1. Clin Exp Allergy 2020;50:508–19.

89. Cheng E, Zhang X, Wilson KS, et al. JAK-STAT6 pathway inhibitors block eotaxin-3 secretion by epithelial cells and fibroblasts from esophageal eosinophilia patients: promising agents to improve inflammation and prevent fibrosis in EoE. PLoS One 2016;11:e0157376.

90. Mendoza Alvarez LB, Liu X, Glover S. Treatment-resistant eosinophilic oesophagitis successfully managed with tofacitinib. BMJ Case Rep 2019;12:e232558.

91. Beck LA, Thaci D, Deleuran M, et al. Dupilumab provides favorable safety and sustained efficacy for up to 3 years in an open-label study of adults with moderate-to-severe atopic dermatitis. Am J Clin Dermatol 2020;21:567–77.

92. Chen ML, Nopsopon T, Akenroye A. Incidence of anti-drug antibodies to monoclonal antibodies in asthma: a systematic review and meta-analysis. J Allergy Clin Immunol Pract 2023;11:1475–84.

93. Aceves SS, Dellon ES, Greenhawt M, et al. Clinical guidance for the use of dupilumab in eosinophilic esophagitis: A yardstick. Ann Allergy Asthma Immunol 2023;130:371–8.

Health-Related Quality of Life in Patients with Eosinophilic Esophagitis

Maria L. van Klink, MD[a,b],*, Albert J. Bredenoord, MD, PhD[a,b]

KEYWORDS

- Quality of life • Health • Eosinophilic esophagitis

KEY POINTS

- Eosinophilic esophagitis (EoE) affects health-related quality of life.
- The main determinants for an impaired quality of life consist of symptom severity and biological and psychological factors.
- Treatment adherence is low in EoE, and improvement could be achieved by educating patients on expectations of symptoms, treatment, and quality of life.

INTRODUCTION

Quality of life (QOL) is a complex and multidimensional construct that can differ among individuals and groups. It refers to an individual's perception of their overall well-being and satisfaction on various domains in life. These domains include physical, psychological, social, and environmental factors.[1] Based on the definition of the World Health Organization, health is defined as a state of complete physical, mental, and social well-being and goes beyond just the absence of illness.[2] QOL is a broad concept covering a wide range of aspects in human life. As changes in health imply changes in QOL, the concept of health-related quality of life (HRQOL) was developed in the 1980s, HRQOL focuses on the effects of illness and particularly how treatment affects QOL.[3] This concept is broadly used in the medical field and has gained increased significance. Assessing HRQOL can provide valuable information about the patients' perception of their health and the impact of treatments.

HRQOL can be measured by different types of instruments: generic and disease-specific questionnaires. Generic instruments, for example, the widely used Short Form-Health Survey (SF-36),[4] aim to assess overall HRQOL across various conditions, enabling comparisons of HRQOL outcomes between different diseases, for example,

[a] Department of Gastroenterology and Hepatology, Amsterdam UMC, Boelelaan 1117, 1081 HV Amsterdam, The Netherlands; [b] Amsterdam UMC, Department of Gastroenterology and Hepatology, Amsterdam Gastroenterology Endocrinology Metabolism, De Boelelaan 1117, 1081 HV Amsterdam, The Netherlands
* Corresponding author.
E-mail address: m.vanklink@amsterdamumc.nl

Immunol Allergy Clin N Am 44 (2024) 265–280
https://doi.org/10.1016/j.iac.2023.12.011
0889-8561/24/© 2024 Elsevier Inc. All rights reserved.

in cost-effectiveness studies. However, disease-specific instruments focus on specific domains related to a particular disease, making them more sensitive to changes that are important to clinicians and patients.[5] In patients with chronic disease, HRQOL is commonly measured to get insights on how disease effects daily living.[6]

A chronic disease that has been recognized the last couple of decades is eosinophilic esophagitis (EoE), and its incidence is rapidly increasing.[7,8] EoE is an immune-mediated, inflammatory disease, characterized by histologic findings of eosinophil-predominant infiltration of the esophageal mucosa in histology.[8,9] The disease has a progressive character, and untreated it can lead to fibrostenotic changes of the esophagus.[10] Clinical symptoms in patients with EoE are a result of esophageal dysfunction, such as dysphagia and food impactions. Therapeutic strategies for EoE focus on reducing symptoms and preventing long-term complications by maintaining histologic and endoscopic remission.[11] Despite the fact that the pathogenesis of EoE is incompletely understood, there is evidence that long-term inflammation is associated with fibrostenotic changes of the esophagus, and patients with EoE are prone to relapse following initial response to therapy.[10,12,13] Current treatment options include dietary interventions, endoscopic dilation, and medical therapies, such as proton pump-inhibitors, swallowed topical corticosteroids, and dupilumab (interleukin-4/ interleukin-13 receptor inhibitor).[11,14–16]

Nowadays, the management of EoE increasingly includes improving QOL, rather than simply relieving clinical symptoms. This is reflected by endpoints used in clinical trials, where instruments to measure changes in HRQOL as outcome measure of treatment efficacy are routinely included. Inclusion of a disease-specific HRQOL instrument as an endpoint has also been recommended by experts as well as regulatory agencies.[17] The physical discomfort, as well as the social and psychological consequences of a food-related disease, can lead to an impaired QOL in patients with EoE.[18,19] This review aims to give an overview of HRQOL and its determinants in adult patients with EoE.

MEASUREMENT OF HEALTH-RELATED QUALITY OF LIFE IN EOSINOPHILIC ESOPHAGITIS

HRQOL has been explored in adult patients with EoE using generic and specific measurements (**Tables 1** and **2**). Several studies evaluated generic HRQOL using the SF-36. This validated instrument measures generic HRQOL through 36 items in 8 domains including: physical functioning, physical role limitations, bodily pain, general health perceptions, vitality, social functioning, emotional role limitations, and mental health.[4] In a study of van Rhijn and colleagues, a total of 74 patients with EoE were included and their SF-36 scores were compared with norm population scores. Physical functioning, general health perceptions, and vitality were lower among patients with EoE compared with average scores of the Dutch population.[20] Another study in patients with EoE showed impaired mental health scores assessed by the SF-36, whereas physical health scores were similar to the general population.[21] It might be expected that there are differences in HRQOL between patients with EoE with active disease and those in remission. Interestingly, this was not found in a study in 147 active and inactive patients with EoE, where the authors found no significant differences in SF-36 scores between both active and inactive cases and scores were in the range of population averages as well. Despite improvement in histologic remission, SF-36 scores did not improve over time.[22]

One could argue the utility of generic instruments to measure HRQOL, such as the SF-36, in patients with EoE, because it might be too general and therefore lacks

Table 1
Generic and disease-specific instruments to measure HRQOL in patients with EoE and the domains they cover

Generic Instruments	Domain	No. of Items	Disease-Specific Instruments[a]	Domain	No. of Items
SF-36[4]	Physical functioning, physical role limitations, bodily pain, general health perceptions, vitality, social functioning, emotional role limitations, and mental health	36	EoE-QoL-A[25]	Eating/diet impact, social impact, emotional impact, disease anxiety, and swallowing anxiety	37, 30, 24[a]
			EoE-IQ[27]	Emotional impact, social impact, productivity, and sleep-related impact	11
			NEQOL[29] [b]	Social function, emotional distress, eating impact, sleep impact, and financial burden	14

[a] Original EoE-QoL-A version consists of 37 items. A refined version consists of 30 items including 6 questions only applicable for patients on empiric elemental diet.
[b] Instrument can be used in several esophageal conditions including EoE.

Table 2
Summary of studies measuring generic and disease-specific HRQOL in adult patients with EoE

Instrument	Study Country	Study Design	Population	Current Treatment	Results
SF-36	Chang et al,[22] 2021 USA	Prospective cohort study	Patients with EoE with active disease (>15 eos/HPF): n = 91 and inactive disease <15 eos/HPF): n = 56	Active vs inactive cases: PPI: 35 (40%) vs 35 (67%) Oral viscous budesonide: 30 (34%) vs 21 (38%) Fluticasone: 5 (6%) vs 10 (18%) Targeted elimination diet: 17 (19%) vs 9 (16%) Empiric elimination diet: 20 (22%) vs 13 (23%) No treatment: 21 (23%) vs 8 (14%)	No differences in SF-36 scores: (active vs inactive cases) PCS (51.0 ± 10.1 vs 51.4 ± 9.3, $P = .80$) MCS (48.8 ± 11.5 vs 50.1 ± 9.5, $P = .49$) Lower MCS in patients treated with elimination diet vs no diet (44.9 vs 50.8; $P = .005$) Dysphagia scores negatively correlated with PCS (r = −0.33; $P<.001$) and MCS (r = −0.18; $P = .03$) No improvement in SF-36 scores over time, despite achieving histologic remission
SF-36	Gonsalves et al,[43] 2012 USA	Prospective clinical trial	Diagnosed patients with EoE (>15 eos/HPF): n = 50	Six-food elimination diet: 50 (100%)	Compared with general population, in patients with EoE slightly improved PCS but slightly decreased MCS (not significant) Increased PCS and MCS after SFED in patients with EoE Individual PCS tended to improve after SFED but individual MCS decreased

Instrument	Study	Study design	Population	Treatment	Results
SF-36	Van Rhijn et al,[20] 2014 Netherlands	Cross-sectional study	Diagnosed patients with EoE n = 74. Controls: n = 1742 (random subjects of a Dutch national reference cohort)	TCS: 13 (18%) PPI: 37 (50%) Diet: 1 (1%)	Decreased QOL in several domains of SF-36: (EcE vs control) Vitality (62.1 ± 22.3 vs 68.6 ± 19.3, $P = .0˜5$) General health (64.4 ± 24.2 vs 70.9 ± 20.6, $P = .024$) Disease duration risk factor for low MCS (OR 1.064 95% CI: 1.003–1.128, $P = .038$)
SF-36, EoE-QoL-A	De Rooij et al,[21] 2022 Netherlands	Cross-sectional study	Diagnosed patients with EoE: n = 147. Controls: n = 1742 (random subjects of a Dutch national reference cohort)	TCS: 35 (24%) PPI: 34 (23%) Combined TCS and dietary restrictions: 14 (10%) Empiric elimination diet: 36 (25%) No treatment: 28 (19%)	Lower MCS in patients with EoE vs population (47.9 ± 10.4 vs 50.1 ± 1.5; $P = .01$) No differences in PCS between patients with EoE vs population (50.5 ± 8.6 vs 51.4 ± 3.2; $P = .244$) Mean overall EoE-QoL-A score of 2.77 ± 0.81 with lower levels in women (vs men $P = .002$) Subdomains with lowest scores: disease anxiety 2.46 ± 1.03 and eating/diet impact (2.47 ± 1.12)
SF-36, EoE-QoL-A	Hewett et al,[34] 2017 United Kingdom	Prospective cross-sectional observational study	Diagnosed patients with EoE (>15 eos/HPF): n = 88. Controls: n = 44	EoE vs control: TCS: 25.7% vs 0% PPI: 20.5% vs 6.8% Antihistamine: 50% vs 2.3%	MCS lower in patients with EoE than controls (52.5, IQR 43.7–56.5 vs 57.6, IQR 52.3–58.8, $P = .002$) No significant difference in PCS between patients with EoE and controls (57.4, IQR 54–59.2 vs 56.9, IQR 54.8–58.1).

(continued on next page)

Table 2
(continued)

Instrument	Study Country	Study Design	Population	Current Treatment	Results
					Dysphagia scores negatively correlated with PCS (r = −0.38, P < .001) and MCS (r = −0.43, P = .01). EoE-QoL-A scores negatively correlated with dysphagia scores (r = −0.66, P < .001). EoE-QoL-A scores positively correlated with MCS (r = 0.59, P < .001) No significant correlation between EoE-QoL-A scores and PCS
SF-36, EORTC QLQOES 18	Larsson et al,[23] 2015 Sweden	Prospective observational study	Diagnosed patients with EoE (>15 eos/HPF): n = 47	2-mo course of mometa-one furoate applied orally as aerosol: 47 (100%)	No significant differences in SF-36 scores between baseline, 2 mo treatment and long-term follow-up Improvement in EORTC QLQOES 18 dysphagia, eating and choking scores after 2 mo of treatment (P = .01, P = .004, P = .003) and dysphagia and eating scores at long-term follow-up (P = .03, P = .005)

EoE-QoL	Lucendo et al,[18] 2018 Spain	Cross-sectional observational study	Diagnosed patients with EoE (>15 eos/HPF): n = 170 Dietary restriction: n = 102 (60%) No dietary restriction: n = 68 (40%)	Dietary restriction vs no dietary restriction: TCS: 40 (39%) vs 33 (49%) PPI: 32 (31%) vs 32 (47%) Montelukast: 4 (4%) vs 0 (0%) Empiric elimination diet: 60 (35%) vs N/A	Mean overall EoE-QoL-A score of 1.4 ± 0.8, no differences between patients on dietary or pharmacologic therapy (1.82 ± 0.8 vs 1.62 ± 0.8, $P = .132$) Emotional impact significantly worse in patients under dietary restrictions Recurrent food impaction, higher educational level, dietary interventions, symptom duration all independent determinant factors for impaired HRQOL. Female gender and empiric elimination diets negatively influenced on diet/eating impact
EoE-QoL-A	Lucendo et al,[45] 2019 Europe	Randomized double-blind placebo controlled clinical trial	Patients with EoE with clinico-histologic active disease (>20 eos/HPF): n = 88 Active treatment: 59 Placebo: 29	Randomly assigned (2:1) to orodispersible budesonide tablet 1 mg 2x/d for 6 wk or placebo	Significant changes from baseline to end of treatment in overall EoE-QoL-A and subdomain in active treatment group Significant changes from baseline to end of treatment on social impact, emotional impact, swallowing anxiety EoE-QoL-A subdomains in placebo group

(continued on next page)

Table 2
(continued)

Instrument	Study Country	Study Design	Population	Current Treatment	Results
EoE-QoL-A	Safroneeva et al,[33] 2015 Switzerland, USA	Prospective study	Patients with EoE: n = 98	EoE specific treatment in last 12 mo: 83 (85%) Hypo-allergenic diet in last 90 d: 11 (11%) TCS in last 90 d: 68 (69%) Dilation in last 12 mo: 13 (13%)	HRQOL strongly correlated with symptom severity ($r = 0.610$, $P < .001$) Symptom severity explained 38% of total variation in overall HRQOL, endoscopic findings 35% and histologic findings 22%
EoE-QoL-A	Safroneeva et al,[44] 2022 USA	Prospective observational	Diagnosed patients with EoE: n = 100 Dilated group: n = 55 (55%) Nondilated group: n = 45 (45%)	Dilated vs nondilated: No treatment: 3 (5.5%) vs 1 (2.2%) Diet: 10 (18.2%) vs 11 (24.4%) PPI: 6 (10.9%) vs 5 (11.1%) TCS: 14 (25.5%) vs 14 (31.1%) Combined therapies: 22 (40.0%) vs 14 (31.1%)	Median EoE-QoL-A score dilated vs nondilated: 26.5 (16.0–47.5) vs 27.0 (15.0–51.0) No significant association between EoE-QoL-A and biologic findings based on dilation status
EoE-QoL-A	Stern et al.[26] 2018 USA	Prospective cohort study	Diagnosed patients with EoE (>15 eos/HPF): n = 167	PPI: 34% TCS: 10% Combined PPI and TCS: 23% Diet: 24% No treatment: 10%	Mean overall EoE-QoL-A score of 2.81 ± 0.83. HRQOL correlated with dysphagia symptom severity ($r = -0.35$) and frequency ($r = -0.32$) (both $P < .001$)
EoE-QoL-A	Straumann et al,[46] 2020 Europe	Randomized, double-blind, placebo controlled clinical trial	Patients with EoE with clinico-histologic active disease (>20 eos/HPF): n = 204 Active treatment 1 mg: n = 68 Active treatment 0.5 mg: n = 68 Placebo: n = 68	Randomly assigned (2:1: to orodispersible budescnide tablet 1 mg 2x/d, 0.5 ng 2x/d or placebo for 48 wk or placebo	Overall EoE-QoL scores and subscores significantly improved from baseline to end of treatment in active treatment groups (1 mg 2x/d and 0.5 mg 2x/d) Overall EoE-QoL scores en most subscores deteriorates from baseline to end of treatment in placebo group

| EoE-IQ | Dellon et al,[27] 2021 USA, Europe Dellon et al,[28] 2022 USA, Europe Rothenberg et al,[47] 2023 USA, Europe | Randomized double-blind placebo controlled clinical trial | Diagnosed patients with EoE (>15 eos/HPF) with active symptoms Part A: n = 81 Active treatment: n = 42 Placebo: n = 39 Part B: n = 240 Active treatment weekly: n = 80 Active treatment every 2 wk: n = 81 Placebo: n = 79 Part A-C: active treatment weekly n = 77 Part B-C: n = 227 Active treatment weekly: n = 111 Active treatment every 2 wk: n = 116 | Part A: Randomly assigned (1:1) to weekly dupilumab subcutaneous injections (300 mg) or placebo for 24 wk Part B: Randomly assigned (1:1:1) to weekly dupilumab subcutaneous injections (300 mg), or every 2 wk dupilumab subcutaneous injections (300 mg) or placebo for 24 wk Part A-C: Patients who completed Part A continued in Part C, all receiving dupilumab subcutaneous injections weekly 300 mg up to 52 wk Part B-C: Patients who completed Part B continued in Part C, all receiving dupilumab subcutaneous injections weekly or every 2 wk on the same dosing regimen as in part B up to 52 wk. Patients who received placebo in part B randomly assigned (1:1) to either weekly dupilumab subcutaneous injections or every 2 wk | Part A: After 24 wk, change from baseline in EoE-IQ score favored weekly dupilumab over placebo (least-squares mean between-group difference of −0.37 points (95% CI, −0.64 to −0.10) Part B: After 24 wk, change from baseline EoE-IQ score between weekly dupilumab and placebo −0.31 points (95% CI, −0.47 to −0.15), and for dupilumab every 2 wk and placebo −0.02 points (95% CI, −0.13–0.15). Part A-C: At wk 52, EoE-IQ improved compared with part A baseline Part B-C: At wk 52, EoE-IQ improved compared with part B baseline Median absolute change from part B baseline to wk 52: • Weekly dupilumab/weekly dupilumab: −1.0 point (IQR −1.4 to −0.4) • Placebo/weekly dupilumab: −0.8 points (−1.3 to −0.4). • Every 2 wk dupilumab/ every 2 wk dupilumab: −0.6 points (IQR −1.0 to −0.4) |

(continued on next page)

Table 2
(continued)

Instrument	Study Country	Study Design	Population	Current Treatment	Results
					• Placebo/every 2 wk dupilumab: −0.8 points (−1.5 to −0.5)
PAGI-QOL	Menard-Katcher et al,[31] 2015 USA	Cross-sectional study	Patients with EoE >18 y diagnosed in childhood (>20 eos/HPF): n = 53	TCS: 3 (6%) Interleukin-5 antagonists: 3 (6%) PPI: 26 (49%) Allergy-directed diets: 40 (76%)	Mean PAGI-QOL score of 4.58/5 with significantly lower score on dietary dimension than total QoL score (P <.01)

Abbreviations: CI, confidence interval; EoE, eosinophilic esophagitis; EoE-QoL-A, adult eosinophilic esophagitis quality of life; EORTC QLQOES 18, European Organization for Research and Treatment of Cancer Quality of Life Questionnaire–Oesophageal Module 18eos/HPF eosinophils per high-power field; eos, eosinophils; HRQOL, health-related quality of life; IQR, interquartile range; MCS, mental component score; NA, not applicable; PAGI-QOL, patient assessment of upper gastrointestinal disorders–quality of life; PCS, physical component score; PPI, proton pump inhibitor; SFED, six-food elimination diet; QoL, quality of life; SF-36, short form-health survey; TCS, topical corticosteroids.

discriminatory effects.[22,23] This is supported by a study of Taft and colleagues, where patients with EoE raised several concerns regarding a generic instrument (SF-36), expressing that it did not sufficiently address their emotional and social challenges related to EoE.[24] Therefore, Taft and colleagues developed a more disease-specific instrument to measure HRQOL.[25] The development of the adult eosinophilic esophagitis quality of life (EoE-QoL-A) questionnaire consisted of a qualitative and quantitative phase. In the qualitative phase, items for the questionnaire were generated through patient interviews, providing valuable information on specific areas of impact experienced by patients with EoE. The original validated questionnaire consisted of 37 items, categorized into 5 subscales: eating/diet impact, social impact, emotional impact, disease anxiety, and swallowing anxiety. Shorter versions of the EoE-QoL-A are used as well.[26]

There are other disease-specific instruments that have been developed to assess HRQOL in EoE as well. For example, the Eosinophilic Esophagitis Impact Questionnaire (EoE-IQ), measuring emotional, social, productivity, and sleep-related impacts of EoE in 11 items.[27,28] Another instrument is the Northwestern Esophageal Quality of Life Scale, developed for use across several esophageal conditions, such as gastroesophageal reflux disease (GERD), achalasia, Barrett esophagus, and EoE.[29] However, the use of these instruments in clinical trials in EoE has been limited so far.

Besides the instruments that were specially developed to assess HRQOL in patients with EoE, several existing instruments that were developed for other upper gastrointestinal conditions have been used in patients with EoE. This applies for the Patient Assessment of Upper Gastrointestinal Disorders–Quality of Life (PAGI-QOL)[30,31] developed for use in patients with GERD, dyspepsia, and gastroparesis and the European Organization for Research and Treatment of Cancer Quality of Life Questionnaire–Oesophageal Module 18 (EORTC QLQ-OES 18)[23,32] developed for use in patients with esophageal cancer.

DETERMINANTS OF QUALITY OF LIFE IN ADULT PATIENTS WITH EOSINOPHILIC ESOPHAGITIS

Various determinants influence patients' perceptions of their well-being. A major determinant is symptom severity. In a prospective trial assessing the impact of symptoms, endoscopic and histologic findings on HRQOL, symptom severity strongly correlated to HRQOL.[33] Symptom severity alone explained 38% of the total variation in overall HRQOL scores, where endoscopic findings explained 35% and histologic findings 22% of total variation. The findings in this study suggest that QOL is determined not only by symptom severity but also by biological disease activity. Another study showed similar results regarding symptom severity correlating to HRQOL, for example, patients who experienced a recent food impaction significantly reported lower QOL.[26] However, in this study, the investigators did not find a correlation between biological disease activity and HRQOL. The influence of symptom severity on HRQOL is further supported by other studies where higher dysphagia scores were negatively correlated to physical and in particular mental components of the SF-36.[22,34] Dysphagia and recurrent food impactions also seem to have a strong influence on the perception of HRQOL.[18,21] In addition, disease duration is another determinant of QOL. One study identified disease duration as a risk factor for lower scores on the mental components of the SF-36 assessment.[20] In another study, patients with long-standing symptoms significantly had worse EoE-QoL-A scores.[18] Moreover, a higher educational level was found to be a determinant of impaired QOL. The effect of gender on QOL shows conflicting results. Some studies show no differences between patients gender[35] ; other studies show that female gender[18,21] can negatively influence QOL. Younger age and in particular young adult patients with EoE experience impaired QOL.[20,21] Other determinants of HRQOL relate to cognitive-affective processes and coping strategies of individual patients. Hypervigilance and symptom-specific anxiety can negatively influence HRQOL and might be more accurate predictive markers of QOL in patients with EoE than histologic and endoscopic disease activity markers.[36] Further, less-effective coping styles (ie, passive/palliative reaction on Utrecht Coping List) are associated with impaired HRQOL.[21]

IMPACT OF TREATMENT ON QUALITY OF LIFE

Dietary interventions have proven to be effective treatments for remission induction of EoE but can impose a substantial psychosocial and financial burden on patients that can subsequently result in an impaired QOL.[37,38] The most effective dietary intervention is the elemental diet, where patients are exclusively fed with amino acid-based formula. In clinical practice, this is not feasible for most patients due to the restrictiveness, poor tolerability, high costs in case of no reimbursement, psychosocial impact, and impaired QOL.[37–39] Other dietary interventions that are often used in clinical practice are the empiric elimination diets. Despite the effectiveness of these diets, adherence is low because of the intensive trajectories, complexity, and numerous restrictions that patients experience.[39–42] Studies have shown that patients following a 6-food elimination diet experience difficulties with avoiding certain food groups, reading food labels, spending time on planning meals and dealing with social situations.[41] Elimination diets can impact mental well-being, with higher diet-related anxiety,[41] and lower mental component scores on generic HRQOL instruments reported in some studies.[22,43] The effect of elimination diets on disease-specific HRQOL can be seen in different domains. In one study, patients on dietary therapy reported worse QOL related to the diet and eating domain measured by the EoE-QoL-A.[26] Another study found that patients with EoE under dietary restriction experienced worse HRQOL in the emotional domain emotional impact on disease-specific QOL as compared with patients with EoE treated with pharmacotherapies but interestingly this did not affect overall EoE-QoL-A scores.[18]

The effect of esophageal dilation on HRQOL has not been evaluated in patients with EoE. There is one study that evaluated the relationship between QOL and histologic and endoscopic findings based on esophageal dilation status, where no significant association was found.[44]

Swallowed topical corticosteroids are effective pharmacologic treatments to induce and maintain remission in adult patients with EoE.[11,14] The effect of swallowed topical corticosteroids on HRQOL has been evaluated in several studies. A 2-month course of swallowed topical corticosteroids (mometasone furoate applied orally as aerosol) improved clinical symptoms of dysphagia and choking but did not show changes in SF-36 scores.[23] The effect of budesonide on HRQOL has also been examined. Lucendo and colleagues investigated the efficacy and safety of an orodispersible budesonide tablet versus placebo in a randomized clinical trial in active patients with EoE.[45] The authors observed that 6 weeks of treatment with 1 mg of budesonide administered twice daily significantly improved HRQOL assessed by EoE-QoL-A in all domains but in the placebo group, HRQOL also improved to a lesser extent on several domains: social impact, emotional impact, and swallowing anxiety. A follow-up of that trial investigated the efficacy of maintenance treatment with the orodispersible budesonide tablet in different dosages (2× per day 1 mg or 0.5 mg) compared with placebo.[46] After 48 weeks of treatment, HRQOL measured with EoE-QoL-A improved significantly in the active treatment groups, in contrast to a decline in the placebo group.

In a 3-part, phase-3 trial, the efficacy and safety of 300 mg dupilumab administered subcutaneously weekly or every 2 weeks compared with placebo was investigated. HRQOL was assessed using the EoE-IQ score. Patients who received weekly dupilumab injections improved more in EoE-IQ scores than the patients who received injections every 2 weeks or placebo.[27,28,47]

The therapeutic objectives of patients with EoE seem to diverge from those of physicians.[48] According to patients, the most crucial therapeutic goals for short-term and long-term treatments are improvement of symptoms and QOL. Patients attribute greater significance to long-term outcomes compared with short-term outcomes. Improvement in biological disease activity is deemed less significant than the relief of symptoms and enhancement of QOL. This is important when physicians prescribe therapies and try to let patients adhere to those therapies. Considering poor adherence rates in patients with EoE to both medical and dietary therapies as found in previous research, there is a strong need to actively promote and educate patients regarding the importance of short-term and long-term treatments.[49]

SUMMARY

In EoE, measurement of HRQOL has gained prominence in both trials and clinical care and can be assessed through various instruments. Current literature shows that EoE has a significant impact on HRQOL. Various factors determine HRQOL in patients with EoE, such as symptom severity and disease duration but also biological factors including endoscopic and histologic activity and psychological factors such as coping mechanisms, hypervigilance and anxiety. Different available treatments can improve symptoms and HRQOL, which are prioritized by patients as most important treatment goals. However, adherence to treatment is suboptimal in patients with EoE. Thus, there is a need to guide and educate patients more and measuring HRQOL can play a crucial role by giving health-care providers a more comprehensive evaluation of patients' health and the specific challenges they face due to EoE. This can lead to an improvement in understanding patients' experiences and facilitating more tailored approaches in health-care management.

CLINICS CARE POINTS

- EoE affects HRQOL.
- Symptom severity and biological and psychological factors are determinants of an impaired quality of life.
- Treatment adherence is low in EoE, and improvement could be achieved by educating patients on expectations of symptoms, treatment, and quality of life.

DISCLOSURE

No sources of funding were used to conduct this study or to prepare this article. M.L. van Klink has no conflicts of interest that are directly relevant to the content of this article, A.J. Bredenoord has received research funding from Nutricia, United States, Norgine, Netherlands, Thelial, Sanofi, United States/Regeneron, SST, and Dr Falk Pharma and received speaker and/or consulting fees from Laborie, Medtronic, Dr Falk Pharma, Calypso Biotech, Eupraxia, Aqilion, Alimentiv, Sanofi/Regeneron,

Reckitt and AstraZeneca. A.J. Bredenoord is supported by Vidi grant 91718300 from the Netherlands Organisation for Scientific Research NWO.

REFERENCES

1. Kuyken W.G., The World Health Organization Quality of Life assessment (WHO-QOL): position paper from the World Health Organization, Soc Sci Med, 41 (10), 1995, 1403–1409.
2. World Health Organization, he first ten years of the World Health, In: Organization, 1958, World Health Organization; Geneva.
3. Lin X-J, Lin IM, Fan S-Y. Methodological issues in measuring health-related quality of life. Tzu Chi Med J 2013/03/01/2013;25(1):8–12.
4. Ware JE Jr, Gandek B. Overview of the SF-36 health survey and the international quality of life assessment (IQOLA) Project. J Clin Epidemiol 1998;51(11):903–12.
5. Patrick DL, Deyo RA. Generic and disease-specific measures in assessing health status and quality of life. Med Care 1989;27(3 Suppl):S217–32.
6. Guyatt GH, Feeny DH, Patrick DL. Measuring health-related quality of life. Ann Intern Med 1993;118(8):622–9.
7. Attwood SE. Overview of eosinophilic oesophagitis. Br J Hosp Med 2019;80(3): 132–8.
8. Muir A, Falk GW. Eosinophilic esophagitis: a review. JAMA 2021;326(13):1310–8.
9. Dellon ES, Hirano I. Epidemiology and natural history of eosinophilic esophagitis. Gastroenterology 2018;154(2):319–32.e3.
10. Warners MJ, Oude Nijhuis RAB, de Wijkerslooth LRH, et al. The natural course of eosinophilic esophagitis and long-term consequences of undiagnosed disease in a large cohort. Am J Gastroenterol 2018;113(6):836–44.
11. Lucendo AJ, Molina-Infante J, Arias Á, et al. Guidelines on eosinophilic esophagitis: evidence-based statements and recommendations for diagnosis and management in children and adults. United European Gastroenterol J 2017;5(3): 335–58.
12. Schoepfer AM, Safroneeva E, Bussmann C, et al. Delay in diagnosis of eosinophilic esophagitis increases risk for stricture formation in a time-dependent manner. Gastroenterology 2013;145(6):1230–6, e1-2.
13. Straumann A, Bussmann C, Zuber M, et al. Eosinophilic esophagitis: analysis of food impaction and perforation in 251 adolescent and adult patients. Clin Gastroenterol Hepatol 2008;6(5):598–600.
14. de Rooij WE, Dellon ES, Parker CE, et al. Pharmacotherapies for the treatment of eosinophilic esophagitis: state of the art review. Drugs 2019;79(13):1419–34.
15. Lucendo AJ. Drug treatment strategies for eosinophilic esophagitis in adults. Expet Opin Pharmacother 2022;23(7):827–40.
16. FDA approves first treatment for eosinophilic esophagitis, a chronic immune disorder. News release. U.S. Food and Drug Administration. 2022. Available at: https://www.fda.gov/news-events/press-announcements/fda-approves-first-treatment-eosinophilic-esophagitis-chronic-immune-disorder. Accessed June 25, 2022.
17. Ma C, Schoepfer AM, Dellon ES, et al. Development of a core outcome set for therapeutic studies in eosinophilic esophagitis (COREOS). J Allergy Clin Immunol 2022;149(2):659–70.
18. Lucendo AJ, Arias-González L, Molina-Infante J, et al. Determinant factors of quality of life in adult patients with eosinophilic esophagitis. United European Gastroenterol J 2018;6(1):38–45.

19. Visaggi P, Savarino E, Sciume G, et al. Eosinophilic esophagitis: clinical, endo-scopic, histologic and therapeutic differences and similarities between children and adults. Therap Adv Gastroenterol 2021;14. https://doi.org/10.1177/17562848209808860. 17562848209808860.

20. van Rhijn BD, Smout AJ, Bredenoord AJ. Disease duration determines health-related quality of life in adult eosinophilic esophagitis patients. Neuro Gastroen-terol Motil 2014;26(6):772–8.

21. de Rooij WE, Evertsz FB, Lei A, et al. General well-being and coping strategies in adult eosinophilic esophagitis patients. J Neurogastroenterol Motil 2022;28(3): 390–400.

22. Chang N, Raja S, Betancourt R, et al. Generic measures of quality of life are not correlated with disease activity in eosinophilic esophagitis. Dig Dis Sci 2021; 66(10):3312–21.

23. Larsson H, Bergman K, Finizia C, et al. Dysphagia and health-related quality of life in patients with eosinophilic esophagitis: a long-term follow-up. Eur Arch Oto-Rhino-Laryngol 2015;272(12):3833–9.

24. Taft TH, Kern E, Keefer L, et al. Qualitative assessment of patient-reported out-comes in adults with eosinophilic esophagitis. J Clin Gastroenterol 2011;45(9): 769–74.

25. Taft TH, Kern E, Kwiatek MA, et al. The adult eosinophilic oesophagitis quality of life questionnaire: a new measure of health-related quality of life. Aliment Pharma-col Ther 2011;34(7):790–8.

26. Stern E, Taft T, Zalewski A, et al. Prospective assessment of disease-specific quality of life in adults with eosinophilic esophagitis. Dis Esophagus 2018; 31(4). https://doi.org/10.1093/dote/dox128.

27. Dellon E, Rothenberg M, Hirano I, et al. Dupilumab improves health-related qual-ity of life (HRQoL) and reduces symptom burden in patients with eosinophilic esophagitis (EoE): results from part a of a randomized, placebo-controlled three-part phase 3 study. J Allergy Clin Immunol 2021;147(2 Supplement):AB91.

28. Dellon ES, Rothenberg ME, Collins MH, et al. Dupilumab in adults and adoles-cents with eosinophilic esophagitis. N Engl J Med 2022;387(25):2317–30.

29. Bedell A, Taft TH, Keefer L, et al. Development of the northwestern esophageal quality of life scale: a hybrid measure for use across esophageal conditions. Am J Gastroenterol 2016;111(4):493–9.

30. De La Loge C, Trudeau E, Marquis P, et al. Responsiveness and interpretation of a quality of life questionnaire specific to upper gastrointestinal disorders. Clin Gastroenterol Hepatol 2004;2(9):778–86.

31. Menard-Katcher P, Marks KL, Liacouras CA, et al. The natural history of eosino-philic oesophagitis in the transition from childhood to adulthood. Aliment Pharma-col Ther 2013;37(1):114–21.

32. Blazeby JM, Conroy T, Hammerlid E, et al. Clinical and psychometric validation of an EORTC questionnaire module, the EORTC QLQ-OES18, to assess quality of life in patients with oesophageal cancer. Eur J Cancer 2003/07/01/2003;39(10): 1384–94. https://doi.org/10.1016/S0959-8049(03)00270-3.

33. Safroneeva E, Coslovsky M, Kuehni CE, et al. Eosinophilic oesophagitis: relation-ship of quality of life with clinical, endoscopic and histological activity. Aliment Pharmacol Ther 2015;42(8):1000–10.

34. Hewett R, Alexakis C, Farmer AD, et al. Effects of eosinophilic oesophagitis on quality of life in an adult UK population: a case control study. Dis Esophagus 2017;30(1):1–7.

35. Schreiner P, Safroneeva E, Rossel JB, et al. Sex impacts disease activity but not symptoms or quality of life in adults with eosinophilic esophagitis. Clin Gastroenterol Hepatol 2022;20(8):1729–38.e1.

36. Taft TH, Carlson DA, Simons M, et al. Esophageal hypervigilance and symptom-specific anxiety in patients with eosinophilic esophagitis. Gastroenterology 2021; 161(4):1133–44.

37. Arias Á, González-Cervera J, Tenias JM, et al. Efficacy of dietary interventions for inducing histologic remission in patients with eosinophilic esophagitis: a systematic review and meta-analysis. Gastroenterology 2014;146(7):1639–48.

38. Kliewer KL, Cassin AM, Venter C. Dietary Therapy for Eosinophilic Esophagitis: Elimination and Reintroduction. Clin Rev Allergy Immunol 2018;55(1):70–87.

39. Molina-Infante J. Nutritional and psychological considerations for dietary therapy in eosinophilic esophagitis. Nutrients 2022;14(8). https://doi.org/10.3390/nu14001588.

40. Votto M, De Filippo M, Lenti MV, et al. Diet therapy in eosinophilic esophagitis. focus on a personalized approach. Front Pediatr 2021;9:820192.

41. Wang R, Hirano I, Doerfler B, et al. Assessing adherence and barriers to long-term elimination diet therapy in adults with eosinophilic esophagitis. Dig Dis Sci 2018;63(7):1756–62.

42. Kliewer KL, Gonsalves N, Dellon ES, et al. One-food versus six-food elimination diet therapy for the treatment of eosinophilic oesophagitis: a multicentre, randomised, open-label trial. Lancet Gastroenterol Hepatol 2023;8(5):408–21.

43. Gonsalves N, Yang GY, Doerfler B, et al. Elimination diet effectively treats eosinophilic esophagitis in adults; food reintroduction identifies causative factors. Gastroenterology 2012;142(7):1451–9.e1.

44. Safroneeva E, Pan Z, King E, et al. Long-lasting dissociation of esophageal eosinophilia and symptoms after dilation in adults with eosinophilic esophagitis. Clin Gastroenterol Hepatol 2022;20(4):766–75.e4.

45. Lucendo AJ, Miehlke S, Schlag C, et al. Efficacy of budesonide orodispersible tablets as induction therapy for eosinophilic esophagitis in a randomized placebo-controlled trial. Gastroenterology 2019;157(1):74–86.e15.

46. Straumann A, Lucendo AJ, Miehlke S, et al. Budesonide orodispersible tablets maintain remission in a randomized, placebo-controlled trial of patients with eosinophilic esophagitis. Gastroenterology 2020;159(5):1672–85.e5.

47. Rothenberg ME, Dellon ES, Collins MH, et al. Efficacy and safety of dupilumab up to 52 weeks in adults and adolescents with eosinophilic oesophagitis (LIBERTY EoE TREET study): a multicentre, double-blind, randomised, placebo-controlled, phase 3 trial. Lancet Gastroenterol Hepatol 2023. https://doi.org/10.1016/S2468-1253(23)00204-2.

48. Safroneeva E, Balsiger L, Hafner D, et al. Adults with eosinophilic oesophagitis identify symptoms and quality of life as the most important outcomes. Aliment Pharmacol Ther 2018;48(10):1082–90.

49. Haasnoot ML, Safi S, Bredenoord AJ. Poor adherence to medical and dietary treatments in adult patients with eosinophilic esophagitis. Am J Gastroenterol 2022;117(9):1412–8.

The Relationship Between Eosinophilic Esophagitis and Immunotherapy

Bridget E. Wilson, MD[a,b,]*, Maria A. Sacta, MD, PhD[c],
Benjamin L. Wright, MD[a,b], Jonathan Spergel, MD, PhD[c],
Nicole Wolfset, MD[c]

KEYWORDS

- Eosinophilic gastrointestinal disease • Adverse effects • Oral immunotherapy
- Allergy shots • Eosinophil

KEY POINTS

- Oral immunotherapy (OIT) for food allergy and sublingual immunotherapy (SLIT) for aeroallergen sensitivity may induce eosinophilic esophagitis (EoE).
- Most patients experience disease remission upon discontinuation of OIT or SLIT.
- Aeroallergens may also trigger EoE.
- Subcutaneous immunotherapy (SCIT) and epicutaneous immunotherapy (EPIT) require further study as potential treatments for EoE.

INTRODUCTION

Eosinophilic esophagitis (EoE) is a chronic disease associated with type 2 inflammation. EoE usually requires long-term surveillance with esophagogastroduodenoscopy (EGD) and treatment with medications or elimination diets. In severe or untreated cases, fibrostenosis and esophageal stricture can occur.[1] The causes of EoE are

Declaration of funding: B.L. Wright receives support from the NIH/NIAID (K23AI158813). J. Spergel receives support from the NIH/NIAID and the Consortium of Eosinophilic Gastrointestinal Disease Researchers (U54 AI117804). N. Wolfset receives support from an NIH T32 training grant (T32GM008562). M.A. Sacta receives support from the Gail B. Slap Department of Pediatrics Fellowship Award.
[a] Division of Allergy, Asthma and Clinical Immunology, Department of Medicine, Mayo Clinic Arizona, 13400 E. Shea Boulevard Scottsdale, AZ 85259, USA; [b] Division of Allergy/Immunology, Phoenix Children's, 1919 E. Thomas Road, Phoenix, AZ 85054, USA; [c] Division of Allergy and Immunology, Children's Hospital of Philadelphia, 3401 Civic Center Boulevard, Philadelphia, PA 19104, USA
* Corresponding author. Division of Allergy, Asthma, and Clinical Immunology, Department of Medicine, Mayo Clinic Arizona, 13400 East Shea Boulevard, Scottsdale, AZ 85259.
E-mail address: wilson.bridget@mayo.edu

Immunol Allergy Clin N Am 44 (2024) 281–291
https://doi.org/10.1016/j.iac.2024.01.001
0889-8561/24/© 2024 Elsevier Inc. All rights reserved.

immunology.theclinics.com

unknown; however, recent studies suggest it may occur in patients receiving treatment with immunotherapy.[2–5]

Immunotherapy has been used for more than a century as a treatment of allergies.[6,7] Although the antigen, route, timing, and mode of delivery may differ, immunotherapy is based on the principle that gradual, incremental allergen exposure induces desensitization. Some forms of immunotherapy are being used as a treatment of EoE,[3,8–11] whereas others may cause or exacerbate it.[2–5] Oral immunotherapy (OIT) specifically induces esophageal eosinophilia, which may be transient or persistent. Once symptoms of esophageal dysfunction occur in association with esophageal eosinophilia, the disease may be reversible with OIT discontinuation or become permanent. The development of esophageal eosinophilia and EoE in the setting of controlled exposure to a trigger antigen may provide unique insights into EoE pathogenesis, as esophageal eosinophilia or reversible disease may be precursors to the chronic disease state. This review examines the relationship between EoE and immunotherapy. We primarily focus on EoE and OIT, because this association is most prevalent in the literature, but we also briefly discuss other forms of immunotherapy.

DEFINITIONS OF IMMUNOTHERAPY

There are multiple forms of immunotherapy, including OIT, subcutaneous (SCIT), sublingual (SLIT), and epicutaneous (EPIT) immunotherapy. OIT is an elective treatment taken daily to reduce the risk of anaphylaxis in IgE-mediated food allergy. SCIT is indicated for patients with allergic rhinoconjunctivitis and/or allergic asthma and is administered monthly after a maintenance dose is reached, requiring 3 to 5 years of injections to maintain aeroallergen desensitization. SLIT is another method for aeroallergen desensitization that is administered as a tablet or liquid extract. SLIT, administered as sublingual drops, and EPIT, applied as a patch, are being studied for food allergen desensitization.

BACKGROUND
Epidemiology of Oral Immunotherapy–Induced Eosinophilic Esophagitis

The estimated incidence and prevalence of EoE during OIT range from 1% to 3.2% and 2.7% to 6.9%, respectively (**Table 1**).[2,12–14] Lucendo and colleagues[2] initially summarized development of EoE in a systematic review reporting a 2.7% incidence among those receiving milk, peanut, and egg OIT over a 9-year period. Twenty patients had EoE confirmed by esophageal biopsy (milk OIT = 10, peanut OIT = 7, egg OIT = 2), whereas one patient developed EoE with multiple allergen OIT.[2] Morales-Cabeza and colleagues[12] analyzed data over a 15-year period in a pediatric Spanish cohort receiving milk, egg, or peanut OIT and reported a prevalence of 2.8%. Of these, 10 and 6 patients were receiving milk and egg OIT, respectively, whereas one patient received milk and egg OIT.[12] Petroni and Spergel[13] assessed symptoms reported during OIT and found that the incidence of biopsy-confirmed EoE was 5.3%. Of these, 4.2% of cases were induced by egg, 5.4% by milk, and 5.2% by peanut OIT. Longitudinal studies focusing on peanut[14] and milk OIT[15] reported an overall incidence of 1% in a cohort of 1217 participants and 6.9% in a cohort of 1545 pooled participants.[14] EoE typically developed in children younger than 18,[2,12–14] with one reported case in a 33-year-old woman; however, there are limited studies of OIT in adults.[14]

The most common symptoms reported included abdominal pain and vomiting,[2,12–14] prompting endoscopy and diagnosis of EoE. The median time to symptom development was 25 months after the up-dosing/build-up phase, with EoE histologically

Table 1
Incidence and prevalence of EoE for patients receiving OIT

Author	Incidence (%)	Prevalence (%)	Total Number of Patients Reported to Have EoE
Lucendo et al,[2] 2014	2.72	2.7	20 out of 711
Morales-Cabeza et al,[12] 2023	—	2.8	17 out of 607
Petroni and Spergel,[13] 2018	—	5.6	35 out of 663, biopsy confirmed
Nilsson et al,[14] 2021	1	—	12 out of 1217
Bognanni et al,[15] 2022	—	6.9	Number of patients with EoE unknown, total patients 1545
Dunlop et al,[17] 2018	3.2	—	6 out of 187

confirmed by 36 months. Although esophageal biopsies were not reported across studies, eosinophilic abscesses, basal cell hyperplasia, and lamina propria fibrosis were noted.[12]

The natural progression of EoE in patients receiving OIT is unclear. Studies are limited by lack of esophageal biopsies before OIT or before symptom manifestation.[2,12–14] As a result, discerning whether eosinophilia existed before OIT initiation or whether OIT exacerbates EoE is challenging. This is due to lack of recognition by patients and symptom screening by providers, along with use of proton pump inhibitors (PPIs) for abdominal discomfort masking symptoms in earlier studies.[2,13] Additionally, whether esophageal barrier dysfunction is present or develops in patients on OIT is unknown. Studies on serial EGDs of patients receiving peanut OIT revealed esophageal barrier dysfunction and eosinophilia. Despite this, not all patients developed EoE and eosinophilia resolved in some.[14] Thus, major questions remain regarding the contribution of OIT toward the development of EoE.

Multiple other factors are associated with EoE development in this subset of patients. Allergic predisposition (eg, asthma, allergic rhinitis, or other food allergies), family history of EoE, and male gender were prevalent in these patients.[2,12–14,16] Importantly, because the disease did not always improve with removal of the allergen from the diet,[12,14,16] intrinsic cellular or genetic factors may also contribute.

Lastly, milk, egg, and peanut OIT are more likely to precipitate the development of EoE, with milk being the most common food trigger. In a study of children receiving milk OIT, 6.9% of patients developed EoE.[15] Likewise, the introduction of baked milk after food challenge in patients with IgE-mediated milk allergy led to the development of EoE in 3.2% of patients.[17] Whether this reflects a greater proportion of patients on milk OIT, compared with other allergen OIT, versus an inherent ability of milk allergens to skew the esophageal inflammatory response toward EoE is unknown. Single-cell studies of T-cell receptor diversity show clonal expansion of pathogenic effector Th2 cells in the esophagus of patients with EoE. A subset of these pathogenic effector T cells in the peripheral blood were reactive to milk antigen, suggesting that the immunogenicity of milk allergens may predispose to EoE.[18] More studies that examine the molecular basis of allergen sensitization in EoE are needed.

DISCUSSION
Potential Explanations for Eosinophilic Esophagitis During Oral Immunotherapy

Preexisting disease
There are several possible explanations for the occurrence of EoE during OIT. First, a patient may have undiagnosed, preexisting EoE at OIT initiation. Inadequate screening

for gastrointestinal symptoms before starting OIT may allow EoE to go undetected.[19] Indeed, baseline gastrointestinal symptoms are common among atopic individuals, and previously undiagnosed EoE has been diagnosed in these patients. Among 100 adults with atopic disease but without known EoE, 44% reported solid food dysphagia greater than or equal to one time per week and/or food impaction for greater than or equal to 30 minutes in the preceding year.[19] Additionally, within the preceding week, participants frequently reported other gastrointestinal symptoms (abdominal pain, 42%; nausea/vomiting, 19%; reflux, 43%). Cytosponge was performed in 5 of 44 patients with dysphagia, and EoE was detected in one. One patient with negative Cytosponge findings was later diagnosed with EoE on EGD. Two participants with other gastrointestinal symptoms were diagnosed with EoE by EGD. In another study of 89 children and adults with history of cow's milk–related anaphylaxis, 37 (42%) reported gastrointestinal symptoms, and 34 (38.2%) had more than 15 eosinophils/high-power field (eos/hpf).[20] Patients with significant esophageal eosinophilia were treated with a PPI for 8 weeks, then underwent a second EGD. After the 8-week PPI trial, 10 still had more than 15 eos/hpf, with 9 of 10 reporting gastrointestinal symptoms.

Some patients may have eosinophilic inflammation in the absence of symptoms of esophageal dysfunction. Asymptomatic esophageal eosinophilia can be an incidental finding when EGD biopsies are performed for another indication. Baseline esophageal eosinophilia (>15 eos/hpf) was noted in 14% (3/21) of adult subjects with IgE-mediated peanut allergy, before peanut OIT initiation in a small, prospective, longitudinal cohort.[21] None reported dysphagia, and some reported mild gastrointestinal symptoms (abdominal pain in 24%, mild reflux not associated with food in 5%), but none of those with symptoms had esophageal eosinophilia. It is possible that patients with asymptomatic esophageal eosinophilia are at higher risk for EoE development during OIT; however, this has not yet been established.

Eosinophilic esophagitis develops independent of oral immunotherapy

Some patients may develop EoE regardless of immunotherapy. EoE prevalence is higher in patients with food allergy, and underlying atopic conditions increase the risk of developing EoE.[22,23] Having greater than or equal to one underlying atopic condition is associated with EoE diagnosis.[23] The prevalence of EoE in children with IgE-mediated food allergy is 4.7%,[22] and estimates of OIT-induced EoE are similar (5.3%).[13] Although these prevalence rates are similar, the temporal relationship between OIT initiation and EoE onset should be considered. Of note, EoE prevalence may be higher in patients receiving OIT due to detection bias, because OIT typically requires clinic visits every 2 weeks and providers maintain a high index of suspicion because of the known association between EoE and OIT.

Oral immunotherapy induces eosinophilic esophagitis development

The final and most probable explanation is that OIT can induce EoE. Specific symptom and laboratory criteria have been proposed to monitor gastrointestinal manifestations during OIT in the absence of biopsies. Goldberg and colleagues[24,25] described a clinical entity, oral immunotherapy-induced gastrointestinal symptoms and eosinophilic responses (OITIGER), defined as abdominal pain or vomiting greater than or equal to 3 days/month, not related to OIT dose timing, with absolute eosinophil count (AEC) greater than or equal to 900 eosinophils/μL.[24,25] In their initial study, more than 8% of OIT patients met symptom criteria for OITIGER.[24] A higher maximum AEC was associated with an increased likelihood of gastrointestinal symptoms. When compared with asymptomatic subjects, those with OITIGER had a higher baseline AEC. All three patients who underwent EGD met histologic EoE criteria.

In a subsequent study, all patients with OITIGER had symptomatic resolution and decreased AEC after cessation or reduction of OIT dosing.[25] Seventeen of 65 patients with OITIGER permanently discontinued OIT. When compared with asymptomatic patients, the OITIGER group were less likely to reach full food allergen desensitization, although more than 70% achieved doses allowing partial desensitization. After restarting OIT, more than 18% had return of OITIGER. OITIGER was more common in patients undergoing milk versus peanut OIT. In milk OIT patients, OITIGER was more likely with a higher initiation dose (>120 mg), increased dose escalation (>4-fold increase higher than the starting dose), and AEC greater than 600 eosinophils/μL. It is important to note that in both studies by Goldberg and colleagues,[24,25] most patients with OITIGER did not undergo EGD, likely underestimating EoE incidence.

Wright and colleagues[26] reported a randomized, double-blind, placebo-controlled study demonstrating a likely causal relationship between EoE and OIT. EGD was performed in subjects receiving peanut OIT versus placebo at baseline, 52 weeks, and 104 weeks. After 52 weeks, esophageal eosinophilia ($\geq$15 eos/hpf) was induced or increased in 57% (4/7) of OIT patients. One subject was formally diagnosed with EoE and withdrew after developing a food impaction. Interestingly, esophageal eosinophilia was usually transient and was dissociated from clinical symptoms. None of the patients treated with placebo met histologic criteria for EoE. In the same cohort, dilated intercellular spaces were noted in all patients at baseline, suggesting patients with IgE-mediated peanut allergy may have esophageal barrier impairment before initiation of OIT.

OUTCOMES AFTER DISCONTINUATION OF ORAL IMMUNOTHERAPY

Response to discontinuation of OIT after the development of EoE is variable. For a subset of patients, removal of the inciting food allergen was sufficient to resolve EoE.[2] In other patients, stopping OIT alone did not lead to remission, and patients required PPIs and/or oral steroids to achieve remission.[12,14,16] For patients choosing to continue OIT, incorporation of PPIs and oral steroids led to remission of disease, which continued through median follow-up at 50 months.[12] In fact, among 17 patients who developed EoE while on milk and egg OIT, 4 patients discontinued OIT without clinical response and required a PPI, whereas 11 patients continued OIT with a PPI. Only one patient required oral steroids before remission.[12] In a separate cohort of patients on peanut OIT, discontinuation of peanut was only implemented for 1 of 12 patients with 10 eventually requiring PPIs and/or oral steroids.[14] In this study, five patients achieved remission, whereas two continued to have active EoE on repeat EGD.[14] Predictors of persistent OIT-induced EoE have not been identified.

AEROALLERGENS AND EOSINOPHILIC ESOPHAGITIS

Animal models first suggested a potential link between aeroallergens and EoE in 2001, when significant esophageal eosinophilia was observed following intranasal exposure of *Aspergillus fumigatus* in mice, resembling the histologic pattern of EoE.[5,27–29] Subsequently, case reports demonstrated a seasonal correlation with EoE symptom exacerbation. One described a 21-year-old woman with asthma and allergic rhinoconjunctivitis, who developed worsening EoE symptoms and esophageal symptoms that correlated temporally with pollen exposure.[28] Additionally, Onbasi and colleagues[30] demonstrated esophageal eosinophilic infiltration in 26% of grass pollen–sensitized patients with allergic rhinitis during the pollen season.

Further substantiating this relationship, a cohort study of 127 adults diagnosed with EoE between January 2006 and November 2008 unveiled a distinct seasonal pattern for newly diagnosed disease. The highest incidence of EoE diagnoses was recorded during the spring (April–June), accounting for 33% of cases (binomial $P = .023$), whereas winter months (January–March) exhibited a marked reduction at 16% (binomial $P = .01$). Diagnoses made during the summer (July–September) and fall (October–December) demonstrated no significant differences, comprising 26% and 24% of cases, respectively.

Ram and colleagues[31] also identified a seasonal trend in EoE exacerbations. In a retrospective review of 1180 pediatric patients with EoE, 160 (14%) exhibited an exacerbation of symptoms triggered by aeroallergens with histologic confirmation of esophageal eosinophilia during pollen seasons in 32 of these patients (20%). Moreover, a positive correlation was identified between the peak grass pollen count and EoE cases during the spring ($r_s = 1.0$; $P < .01$). The precise nature of aeroallergen involvement in EoE pathogenesis is uncertain. It is unclear whether individuals with preexisting EoE experience worsened symptoms during periods of elevated outdoor pollen concentrations or if these instances represent entirely new EoE diagnoses.[27]

Aeroallergen Subcutaneous Immunotherapy and Eosinophilic Esophagitis

Published case reports have advocated for the consideration of SCIT as a potential therapy for a specific subset of patients with EoE and allergic rhinoconjunctivitis or oral allergy syndrome.[10,32] In some of these cases, SCIT initially exacerbated symptoms and eosinophilic inflammation; however, continuation led to gradual symptomatic improvement and possible disease remission over time.[32] Ramirez and Jacobs[10] also described a 4-year-old boy with refractory EoE and allergic rhinoconjunctivitis who underwent dust mite SCIT followed by resolution of persistent emesis over the ensuing 2 years. EoE remission was confirmed by biopsy.[10] In adults, Perez and Guarderas[9] described a 65-year-old man with EoE and seasonal allergies who demonstrated resolution of EoE symptoms after 5 years of SCIT intended for uncontrolled environmental allergies.[8,31,32]

Robey and colleagues[11] examined the use of SCIT in the setting of EoE in a retrospective cohort study. Ten adult patients with EoE who underwent SCIT (EoE + SCIT) were compared with 667 patients with EoE who did not undergo SCIT (EoE − SCIT). Both groups had similar baseline characteristics and endoscopic features, but the EoE + SCIT group exhibited longer duration of symptoms before EoE diagnosis (13.8 vs 7.3 years; $P = 0.046$) and had more atopic disease.[11] Initial EoE treatment with swallowed steroids in the EoE + SCIT group resulted in a symptomatic response in 60% and histologic response in 30% of the patients. After the introduction of SCIT, of the five patients who had follow-up data and were concurrently treated with SCIT, 40% had symptomatic response and 40% had histologic response. There were no adverse events reported in the EoE + SCIT cohort. This study suggests that SCIT in patients with EoE is safe and may be worth considering in some patients.[11] Together, this literature suggests a link between aeroallergens and EoE, with the potential consideration for SCIT as an avenue for select patients; however, controlled studies are needed to validate these findings.

Aeroallergen Sublingual Immunotherapy–Induced Eosinophilic Esophagitis

Significant advancements have been achieved in the development of therapeutic strategies for atopic conditions, notably SLIT. However, advancements are occasionally accompanied with unanticipated outcomes, and a recognized link between EoE and aeroallergen SLIT has raised clinical concerns. As a result, EoE is a contraindication to the administration of SLIT therapy.[4,29]

The first report of eosinophilic gastrointestinal disease (EGID) following SLIT was in 2013, involving a 44-year-old woman with new-onset dysphagia 4 weeks after starting SLIT for hazelnut, birch, and alder. EoE was confirmed on biopsy. She experienced resolution of symptoms and esophageal eosinophilia within 4 weeks of SLIT discontinuation with sustained symptom resolution by 12 weeks. This case stands as a significant milestone in highlighting the potential interplay between SLIT and the development of EoE.[3,4]

Since then, additional reports have emerged detailing a similar connection. Cafone and colleagues[4] and Votto and colleagues[3] summarized case reports of SLIT and EoE development. These reports included patients ages 9 to 53 years and observed that the onset of EoE occurred during the up-dosing and maintenance phases of SLIT. After histologic confirmation of EoE, subsequent remission occurred 1 to 16 months following discontinuation of SLIT. These reports emphasize the clinical relevance of EoE and SLIT, underscoring the importance of individualized consideration before treatment with SLIT. In cases where gastrointestinal symptoms manifest during SLIT treatment, timely assessment is imperative to ensure prompt diagnosis, appropriate treatment, and discontinuation of potentially problematic therapy.[3]

PROPOSED OPTIONS FOR MANAGEMENT
General Considerations

The generally accepted clinical practice is to discontinue OIT or SLIT in patients newly diagnosed with EoE. However, recent publications report simultaneous OIT continuation with EoE treatment.[33–35] In a pediatric OIT cohort, 13 of 1994 (0.7%) patients developed EoE.[34] Of these, 12 (92%) continued OIT. One discontinued OIT because of OIT-associated anaphylaxis and had spontaneous EoE resolution. Another did not receive EoE treatment, continued OIT, and had symptomatic and histologic EoE resolution on follow-up EGD. Eleven patients were treated with high-dose PPI monotherapy, and five achieved EoE remission. Of the remaining six patients, two received swallowed topical corticosteroids, two continued low-dose PPI, and two discontinued OIT. One patient receiving swallowed topical corticosteroids had complete symptomatic and histologic remission. The other patients had clinical resolution and only partial histologic resolution.

Because gastrointestinal symptoms during OIT are common and may or may not indicate underlying EoE/EGID, Chua and colleagues[35] developed an algorithm to manage and risk-stratify these patients. If symptoms are moderate/severe or if EGD is readily available, and the caregiver is in agreement, OIT dosing should be paused until gastroenterology evaluation. If this is not the case, a PPI trial may be initiated and OIT dosing may be paused versus continued at the same or reduced dose. If effective, PPIs can be discontinued, and OIT dosing is increased more gradually. Pending further research evaluating long-term outcomes of OIT continuation after EoE diagnosis, the decision to deviate from current standards of care should be carefully considered after shared decision-making between the patient/caregiver and provider.[36]

Milk Epicutaneous Immunotherapy for Milk-Induced Eosinophilic Esophagitis

EPIT has been used to treat IgE-mediated food allergy through delivery of antigen through a transdermal patch. Cutaneous reactions are the most common side effect, and EPIT-induced EoE has not been reported. In fact, milk EPIT has been proposed for management of milk-induced EoE. Following evidence of successful reduction of EGID with EPIT in mice and pig models, Spergel and colleagues[37] performed a randomized placebo-controlled trial to study the efficacy of Viaskin milk-EPIT (500 mg of milk protein) in 20 children with milk-induced EoE. Subjects were randomized in a 3:1 ratio (Viaskin milk to placebo) and were on a milk-free diet for 9 months, followed by a milk-containing diet for 2 months. Histologic end points demonstrated no significant difference in mean eos/hpf in the Viaskin milk group (50.1 ± 43.97) compared with placebo (48.20 ± 56.98) in the intent-to-treat population (Viaskin milk n = 15, placebo n = 5). The failed response in the intent-to-treat population may have been confounded by protocol violations in both arms regarding diet and PPI use. In the per protocol analysis (Viaskin milk n = 7, placebo n = 2), subjects in the Viaskin milk group demonstrated significantly lower mean eos/hpf (25.57 ± 31.19) compared with placebo (95.00 ± 63.64) (P = .038). After continuation with open label Viaskin milk for 11 months in 19 patients, six had less than 6 eos/hpf (32%) and three had 7 to 14 eos/hpf (16%), for a total response rate of 47%.[37]

Follow-up from this pilot study suggests that the treatment effect of EPIT on EoE can persist for 2 years after stopping therapy. Six of seven patients in the complete responder (<6 eos/hpf) and partial responder (6–14 eos/hpf) groups successfully continued with two servings of milk per day without exacerbation of symptoms. Of these patients, one complete responder had zero eosinophils and one partial responder had 6 to 14 eos/hpf on follow-up esophageal biopsies.[38] Further investigations on efficacy and long-term data are needed to enhance the understanding of the potential role of EPIT in the treatment of EoE.

SUMMARY

Immunotherapy may have mixed effects on EoE development and disease depending on the route, dose, nature of the antigens, and status of the epithelium. Data are uncertain regarding improvement in EoE disease activity with aeroallergen SCIT, and SLIT may induce EoE. OIT for IgE-mediated food allergy may unmask and/or induce EoE; whereas, EPIT for non-IgE-mediated, milk-induced EoE has been investigated as a therapeutic. Different EoE outcomes are likely related to mode of administration and immune mechanism. For example, in OIT, a potentially compromised esophageal epithelial barrier is directly exposed to allergens known to cause IgE-mediated effects; whereas in EPIT for EoE, a presumably intact skin barrier is exposed to an EoE food trigger. The presentation of EoE during immunotherapy presents several ethical dilemmas; therefore, the risks and benefits of continuing immunotherapy must be weighed for each patient. Additional studies are needed to identify the cellular and molecular mechanisms underlying the relationship between EoE and immunotherapy to identify those patients who are at risk for this complication.

CLINICS CARE POINTS

- OIT induces esophageal eosinophilia, which may be transient and asymptomatic.
- OIT and SLIT may induce EoE.
- Most patients experience disease remission upon discontinuation of OIT or SLIT.
- Aeroallergens may trigger EoE.
- Additional studies are needed to determine whether SCIT decreases EoE disease activity in patients with aeroallergen sensitivity.
- EPIT is being investigated as a treatment of EoE.

DISCLOSURE

B.L. Wright has received in-kind support from Regeneron in the form of study drug for an ongoing clinical trial investigating the role of dupilumab as an adjunct to milk oral immunotherapy. J. Spergel has consulting agreements with Regeneron, Sanofi, Novartis, and Alladapt, and he has royalties with UpToDate. J. Spergel and N. Wolfset have received in-kind support from Regeneron, United States in the form of study drug for an ongoing clinical trial investigating the role of dupilumab in eosinophilic esophagitis. All other authors report no conflicts of interest.

REFERENCES

1. Philpott H, Dellon ES. The role of maintenance therapy in eosinophilic esophagitis: who, why, and how? J Gastroenterol 2018;53(2):165–71.
2. Lucendo AJ, Arias A, Tenias JM. Relation between eosinophilic esophagitis and oral immunotherapy for food allergy: a systematic review with meta-analysis. Ann Allergy Asthma Immunol 2014;113(6):624–9.
3. Votto M, De Filippo M, Caminiti L, et al. Eosinophilic gastrointestinal disorders and allergen immunotherapy: lights and shadows. Pediatr Allergy Immunol 2021;32(5):814–23.
4. Cafone J, Capucilli P, Hill DA, et al. Eosinophilic esophagitis during sublingual and oral allergen immunotherapy. Curr Opin Allergy Clin Immunol 2019;19(4):350–7.
5. Wells R, Fox AT, Furman M. Recurrence of eosinophilic oesophagitis with subcutaneous grass pollen immunotherapy. BMJ Case Rep 2018;15:2018.
6. Fitzhugh DJ, Lockey RF. History of immunotherapy: the first 100 years. Immunol Allergy Clin North Am 2011;31(2):149–57.
7. Lanser BJ, Wright BL, Orgel KA, et al. Current options for the treatment of food allergy. Pediatr Clin North Am 2015;62(6):1531–49.
8. Iglesia EGA, Commins SP, Dellon ES. Complete remission of eosinophilic esophagitis with multi-aeroallergen subcutaneous immunotherapy: a case report. J Allergy Clin Immunol Pract 2021;9(6):2517–9.e2.
9. Perez JEPT, Guarderas J. Allergen specific immunotherapy as a treatment for eosinophilic esophagitis. World Allergy Organ J 2012;5(Suppl 2):S146.
10. Ramirez RM, Jacobs RL. Eosinophilic esophagitis treated with immunotherapy to dust mites. J Allergy Clin Immunol 2013;132(2):503–4.
11. Robey BS, Eluri S, Reed CC, et al. Subcutaneous immunotherapy in patients with eosinophilic esophagitis. Ann Allergy Asthma Immunol 2019;122(5):532–3.e3.
12. Morales-Cabeza C, Infante S, Cabrera-Freitag P, et al. Oral immunotherapy and risk of eosinophilic esophagitis in children: 15 years' experience. J Pediatr Gastroenterol Nutr 2023;76(1):53–8.
13. Petroni D, Spergel JM. Eosinophilic esophagitis and symptoms possibly related to eosinophilic esophagitis in oral immunotherapy. Ann Allergy Asthma Immunol 2018;120(3):237–40.e4.
14. Nilsson C, Scurlock AM, Dellon ES, et al. Onset of eosinophilic esophagitis during a clinical trial program of oral immunotherapy for peanut allergy. J Allergy Clin Immunol Pract 2021;9(12):4496–501.
15. Bognanni A, Chu DK, Firmino RT, et al. World allergy organization (WAO) diagnosis and rationale for action against cow's milk allergy (DRACMA) guideline update - XIII - oral immunotherapy for CMA: systematic review. World Allergy Organ J 2022;15(9):100682.

16. Hamant L, Freeman C, Garg S, et al. Eosinophilic esophagitis may persist after discontinuation of oral immunotherapy. Ann Allergy Asthma Immunol 2021; 126(3):299–302.

17. Dunlop JH, Keet CA, Mudd K, et al. Long-term follow-up after baked milk introduction. J Allergy Clin Immunol Pract 2018;6(5):1699–704.

18. Morgan DM, Ruiter B, Smith NP, et al. Clonally expanded, GPR15-expressing pathogenic effector T(H)2 cells are associated with eosinophilic esophagitis. Sci Immunol 2021;6(62). https://doi.org/10.1126/sciimmunol.abi5586.

19. Eid R, Noonan E, Borish L, et al. High prevalence of gastrointestinal symptoms and undiagnosed eosinophilic esophagitis among allergic adults. J Allergy Clin Immunol Pract 2022;10(12):3325–7.e1.

20. Barbosa AC, Castro FM, Meireles PR, et al. Eosinophilic esophagitis: latent disease in patients with anaphylactic reaction to cow's milk. J Allergy Clin Immunol Pract 2018;6(2):451–6.e1.

21. Wright BL, Fernandez-Becker NQ, Kambham N, et al. Baseline gastrointestinal eosinophilia is common in oral immunotherapy subjects with IgE-mediated peanut allergy. Front Immunol 2018;9:2624.

22. Hill DA, Dudley JW, Spergel JM. The prevalence of eosinophilic esophagitis in pediatric patients with IgE-mediated food allergy. J Allergy Clin Immunol Pract 2017; 5(2):369–75.

23. Hill DA, Grundmeier RW, Ramos M, et al. Eosinophilic esophagitis is a late manifestation of the allergic march. J Allergy Clin Immunol Pract 2018;6(5):1528–33.

24. Goldberg MR, Elizur A, Nachshon L, et al. Oral immunotherapy-induced gastrointestinal symptoms and peripheral blood eosinophil responses. J Allergy Clin Immunol 2017;139(4):1388–90.e4.

25. Goldberg MR, Nachshon L, Levy MB, et al. Risk factors and treatment outcomes for oral immunotherapy-induced gastrointestinal symptoms and eosinophilic responses (OITIGER). J Allergy Clin Immunol Pract 2020;8(1):125–31.

26. Wright BL, Fernandez-Becker NQ, Kambham N, et al. Gastrointestinal eosinophil responses in a longitudinal, randomized trial of peanut oral immunotherapy. Clin Gastroenterol Hepatol 2021;19(6):1151–9.e14.

27. Moawad FJ, Veerappan GR, Lake JM, et al. Correlation between eosinophilic oesophagitis and aeroallergens. Aliment Pharmacol Ther 2010;31(4):509–15.

28. Fogg MI, Ruchelli E, Spergel JM. Pollen and eosinophilic esophagitis. J Allergy Clin Immunol 2003;112(4):796–7.

29. Egan M, Atkins D. What is the relationship between eosinophilic esophagitis (EoE) and aeroallergens? Implications for allergen immunotherapy. Curr Allergy Asthma Rep 2018;18(8):43.

30. Onbasi K, Sin AZ, Doganavsargil B, et al. Eosinophil infiltration of the oesophageal mucosa in patients with pollen allergy during the season. Clin Exp Allergy 2005;35(11):1423–31.

31. Ram G, Lee J, Ott M, et al. Seasonal exacerbation of esophageal eosinophilia in children with eosinophilic esophagitis and allergic rhinitis. Ann Allergy Asthma Immunol 2015;115(3):224–8.e1.

32. De Swert L, Veereman G, Bublin M, et al. Eosinophilic gastrointestinal disease suggestive of pathogenesis-related class 10 (PR-10) protein allergy resolved after immunotherapy. J Allergy Clin Immunol 2013;131(2):600–2, e1-3.

33. Chu DK, Spergel JM, Vickery BP. Management of eosinophilic esophagitis during oral immunotherapy. J Allergy Clin Immunol Pract 2021;9(9):3282–7.

34. Epstein-Rigbi N, Elizur A, Levy MB, et al. Treatment of oral immunotherapy-associated eosinophilic esophagitis. J Allergy Clin Immunol Pract 2022. https://doi.org/10.1016/j.jaip.2022.11.010.

35. Chua GT, Chan ES, Invik R, et al. How we manage gastrointestinal symptoms during oral immunotherapy through a shared decision-making process-a practical guide for the community practitioner. J Allergy Clin Immunol Pract 2023;11(4): 1049–55.

36. Wilson BE, Meltzer EC, Wright BL. Ethical implications of continuing oral immunotherapy after the development of eosinophilic esophagitis. J Allergy Clin Immunol Pract 2023. https://doi.org/10.1016/j.jaip.2023.08.012.

37. Spergel JM, Elci OU, Muir AB, et al. Efficacy of epicutaneous immunotherapy in children with milk-induced eosinophilic esophagitis. Clin Gastroenterol Hepatol 2020;18(2):328–36.e7.

38. Spergel JM, Muir AB, Liacouras CA, et al. Sustained milk consumption after 2 years post-milk epicutaneous immunotherapy for eosinophilic esophagitis. Allergy 2021;76(5):1573–6.

Embracing Diversity, Equity, Inclusion, and Accessibility in Eosinophilic Gastrointestinal Diseases

Amanda B. Muir, MD, MSTR[a], Dominique D. Bailey, MD[b], Pooja Mehta, MD, MSCS[c],*

KEYWORDS

- Eosinophilic esophagitis • Eosinophilic gastroenteritis • Disparities • Inequities
- Diversity

KEY POINTS

- Eosinophilic gastrointestinal disorders are growing in incidence and prevalence and are currently thought to predominantly affect people who are White and from more affluent backgrounds.
- Studies on the impact of racism and social determinants of health on patients with eosinophilic gastrointestinal diseases are limited.
- Current research suggests that there may be disparities in care between rural and urban settings and that race and socioeconomic status affect eosinophilic esophagitis diagnosis and management.

INTRODUCTION

Pervasive racial and ethnic inequities in health care have been widely documented, impacting diagnosis, treatment, and patient outcomes across all disciplines. The recent Black Lives Matter movement further highlighted the far-reaching consequences of structural racism and its role in impeding health equity. A comprehensive understanding of these disparities is required to better inform future research in eosinophilic gastrointestinal disorders (EGIDs) and improve inequities that exist in diagnosis and treatment.

Financial support: None.

[a] Division of Gastroenterology, Hepatology, and Nutrition, Department of Pediatrics, Children's Hospital of Philadelphia, 2057 Lombard Street, Philadelphia, PA 19146, USA; [b] Division of Pediatric Gastroenterology, Hepatology, and Nutrition, Department of Pediatrics, Columbia University Vagelos College of Physicians and Surgeons/New York-Presbyterian Morgan Stanley Children's Hospital, 3959 Broadway, New York, NY 10032, USA; [c] Section of Gastroenterology, Hepatology, and Nutrition, Department of Pediatrics, Children's Hospital Colorado, University of Colorado School of Medicine, 13123 East 16th Avenue, B290, Aurora, CO 80045, USA
* Corresponding author.
E-mail address: Pooja.Mehta@childrenscolorado.org

Immunol Allergy Clin N Am 44 (2024) 293–298
https://doi.org/10.1016/j.iac.2024.01.002
0889-8561/24/© 2024 Elsevier Inc. All rights reserved.

immunology.theclinics.com

EGID is an all-encompassing term used to describe disorders of abnormal eosinophilic infiltration of the gastrointestinal tract after all other potential etiologies have been excluded. Eosinophilic esophagitis (EoE), first described in the early 1990s, is the most common EGID.[1,2] EoE is a chronic inflammatory disorder in which eosinophils as well as other inflammatory cells invade the esophageal mucosa, causing tissue damage. This leads to symptoms of vomiting, poor feeding, abdominal pain, and dysphagia. Eosinophilic inflammation in other parts of the GI tract is referred to based on the location of the inflammation and includes eosinophilic gastritis, enteritis, and colitis (EoG, EoN and EoC, respectively). These entities, although less common,[3] may be increasing in incidence. Depending on the affected organ, symptomatology of EGIDs may vary but include vomiting, abdominal pain, or diarrhea. For all EGIDs, diagnosis requires clinical symptoms as well as a histologic diagnosis, requiring endoscopy with biopsy. Because diagnosis requires a visit to a subspecialist, as well as an endoscopy requiring anesthesia, access to care may play a role in our current understanding of EGID demographics.[4,5]

In this review, we will discuss pre-eminent issues related to diversity, equity, inclusion, and accessibility in EGIDs. The authors evaluate the deficiencies in the literature and where future research should focus.

IMPACT OF RACE, ETHNICITY, AND SOCIOECONOMIC FACTORS ON EOSINOPHILIC GASTROINTESTINAL DISEASES

While the incidence and prevalence of EGIDS has increased rapidly over the course of the past 25 years, most population-based epidemiologic studies have been conducted in North America and Europe.[6-16] Based on these epidemiologic studies, EGIDS are thought to affect predominantly White males.[17] Despite this reported prevalence, a growing recognition that race and ethnicity may impact EGID diagnosis and management is emerging in the EGID literature. In fact, a recent multi-state consortium study of nearly 220,000 children found that approximately 40% of children with EoE were of non-White race.[18] Several studies have also cited differences in symptoms and endoscopic features based on race[19-23]; however, most of these studies have had a relatively small sample size and did not account for other socioeconomic variables that can influence the relationship between race, ethnicity, and disease history. Two studies showed that Black children with EoE undergo endoscopy for disease surveillance less frequently than White children with EoE and raise concern for both the impact of historical racism as well as implicit bias.[4,20] Notably, in studies that have included more diverse populations, the prevalence of EGIDS is higher in Black patients than previously reported.[20,24] Although our understanding of how race and ethnicity impact EGIDS is incomplete, there is increasing awareness of the importance of these important factors in patient care and outcomes.[25]

Though race, ethnicity, and socioeconomic status are often interconnected due to structural inequities and historical factors,[26] several studies have exposed socioeconomic status as an independent risk factor for disparate outcomes in allergic diseases. Lower socioeconomic status is associated with persistent asthma, higher allergic risk, and greater severity of atopic dermatitis.[27,28] Among EGIDS, children from lower socioeconomic status have greater EoE disease severity, less radiographic evaluation of their disease, and are seen less frequently in multidisciplinary clinics.[29] Moreover, not only is the economic burden of EGIDS high, but also economic uncertainty is associated with worse quality of life.[30-33] This may be especially pronounced in patients with lower incomes given high out-of-pocket costs associated with EGIDS including the prohibitive costs associated with both pharmacologic and dietary elimination therapies.[34-39]

DISPARITIES IN RURAL COMMUNITIES

Population-based studies reported that population density and diagnosis of EoE were inversely related. Specifically, utilizing a pathology database of close to 300,000 unique subjects, the odds of having EoE was significantly increased in the lowest quintile population density (OR 1.27, 95% confidence interval (CI): 1.18, 1.36). However, this study included less than 3% pediatric patients.[40] ICD9 coding from the 2012 Medicaid database demonstrated in pediatrics the odds of being diagnosed with EoE in a rural location was lower (OR 0.68, 95% CI0.59–0.78).[41] The opposing results in pediatric and adult population studies may signify lack of access to pediatric subspecialty care in rural areas. Utilizing geographic information from the pediatric gastroenterologist society (n = 1496) as well as 18,452,886 children enrolled in Medicaid, the distance between subjects and providers demonstrated that the protective effect of rural environment was explained by distance to provider.[36] This study highlights the disparity in care for pediatric subspecialists and highlights that lack of access to care may be influencing our understanding of EoE demographics.

FUTURE DIRECTIONS: WHERE DO WE GO FROM HERE?

Dismantling structural racism and achieving both economic equality and equal access to care is the most important step promoting equity in health care.[42] While much progress still needs to be made in this arena, there are several concrete steps that EGID researchers and health care providers can take to start to meet this goal. First, medical education can include specific education on combating the systemic racism and bias that are pervasive inio medicine. Dedicated diversity, equity, and inclusion-related trainings has become increasingly part of medical education including not only knowledge-based seminars and courses but also more tangible and specific actions like how to reduce microaggressions and decrease stigmatizing language in the medical record.[43–46] Furthermore, promoting equity in both health care and research should be included in routine day-to-day practice regardless of years since completing training. For example, the NIH-funded Consortium of Eosinophilic Gastrointestinal Disease Researchers recently published a manuscript describing their diversity committee.[25] This committee was established to examine systemic racism and implicit bias in the care and research of EGIDS and can serve as a model for future work in this arena.[25] Finally, combatting disparities must include diversifying representation among EGID clinicians, researchers, and hospital administration/leadership. Fostering an inclusive and diverse workforce not only increases participation in research but also improves access to care and health care quality among marginalized communities.[47,48]

SUMMARY

Social and racial inequities permeate medicine. As clinicians and researchers studying these rare diseases, it is imperative to strive for diversity in research, work to ensure care for all patients with suspected EGIDs, and enable access to therapy and medical foods.

CLINICS CARE POINTS

- Previous studies evaluating race and ethnicity in EGIDs are limited by their lack of evaluation of socioeconomic factors.
- There may exist disparities in care between rural and urban settings, especially for pediatric EGID patients.

- Future work should include dedicated DEIA training and improved representation across EGID clinicians and researchers.

DISCLOSURES

A.B. Muir serves on medical advisory board for Nexstone immunology, Bristol Meyers Squibb, Regeneron/Sanofi; Receives research support from Allakos and Morphic.

REFERENCES

1. Kelly KJ, Lazenby AJ, Rowe PC, et al. Eosinophilic esophagitis attributed to gastroesophageal reflux: Improvement with an amino acid-based formula. Gastroenterology 1995;109:1503–12.
2. Muir A, Falk GW. Eosinophilic Esophagitis: A Review. JAMA 2021;326:1310–8.
3. Jensen ET, Martin CF, Kappelman MD, et al. Prevalence of Eosinophilic Gastritis, Gastroenteritis, and Colitis: Estimates From a National Administrative Database. J Pediatr Gastroenterol Nutr 2016;62:36–42.
4. Sabet C, Klion AD, Bailey D, et al. Do rural health disparities affect prevalence data in pediatric eosinophilic esophagitis? J Allergy Clin Immunol Pract 2021;9: 2549–51.
5. McGowan EC, Keller JP, Muir AB, et al. Distance to pediatric gastroenterology providers is associated with decreased diagnosis of eosinophilic esophagitis in rural populations. J Allergy Clin Immunol Pract 2021;9:4489–92.e2.
6. Dellon ES, Erichsen R, Baron JA, et al. The increasing incidence and prevalence of eosinophilic oesophagitis outpaces changes in endoscopic and biopsy practice: National population-based estimates from Denmark. Aliment Pharmacol Ther 2015;41:662–70.
7. Giriens B, Yan P, Safroneeva E, et al. Escalating incidence of eosinophilic esophagitis in Canton of Vaud, Switzerland, 1993-2013: A population-based study. Allergy: European Journal of Allergy and Clinical Immunology 2015;70(12):1633–9.
8. Hruz P, Straumann A, Bussmann C, et al. Escalating incidence of eosinophilic esophagitis: a 20-year prospective, population-based study in Olten County, Switzerland. J Allergy Clin Immunol 2011;128:1349–50.e5.
9. Prasad GA, Alexander JA, Schleck CD, et al. Epidemiology of eosinophilic esophagitis over three decades in Olmsted County, Minnesota. Clin Gastroenterol Hepatol 2009;7:1055–61.
10. Dalby K, Nielsen RG, Kruse-Andersen S, et al. Eosinophilic oesophagitis in infants and children in the region of southern Denmark: a prospective study of prevalence and clinical presentation. J Pediatr Gastroenterol Nutr 2010;51:280–2.
11. van Rhijn BD, Verheij J, Smout AJPM, et al. Rapidly increasing incidence of eosinophilic esophagitis in a large cohort. Neuro Gastroenterol Motil 2013;25: 47–52.e5.
12. Arias Á, Lucendo AJ. Prevalence of eosinophilic oesophagitis in adult patients in a central region of Spain. Eur J Gastroenterol Hepatol 2013;25:208–12.
13. Warners MJ, de Rooij W, van Rhijn BD, et al. Incidence of eosinophilic esophagitis in the Netherlands continues to rise: 20-year results from a nationwide pathology database. Neuro Gastroenterol Motil 2018;30. https://doi.org/10.1111/nmo.13165.

14. Arias A, Pérez-Martínez I, Tenías JM, et al. Systematic review with meta-analysis: The incidence and prevalence of eosinophilic oesophagitis in children and adults in population-based studies. Aliment Pharmacol Ther 2016;43(1):3–15.
15. Pesek RD, Reed CC, Muir AB, et al. Increasing Rates of Diagnosis, Substantial Co-Occurrence, and Variable Treatment Patterns of Eosinophilic Gastritis, Gastroenteritis, and Colitis Based on 10-Year Data Across a Multicenter Consortium. Am J Gastroenterol 2019;114:984–94.
16. Licari A, Votto M, Scudeller L, et al. Epidemiology of Nonesophageal Eosinophilic Gastrointestinal Diseases in Symptomatic Patients: A Systematic Review and Meta-Analysis. J Allergy Clin Immunol Pract 2020;8:1994–2003.e2.
17. Dellon ES, Hirano I. Epidemiology and Natural History of Eosinophilic Esophagitis. Gastroenterology 2018;154(1):319–32.e3.
18. Gabryszewski SJ, Dudley J, Shu D, et al. Patterns in the Development of Pediatric Allergy. Pediatrics 2023;152. https://doi.org/10.1542/peds.2022-060531.
19. Sperry SL, Woosley JT, Shaheen NJ, et al. Influence of race and gender on the presentation of eosinophilic esophagitis. Am J Gastroenterol 2012;107:215–21.
20. Weiler T, Mikhail I, Singal A, et al. Racial differences in the clinical presentation of pediatric eosinophilic esophagitis. J Allergy Clin Immunol Pract 2014;2:320–5.
21. Gill RK, Al-Subu A, Elitsur Y, et al. Prevalence and characteristics of eosinophilic esophagitis in 2 ethnically distinct pediatric populations. J Allergy Clin Immunol 2014;133:576–7.
22. Chehade M, Jones SM, Pesek RD, et al. Phenotypic Characterization of Eosinophilic Esophagitis in a Large Multicenter Patient Population from the Consortium for Food Allergy Research. J Allergy Clin Immunol Pract 2018;6:1534–44.e5.
23. Hiremath G, Yazdian A, Onuh I, et al. Race and Gender Influences the Presentation of Eosinophilic Esophagitis. Dysphagia 2023. https://doi.org/10.1007/s00455-023-10577-y.
24. Chatham D, Cavender CP, Lieberman JA. Racial disparity in eosinophilic esophagitis from a single, defined population. Ann Allergy Asthma Immunol 2014;113:489–91.
25. Chehade M, Furuta G, Klion A, et al. Enhancing diversity, equity, inclusion, and accessibility in eosinophilic gastrointestinal disease research: the consortium for eosinophilic gastrointestinal disease researchers' journey. Ther Adv Rare Dis 2023;4. 26330040231180896.
26. Bailey ZD, Krieger N, Agénor M, et al. Structural racism and health inequities in the USA: evidence and interventions. Lancet 2017;389:1453–63.
27. Hossenbaccus L, Linton S, Ramchandani R, et al. Insights into allergic risk factors from birth cohort studies. Ann Allergy Asthma Immunol 2021;127:312–7.
28. Silverberg JI, Simpson EL. Associations of childhood eczema severity: a US population-based study. Dermatitis 2014;25:107–14.
29. Mehta P, Pan Z, Zhou W, et al. Examining Disparities in Pediatric Eosinophilic Esophagitis. J Allergy Clin Immunol Pract 2023. https://doi.org/10.1016/j.jaip.2023.06.011.
30. Dellon ES. Cost-effective care in eosinophilic esophagitis. Ann Allergy Asthma Immunol 2019;123(8):166–72.
31. Hannan N, McMillan SS, Tiralongo E, et al. Treatment Burden for Pediatric Eosinophilic Esophagitis: A Cross-Sectional Survey of Carers. J Pediatr Psychol 2021;46:100–11.
32. Mukkada V, Falk GW, Eichinger CS, et al. Health-Related Quality of Life and Costs Associated With Eosinophilic Esophagitis: A Systematic Review. Clin Gastroenterol Hepatol 2018;16:495–503.e8.

33. Jensen ET, Kappelman MD, Martin CF, et al. Health-care utilization, costs, and the burden of disease related to eosinophilic esophagitis in the United States. Am J Gastroenterol 2015;110:626–32.

34. Hiremath G, Kodroff E, Strobel MJ, et al. Individuals affected by eosinophilic gastrointestinal disorders have complex unmet needs and frequently experience unique barriers to care. Clin Res Hepatol Gastroenterol 2018;42:483–93.

35. Wechsler JB, Schwartz S, Amsden K, et al. Elimination diets in the management of eosinophilic esophagitis. J Asthma Allergy 2014;7:85–94.

36. Joshi S, Rubenstein JH, Dellon ES, et al. Variability in Practices of Compounding Budesonide for Eosinophilic Esophagitis. Am J Gastroenterol 2021;116:1336–8.

37. Parasher AK, Gliksman M, Segarra D, et al. Economic Evaluation of Dupilumab Versus Endoscopic Sinus Surgery for the Treatment of Chronic Rhinosinusitis With Nasal Polyps. Int Forum Allergy Rhinol 2022;12:813–20.

38. Zimmermann M, Rind D, Chapman R, et al. Economic Evaluation of Dupilumab for Moderate-to-Severe Atopic Dermatitis: A Cost-Utility Analysis. J Drugs Dermatol 2018;17:750–6.

39. Asher Wolf W, Huang KZ, Durban R, et al. The Six-Food Elimination Diet for Eosinophilic Esophagitis Increases Grocery Shopping Cost and Complexity. Dysphagia 2016;31:765–70.

40. Jensen ET, Hoffman K, Shaheen NJ, et al. Esophageal eosinophilia is increased in rural areas with low population density: results from a national pathology database. Am J Gastroenterol 2014;109:668–75.

41. McGowan EC, Keller JP, Dellon ES, et al. Prevalence and geographic distribution of pediatric eosinophilic esophagitis in the 2012 US Medicaid population. J Allergy Clin Immunol Pract 2020;8:2796–8.e4.

42. Lavizzo-Mourey RJ, Besser RE, Williams DR. Understanding and Mitigating Health Inequities - Past, Current, and Future Directions. N Engl J Med 2021; 384:1681–4.

43. Simpson T, Evans J, Goepfert A, et al. Implementing a graduate medical education anti-racism workshop at an academic university in the Southern USA. Med Educ Online 2022;27:1981803.

44. York M, Langford K, Davidson M, et al. Becoming Active Bystanders and Advocates: Teaching Medical Students to Respond to Bias in the Clinical Setting. MedEdPORTAL 2021;17:11175.

45. Walker VP, Hodges L, Perkins M, et al. Taking the VITALS to Interrupt Microaggressions. MedEdPORTAL 2022;18:11202.

46. Raney J, Pal R, Lee T, et al. Words Matter: An Antibias Workshop for Health Care Professionals to Reduce Stigmatizing Language. MedEdPORTAL 2021;17:11115.

47. Salsberg E, Richwine C, Westergaard S, et al. Estimation and Comparison of Current and Future Racial/Ethnic Representation in the US Health Care Workforce. JAMA Netw Open 2021;4:e213789.

48. Getz K, Florez M, Botto E, et al. Global Investigative Site Personnel Diversity and Its Relationship with Study Participant Diversity. Ther Innov Regul Sci 2022;56: 777–84.

Pathophysiology of Non-Esophageal Eosinophilic Gastrointestinal Disorders

Julia L.M. Dunn, PhD[a], Lisa A. Spencer, PhD[a],*

KEYWORDS

- Eosinophilic gastritis (EoG) • Eosinophilic enteritis (EoN)
- Eosinophilic duodenitis (EoD) • Eosinophilic colitis (EoC)
- Eosinophilic gastroenteritis • Eosinophilic gastrointestinal disorder (EGID)

KEY POINTS

- Non-esophageal eosinophilic gastrointestinal disorders (EGIDs) are challenging to diagnose and treat due to their rarity, non-specific symptoms, lack of diagnostic guidelines, incomplete understanding of pathogenesis, and paucity of standardized data on treatment options and outcomes.
- Recently developed consensus nomenclature systematizes EGIDs coding based on the specific site(s) of gastrointestinal eosinophilia, enabling data sharing across centers to exponentiate research efforts and improve patient care.
- Shared aspects of EGIDs localized to the esophagus, stomach, and small bowel include an allergic etiology and molecular pathophysiology suggestive of an overarching chronic, food allergen-driven, Th2-mediated immune response.
- EGIDs localized to the colon may follow a distinct pathophysiology compared to the other EGIDs.

INTRODUCTION

Eosinophilic gastrointestinal disorder (EGID) is an umbrella term encompassing a group of chronic, immune-mediated disorders characterized by eosinophil-rich inflammation affecting one or more segments of the gastrointestinal (GI) tract in the absence of another known cause for the eosinophilia (eg, hypereosinophilic syndrome (HES), parasitic infection, drug reactions, or malignancy). The most commonly recognized EGID is eosinophilic esophagitis (EoE), which is to date also the most well-studied. Non-EoE EGIDs are rare,

[a] Department of Pediatrics, Section of GI, Hepatology, and Nutrition, University of Colorado School of Medicine, and Digestive Health Institute, Children's Hospital Colorado, Aurora, CO 80045, USA
* Corresponding author. University of Colorado School of Medicine, 12700 East 19th Avenue, Research Complex 2, Mailstop C226, Aurora, CO 80016.
E-mail address: lisa.spencer@cuanschutz.edu

Immunol Allergy Clin N Am 44 (2024) 299–309
https://doi.org/10.1016/j.iac.2024.01.003
0889-8561/24/© 2024 Elsevier Inc. All rights reserved.

and can involve the stomach, small bowel, and/or colon. Varied and non-specific symptoms and lack of consensus diagnostic criteria contribute to diagnostic delays and under-diagnosis. Lack of consensus in nomenclature had further hindered progress in delineating their pathophysiology. However, a recent consensus in nomenclature and emerging data made possible through multi-center consortia are beginning to unravel the molecular and cellular underpinnings of EGIDs below the esophagus. These emerging findings are revealing both overarching commonalities related to a food allergen-driven, chronic, Th2-mediated immune response as well as location-specific nuances in the pathophysiology of the collective EGIDs. Altogether, these advances offer promise for improved diagnoses and more efficacious interventional strategies.

DEFINITIONS AND CHALLENGES

Non-esophageal EGIDs are challenging to diagnose. Symptoms (eg, abdominal pain, vomiting, and diarrhea) are non-specific and may not warrant biopsy. Symptoms also vary, both by age, and the specific GI segment (ie, stomach, small bowel, colon) and tissue layer (ie, mucosal, muscular, serosal) affected. Likewise, a range of endoscopic abnormalities (eg, erosion, erythema, edema, or nodules) can be present, and may be subtle. Due to the lack of a validated scoring instrument, endoscopic findings on their own offer limited value for detection and diagnosis. However, a recent prospective assessment of an Eosinophilic Gastritis Endoscopic Reference System in a multi-site cohort has offered deeper insights into endoscopic abnormalities encountered in eosinophilic gastritis (EoG).[1] Histologic assessment rests largely upon quantifying eosinophilic inflammation. This is complicated by the fact that, unlike the esophagus, eosinophils are a normal cellular component of the healthy stomach, small bowel, and colon. Normal ranges of GI tissue eosinophils are broad, levels vary along the length of the GI tract, and eosinophilic distribution can be patchy, collectively complicating the establishment of threshold values.[2] Currently, specific thresholds for the stomach ($\geq$30 eos/hpf), duodenum ($\geq$52 eos/hpf), ileum ($\geq$56 eos/hpf), right colon (>100 eos/hpf), transverse and descending colon (>84 eos/hpf), and rectosigmoid colon (>64 eos/hpf) have been recommended.[3] Further complicating diagnoses, GI tract eosinophilia is not unique to EGIDs; rather, eosinophils are often elevated in other more common conditions, including inflammatory bowel disease and celiac disease.

EPIDEMIOLOGY

Gastric or intestinal EGIDs are rare, with estimated US prevalences of 6.3, 5.1 to 8.4, and 2.1 to 3.1 per 100,000 individuals for eosinophilic gastritis, eosinophilic gastroenteritis, and eosinophilic colitis, respectively.[4,5] Although, due to the aforementioned diagnostic challenges, non-esophogeal EGIDs are likely under-identified.[6] In contrast to the male predominance of EoE, non-esophageal EGIDs are reported either equally across both genders or more commonly in females, with female predominance most notable in EoG.[5] Although etiologic risk factors have not yet been well described, early life factors (eg, antenatal or prenatal pregnancy complications and antibiotics within the first year of life) are associated with an increased risk for developing an EGID,[7] and enrichment of *Prevotella* taxa in gastric biopies of EoG patients suggests contributions of the microbiome.[8]

NOMENCLATURE

Rapid advancement in the diagnosis, treatment, and overall understanding of rare diseases relies upon multi-center collaboration. However, lack of consensus terminology had stymied efforts to advance understanding of the non-EoE EGIDs by preventing aggregated analyses across sites. Prior to 2022, there was substantial variability in the terminology used to indicate EGIDs with extra-esophageal involvement, with the non descript term "eosinophilic gastroenteritis" commonly utilized as the catchall phrase in clinical coding and research descriptions. This lack of clarity and precision with respect to the specific involved area(s) of the GI tract (ie, gastric, smalland/or large bowel) made data collation and comparison across studies and centers challenging. Recent efforts that drew input from an international group of over 85 experts utilized iterative Delphi methodology to reach a consensus on EGID nomenclature.[9] As described in **Table 1**, consensus nomenclature now identifies each specific EGID based on the involved area(s) of the GI tract, such that eosinophilic gastritis (EoG), eosinophilic enteritis (EoN), and eosinophilic colitis (EoC) now distinguish EGIDs with predominant eosinophilic infiltration of the stomach, small bowel, and colon, respectively. EoN may be further divided into eosinophilic duodenitis (EoD), jejunitis (EoJ), and ileitis (EoI) when more granular context is available. Importantly, when multiple segments of the GI tract are involved, naming each of the involved areas is recommended. Systematization enabled through adoption of the consensus nomenclature is exponentially improving clinical and research comparisons across sites and studies and, as detailed later, is revealing both overarching commonalities and location-specific nuances in the pathophysiology of non-EoE EGIDs.

ALLERGIC ETIOLOGY

Similar to EoE, an allergic etiology of non-EoE EGIDs localized to gastric or small intestinal tissues is supported by their association with allergic disorders, success of dietary elimination strategies to improve symptoms and histologic scores in some patients, and evidence for local and systemic type 2 immunity. In contrast, an allergic etiology is less clear in EoC. **Table 2** provides an overview comparing features of EoE and non-esophageal EGIDs.

Association with Allergic Diseases

Data from 3 database studies, which predated consensus nomenclature recommendations, have provided insights into the occurrence of allergic co-morbidities in EGIDs patients. Guajardo and colleagues reported on 107 patients by collecting patient/caregiver-provided questionnaires through a web-based registry. EoG and EoD were collectively captured as an "EGE" cohort (n = 57) in this study, and also included patients with concomitant EoE.[10] Jensen and colleagues utilized ICD-9 codes to

Table 1
Consensus nomenclature recommendations for esophageal gastrointestinal disorders

Gastrointestinal Segment Involved	Standardized Nomenclature	Abbreviation
Esophagus	Eosinophilic esophagitis	EoE
Stomach	Eosinophilic gastritis	EoG
Small bowel	Eosinophilic enteritis	EoN
Duodenum	Eosinophilic duodenitis	EoD
Jejunum	Eosinophilic jejunitis	EoJ
Ileum	Eosinophilic ileitis	EoI
Colon	Eosinophilic colitis	EoC

Table 2
Shared and divergent features across esophageal gastrointestinal disorders pathophysiology

	EoE	EoG	EoN	EoC
Prevalence (per 100,000	50–100[a]	6.3	2.1–3.1[b]	2.1–3.1
Sex bias	M > F	F ≥ M	F ≥ M	F ≥ M
Peripheral eosinophilia	–/+	+	+	–/+
Eosinophils/hpf thresholds	≥ 15	≥ 30	≥ 52 (duodenum) ≥ 56 (ileum)	≥ 100 (right) ≥ 84 (descending) ≥ 64 (rectosigmoid)
Allergic etiology	++	++	++	–/+
Local tissue type 2 response	++	++	++	–/+
Association with local tissue IgG4	+	+	+	ND
Epithelial proliferative response	+	+	+	-

Abbreviation: ND, not determined.
[a] Dellon and Hirano, *Gastroenterology,* 2018; 154(2):319. https://doi.org/10.1053/j.gastro.2017.06.067.
[b] Based on reported prevalence under the term "gastroenteritis"; see text.
Evan S. Dellon, Ikuo Hirano, Epidemiology and Natural History of Eosinophilic Esophagitis, Gastroenterology, 154 (2), 2018, 319-332.e3, https://doi.org/10.1053/j.gastro.2017.06.067.

extract data on EoG (n = 774), EGE (n = 954), and EoC (n = 404) from a US national administrative database,[5] and using a separate US electronic health record database Mansoor and colleagues reported on n = 1820 EGE cases.[4] These studies reported prevalences higher than in the general population for co-morbid allergic conditions, including allergic rhinitis (30%–63%), asthma (19%–39%), and food allergic responses (3%–26%) in EGE cases.[4,5,10] Of note, drug allergies were also commonly encountered in EGE (49%–53%),[4,10] more so than in EoE alone (53% vs 26%; $P < .01$).[10] Data surrounding EoC are the most nebulous, with reported associations with any allergic condition ranging from 18% to 42%.[5,11] Collectively, these data reveal co-existing allergic conditions to be relatively common in non-EoE EGIDs, particularly localized to the stomach and/or small intestine, with drug allergies and allergic rhinitis the most commonly reported.

Insights from Dietary Elimination

Empirical food elimination approaches are effective to achieve histologic remission in EoE with milk emerging as the most common allergen trigger,[12] prompting incorporation of dietary intervention into the treatment of some non-EoE EGID patients. Over 20 manuscripts reporting on single patient case studies or small case series report symptomatic improvements in EoG/EoN in response to dietary therapy involving single-food or multi-food elimination (reviewed in[13]). Although largely anecdotal, these data point to food allergen triggers as a shared feature across EoE and EoG/EoN. More objective support is emerging from a prospective trial of adult EoG/EoN patients adhering to 6 food elimination (SFED; milk, eggs, wheat, soy, peanuts/tree nuts, and fish/shellfish) or elemental diets that has reported resolution of both symptoms and histologic and peripheral eosinophilia, with reversal of improvements upon reintroduction of foods.[14,15]

Evidence of Th2-Driven Disease

Non-esophageal EGIDs are commonly associated with elevated serum immunoglobulin (Ig)E, increased numbers of peripheral blood eosinophils and peripheral Th2 cells, and elevated levels of circulating eotaxin 3 (CCL26), thymus and activation-regulated chemokine (TARC), interleukin (IL)-5, and thymic stromal lymphopoietin (TSLP).[16,17] These attributes are collectively indicative of a systemic allergic Th2-type immune response. (Of note, a scoring system based on combined assessments of circulating CCL26, TARC, IL-5, and TSLP delineated EoG from non-EoG controls presenting with similar digestive symptoms.[17]).

Transcriptomic and intra-cellular analyses of gastric or duodenal biopsies from EoG and EoD patients, respectively, likewise revealed gene profiles redolent of local Th2-driven disease, including elevated T regulatory (T_{reg}) and Th2 cells, type 2 cytokines (ie, IL-4, IL-5 and IL-13), and increased eosinophils and mast cells.[18–20] Moreover, levels of Th2 cytokines were positively correlated with histopathologic and endoscopic features of disease.[18] In marked contrast, in a multi-site study, the EoC transcriptome lacked evidence of a strong allergic type 2 signature, with no induction of type 2 cytokines relative to biopsies from control or Crohn's disease patients,[21] suggesting distinct molecular mechanisms underly EoC relative to the other EGIDs.

CELLULAR AND MOLECULAR PATHOPHYSIOLOGY

Of the EGIDs, the pathogenesis of EoE has been best described[22] and is therefore the comparative standard for non-esophageal EGIDs. EoE is thought to involve aero-allergen or food-allergen-driven inflammation downstream of epithelial barrier dysfunction that triggers release of alarmins (eg, TSLP). The resultant cellular cascade involves type 2 innate lymphoid cells (ILC2s), Th2 cells, eosinophils, and mast cells, is dominated by type 2 cytokines (ie, IL-4, IL-5, and IL-13), and drives epithelial basal zone hyperplasia and differentiation defects. Molecular and cellular analyses of patient biopsies strongly suggest the same overarching theme of Th2-driven eosinophilic inflammation and epithelial proliferation in EoG and EoD. As expounded upon in the sections later, these features include a dominant type 2 cytokine signature, IL-13/IL-4-driven gene pathways, and local infiltration of Th2 lymphocytes, mast cells, IgG4-secreting plasma cells, and eosinophils. **Fig. 1** summarizes a current model of EoG/EoN pathophysiology extrapolated largely from transcriptomic tissue signatures. In marked contrast, the local transcriptome of EoC shares fewer common features with the other EGIDs, with diminished epithelial cell proliferation and minimal evidence of type 2 immunity.[20,21]

Despite strong overlap in type 2 pathways, the EoG and EoD transcriptomes also reveal gene programs that are distinct, both from EoE and from each other. Non-overlapping, differentially expressed gene sets include tissue segment-specific pathways suggestive of loss of tissue identity.[20] These findings may help to explain how a common pathogenic process may elicit different GI segment-specific endoscopic and histologic features and highlight the importance of EoG, EoN, and EoC site-specific studies.

Epithelium

Food allergen triggers are likely drivers of EGIDs, with their first tissue contact being the epithelium. Unlike the multi-layered squamous epithelium of the esophagus, the barrier protecting the GI tract below the esophagus is a single layer, simple columnar epithelium that is concurrently engaged in nutrient absorption. Despite their architectural and functional dissimilarities, several aspects of the epithelial transcriptome are consistent between EoE and EoG/EoD, including evidence of a proliferative response and overexpression of cadherin 26 (*CDH26*).[19,23] Epithelial CDH26 is often associated with allergic diseases including asthma[24] and has been implicated in regulation of

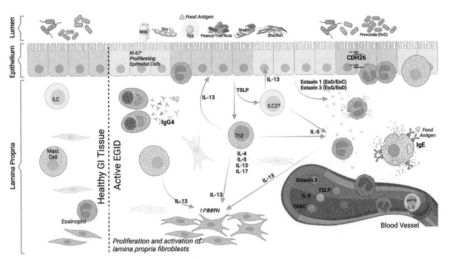

Fig. 1. Proposed pathogenesis of eosinophilic gastritis (EoG) and eosinophilic enteritis (EoN). EGID, eosinophilic gastrointestinal disorder; EoD, eosinophilic duodenitis; EoG, eosinophilic gastritis; EoN, eosinophilic enteritis; Ig, immunoglobulin; ILC2, innate lymphoid cell type 2; IL, interleukin; peTh2, pathogenic effector Th2; POSTN, periostin; Th2, T helper cell type 2; TSLP, thymsic stromal lymphopoietin; TARC, thymus and activation-regulated chemokine. (Created with BioRender.com.)

leukocyte migration[23] and amplification of IL-4R-mediated epithelial functions.[25] Upregulation of epithelial-derived alarmins such as TSLP, and members of the eotaxin family of eosinophil chemoattractants are also features shared between EoE, EoG, and EoD.[18–20,26] Of note, EoE and EoG are associated with strong induction of CCL26 (eotaxin 3), EoD with CCL26 and CCL11 (eotaxin 1), and EoC with CCL11,[21] suggesting underlying eosinophilia in EGIDs is regulated by different eotaxin family members along the length of the GI tract. In contrast to the proliferative epithelial signatures observed in the other EGIDs, EoC was associated with decreased epithelial proliferation.[21]

Cytokines

Similar to EoE, type 2 cytokines (IL-4, IL-5, and IL-13) are strongly upregulated in EoG and EoD. IL-5 is a cytokine central to the expansion of eosinophil-committed progenitors within bone marrow and provides activation and survival signals to mature eosinophils in circulation and tissues. Blockade of IL-5 or its receptor effectively depletes eosinophils. IL-13 drives gene programs readily observed in the EoG/EoD transcriptomes, including epithelial-derived eotaxins and fibroblast-derived periostin, the latter an extracellular matrix protein broadly associated with allergic diseases as well as inflammatory bowel diseases. Of note, IL-17 is also elevated in EoG, reminiscent of the mixed cytokine profile of asthma and eczema. In contrast, type 2 cytokines are not uniformly elevated in EoC.[21]

Innate Immune Cells

Eosinophils are the cardinal diagnostic cellular feature of EGIDs across all GI segments, although their specific functional contributions to the pathophysiology of any EGID are not yet fully understood. Activated eosinophils can promote barrier disruption, exacerbate pro-allergic inflammatory responses, and encourage tissue fibrosis through deposition of granule proteins, release of oxidative products, and secretion of a vast array of pro-inflammatory and pro-fibrotic mediators.[27,28] Eosinophilic inflammation in EGID may be localized to different tissue layers (eg, mucosal, muscular, or serosal), and may contribute different pathologic functions based on their localization. Unlike the esophagus, which is normally devoid of eosinophils, eosinophils naturally home to the GI tract mucosa from stomach to anus in health. Basal homing to the GI tract might offer at least a partial explanation as to why non-EoE EGIDs (relative to EoE) are more often associated with peripheral eosinophilia. In contrast to their potential pathologic functions in allergic inflammation, resident GI tissue eosinophils contribute to immune, tissue, and metabolic homeostasis.[29] Therefore, in addition to complicating the histologic diagnosis that relies primarily on tissue eosinophil counts, the presence of basal, presumably "homeostatic" intestinal eosinophils raises the question of whether functionally distinct tissue eosinophil subsets might co-exist, and may challenge the choice of therapeutic regimens designed to ablate all eosinophils. A burgeoning literature in mouse models that supports the existence of distinct homeostatic and inflammatory eosinophil states[30–33] is awaiting elaboration and translation to humans.

Increased numbers of tissue mast cells and evidence of their activation is also a common feature across EGIDs.[34–36] Like eosinophils, mast cells are normal cellular constituents of the GI tract and their increased numbers in EoD correlate with mean tissue eosinophil levels.[34] Mast cells can be significant sources of the type 2 cytokines IL-13 and IL-5,[37,38] and pro-fibrotic mediators.[39] A separate chapter within this EGIDs issue takes a deeper look at the potential roles of mast cells in non-EoE EGIDs.

Type 2 innate lymphoid cells (ILC2s) are innate immune cells that exhibit lymphoid characteristics but lack antigen-specific receptors. ILC2s function as a bridge between the epithelium and the immune system by rapidly proliferating and secreting IL-13 and IL-5 in response to the epithelial cell-derived alarmins IL-25, IL-33, and TSLP. Therefore, it is probable that ILC2s contribute to the pathogenesis of EoG/EoN, as has been reported in EoE.[40] However, this remains to be confirmed.

Adaptive Immune Cells and Tissue IgG4

A systemic Th2 response in non-EoE EGIDs has been recognized since the mid 1990s, when restimulation of peripheral blood T cells from patients with eosinophilic gastroenteritis elicited higher levels of IL-4 and IL-5, and lower levels of IFN-γ, relative to T cells from non-EGID controls.[16] More recent work has shown that CRTH2$^+$CD161$^+$ pathogenic effector Th2 cells (peTh2), also elevated in food allergic patients, are more highly detected in the peripheral circulation of EGID patients relative to healthy controls. However, unlike peTh2 cells found in food allergic patients, peTh2 cells in EGIDs express IL-5.[41,42] Within the local gastric tissue in EoG, numbers of GATA3$^+$ Th2 cells and FOXP3$^+$ T regulatory (T$_{reg}$) cells are elevated 10-fold and 2-fold, respectively, with a higher percentage of those Th2 cells expressing IL-4, IL-5, and IL-13. Importantly, total Th2 and T$_{reg}$ cells correlated with peak gastric eosinophil levels and endoscopic and histologic features of disease.[18] These data strongly implicate both a systemic and local Th2-dominated immune response in EoG/EoN.

IgE is not thought to be a primary effector of EGID pathophysiology, although total IgE is often elevated in EGID patients[43] and treatment with omalizumab lowered gastric and duodenal tissue eosinophil counts and improved symptoms in some patients in a small open-label, non-placebo controlled clinical trial.[44] Rather, EGIDs are thought to lie in the space between pure IgE-mediated and delayed Th2-type immune responses. Elevated peripheral and local tissue IgG4 (both secreted and plasma cell-associated) is a shared feature of EoE and EoG/EoN, in both adult and pediatric patients.[45–47] Numbers of local tissue IgG4+ plasma cells correlated with peak eosinophil counts and presence of endoscopic abnormalities in pediatric patients with active EoG or EoD, and were decreased in both treatment-induced and spontaneous remission.[45] If and how tissue IgG4 might participate in the pathophysiology of EGIDs remains unclear and is an area of active investigation. Due to its relatively poor capacity for allergen crosslinking and weak propensity for inducing antibody-dependent or complement-dependent cellular cytotoxicity,[48] IgG4 had been considered a beneficial isotype that sequesters allergen from IgE within the context of allergic inflammation. Moreover, IgG4 binding to the inhibitory receptor FcγRIIb can further suppress IgE-mediated hypersensitivity.[49] However, positive correlations between IgG4 levels and disease indices in some allergic diseases (eg, eosinophilic chronic rhinosinusitis and EGIDs) and observations of IgG4+ immune complexes in EoE biopsies challenge this dogma and suggest there are further nuances to be unraveled.[50]

SUMMARY

Despite their rarity and complicated diagnosis, significant strides have been made in recent years toward the understanding of non-esophageal EGIDs due in large part to establishment of a consensus nomenclature and data-sharing in multi-site consortia. Transcriptomic analysis is enabling direct comparisons with the more fully characterized EoE, accelerating insight into the cellular and mechanistic underpinnings of non-esophageal EGIDs. The emerging pathophysiologic picture for EoG/EoN is one of a chronic, food allergen-driven, Th2-type immune response that shares many cellular and molecular features with EoE. In contrast to EoG/EoN, emerging data suggest EoC may share fewer commonalities with the other EGIDs.

Key knowledge gaps in delineating EGID pathophysiology include (1) specific role(s) of eosinophils in tissue changes that accompany EGID progression and the potential for functionally distinct "homeostatic" versus "inflammatory" eosinophils to evoke distinct outcomes; (2) contributions of mast cells to disease progression; (3) mechanisms whereby food allergens trigger disease; (4) significance of local tissue-derived food-specific IgG4; (5) delineation of early life factors and genetic susceptibilities that predispose to EGID development; and (6) elucidation of GI segment and tissue layer-specific variations in disease manifestations. Filling these gaps will likely reduce the time from presentation to diagnosis, and inform implementation of treatment modalities that target different cellular or molecular aspects of Th2-type immunity.

CLINICS CARE POINTS

- EGIDs localized to different segments of the GI tract exhibit both overlapping and unique pathophysiologic features.
- EGIDs localized to the stomach or small bowel share many cellular and molecular features with EoE, including an allergic etiology and both local and systemic evidence of a type 2 immune response.
- In contrast, the pathophysiology of eosinophilic colitis may be less similar to that of the other EGIDs.

FUNDING

NIH grant R01AI168134 to LAS.

DISCLOSURE

None.

REFERENCES

1. Hirano I, Collins MH, King E, et al. Prospective Endoscopic Activity Assessment for Eosinophilic Gastritis in a Multisite Cohort. Am J Gastroenterol 2022;117: 413–23.
2. Turner KO, Collins MH, Walker MM, et al. Quantification of Mucosal Eosinophils for the Histopathologic Diagnosis of Eosinophilic Gastritis and Duodenitis: A Primer for Practicing Pathologists. Am J Surg Pathol 2022;46:557–66.
3. Collins MH. Histopathologic features of eosinophilic esophagitis and eosinophilic gastrointestinal diseases. Gastroenterol Clin N Am 2014;43:257–68.
4. Mansoor E, Saleh MA, Cooper GS. Prevalence of Eosinophilic Gastroenteritis and Colitis in a Population-Based Study, From 2012 to 2017. Clin Gastroenterol Hepatol 2017;15:1733–41.
5. Jensen ET, Martin CF, Kappelman MD, et al. Prevalence of Eosinophilic Gastritis, Gastroenteritis, and Colitis: Estimates From a National Administrative Database. J Pediatr Gastroenterol Nutr 2016;62:36–42.
6. Genta RM, Dellon ES, Turner KO. Non-oesophageal eosinophilic gastrointestinal diseases are undersuspected clinically and underdiagnosed pathologically. Aliment Pharmacol Ther 2022;56:240–50.
7. Jensen ET, Dai X, Kodroff E, et al. Early life exposures as risk factors for non-esophageal eosinophilic gastrointestinal diseases. Clin Res Hepatol Gastroenterol 2023;47:102170.
8. Furuta GT, Fillon SA, Williamson KM, et al. Mucosal Microbiota Associated With Eosinophilic Esophagitis and Eosinophilic Gastritis. J Pediatr Gastroenterol Nutr 2023;76:347–54.
9. Dellon ES, Gonsalves N, Abonia JP, et al. International Consensus Recommendations for Eosinophilic Gastrointestinal Disease Nomenclature. Clin Gastroenterol Hepatol 2022. https://doi.org/10.1016/j.cgh.2022.02.017.
10. Guajardo JR, Plotnick LM, Fende JM, et al. Eosinophil-associated gastrointestinal disorders: a world-wide-web based registry. J Pediatr 2002;141:576–81.
11. Diaz Del Arco C, Taxonera C, Olivares D, et al. Eosinophilic colitis: Case series and literature review. Pathol Res Pract 2018;214:100–4.
12. Kliewer KL, Gonsalves N, Dellon ES, et al. One-food versus six-food elimination diet therapy for the treatment of eosinophilic oesophagitis: a multicentre, randomised, open-label trial. Lancet Gastroenterol Hepatol 2023;8:408–21.
13. Lucendo AJ, Serrano-Montalban B, Arias A, et al. Efficacy of Dietary Treatment for Inducing Disease Remission in Eosinophilic Gastroenteritis. J Pediatr Gastroenterol Nutr 2015;61:56–64.
14. Gonsalves N, Doerfler B, Yang Guang, et al. Ikuo A Prospective Clinical Trial of Six Food Elimination Diet or Elemental Diet in the Treatment of Adults with Eosinophilic Gastroenteritis. Gastroenterology 2009. https://doi.org/10.1016/S0016-5085(09)61276-2. S-1861.
15. Gonsalves N, Doerfler B, Zalewski A, et al. Prospective study of an amino acid-based elemental diet in an eosinophilic gastritis and gastroenteritis nutrition trial. J Allergy Clin Immunol 2023;152:676–88.
16. Jaffe JS, James SP, Mullins GE, et al. Evidence for an abnormal profile of interleukin-4 (IL-4), IL-5, and gamma-interferon (gamma-IFN) in peripheral blood

T cells from patients with allergic eosinophilic gastroenteritis. J Clin Immunol 1994;14:299–309.

17. Shoda T, Wen T, Caldwell JM, et al. Molecular, endoscopic, histologic, and circulating biomarker-based diagnosis of eosinophilic gastritis: Multi-site study. J Allergy Clin Immunol 2020;145:255–69.

18. Ben-Baruch Morgenstern N, Shoda T, Rochman Y, et al. Local type 2 immunity in eosinophilic gastritis. J Allergy Clin Immunol 2023;152:136–44.

19. Caldwell JM, Collins MH, Stucke EM, et al. Histologic eosinophilic gastritis is a systemic disorder associated with blood and extragastric eosinophilia, TH2 immunity, and a unique gastric transcriptome. J Allergy Clin Immunol 2014;134: 1114–24.

20. Shoda T, Rochman M, Collins MH, et al. Molecular analysis of duodenal eosinophilia. J Allergy Clin Immunol 2023;151:1027–39.

21. Shoda T, Collins MH, Rochman M, et al. Evaluating Eosinophilic Colitis as a Unique Disease Using Colonic Molecular Profiles: A Multi-Site Study. Gastroenterology 2022;162:1635–49.

22. O'Shea KM, Aceves SS, Dellon ES, et al. Pathophysiology of Eosinophilic Esophagitis. Gastroenterology 2018;154:333–45.

23. Caldwell JM, Collins MH, Kemme KA, et al. Cadherin 26 is an alpha integrin-binding epithelial receptor regulated during allergic inflammation. Mucosal Immunol 2017;10:1190–201.

24. Woodruff PG, Boushey HA, Dolganov GM, et al. Genome-wide profiling identifies epithelial cell genes associated with asthma and with treatment response to corticosteroids. Proc Natl Acad Sci U S A 2007;104:15858–63.

25. Feng Y, Chen S, Xiong L, et al. Cadherin-26 Amplifies Airway Epithelial IL-4 Receptor Signaling in Asthma. Am J Respir Cell Mol Biol 2022;67:539–49.

26. Sato M, Shoda T, Shimizu H, et al. Gene Expression Patterns in Distinct Endoscopic Findings for Eosinophilic Gastritis in Children. J Allergy Clin Immunol Pract 2017;5:1639–1649 e1632.

27. Furuta GT, Nieuwenhuis EES, Karhausen J, et al. Eosinophils alter colonic epithelial barrier function: role for major basic protein. Am J Physiol Gastrointest Liver Physiol 2005;289:G890–7.

28. Weller PF, Spencer LA. Functions of tissue-resident eosinophils. Nat Rev Immunol 2017;17:746–60.

29. Masterson JC, Menard-Katcher C, Larsen LD, et al. Heterogeneity of Intestinal Tissue Eosinophils: Potential Considerations for Next-Generation Eosinophil-Targeting Strategies. Cells 2021. https://doi.org/10.3390/cells10020426.

30. Gurtner A, Borrelli C, Gonzalez-Perez I, et al. Active eosinophils regulate host defense and immune responses in colitis. Nature 2022. https://doi.org/10.1038/s41586-022-05628-7.

31. Wang WL, Kasamatsu J, Joshita S, et al. The aryl hydrocarbon receptor instructs the immunomodulatory profile of a subset of Clec4a4(+) eosinophils unique to the small intestine. Proc Natl Acad Sci U S A 2022;119. e2204557119.

32. Larsen LD, Dockstader K, Olbrich CL, et al. Modulation of surface CD11c expression tracks plasticity in murine intestinal tissue eosinophils. J Leukoc Biol 2022; 111:943–52.

33. Xenakis JJ, Howard ED, Smith KM, et al. Resident intestinal eosinophils constitutively express antigen presentation markers and include two phenotypically distinct subsets of eosinophils. Immunology 2018;154:298–308.

34. Reed CC, Genta RM, Youngblood BA, et al. Mast Cell and Eosinophil Counts in Gastric and Duodenal Biopsy Specimens From Patients With and Without Eosinophilic Gastroenteritis. Clin Gastroenterol Hepatol 2021;19:2102–11.

35. Youngblood BA, Brock EC, Leung J, et al. Siglec-8 antibody reduces eosinophils and mast cells in a transgenic mouse model of eosinophilic gastroenteritis. JCI Insight 2019;4. https://doi.org/10.1172/jci.insight.126219.

36. Mir SA, Scfy D, Olive AP, et al. Mucosal mast cell counts in pediatric eosinophilic gastrointestinal disease. Pediatr Allergy Immunol 2014;25:94–5.

37. Lorentz A, Schwengberg S, Mierke C, et al. Human intestinal mast cells produce IL-5 in vitro upon IgE receptor cross-linking and in vivo in the course of intestinal inflammatory disease. Eur J Immunol 1999;29:1496–503.

38. Ben-Baruch Morgenstern N, Ballaban AY, Wen T, et al. Single-cell RNA sequencing of mast cells in eosinophilic esophagitis reveals heterogeneity, local proliferation, and activation that persists in remission. J Allergy Clin Immunol 2022;149:2062–77.

39. Berton A, Levi-Schaffer F, Emonard H, et al. Activation of fibroblasts in collagen lattices by mast cell extract: a model of fibrosis. Clin Exp Allergy 2000;30:485–92.

40. Doherty TA, Baum R, Newbury RO, et al. Group 2 innate lymphocytes (ILC2) are enriched in active eosinophilic esophagitis. J Allergy Clin Immunol 2015;136:792–794 e793.

41. Prussin C, Lee J, Foster B. Eosinophilic gastrointestinal disease and peanut allergy are alternatively associated with IL-5+ and IL-5(-) T(H)2 responses. J Allergy Clin Immunol 2009;124:1326–1332 e1326.

42. Makiya MA, Brown T, Holland N, et al. Distinct CRTH2+CD161+ (peTh2) memory CD4+ T-cell cytokine profiles in food allergy and eosinophilic gastrointestinal disorders. Clin Exp Allergy 2023;53:1031–40.

43. Ishimura N, Furuta K, Sato S, et al. Limited role of allergy testing in patients with eosinophilic gastrointestinal disorders. J Gastroenterol Hepatol 2013;28:1306–13.

44. Foroughi S, Foster B, Kim N, et al. Anti-IgE treatment of eosinophil-associated gastrointestinal disorders. J Allergy Clin Immunol 2007;120:594–601.

45. Quinn L, Nguyen B, Menard-Katcher C, et al. IgG4+ cells are increased in the gastrointestinal tissue of pediatric patients with active eosinophilic gastritis and duodenitis and decrease in remission. Dig Liver Dis 2023;55:53–60.

46. Masuda MY, LeSuer WE, Horsley-Silva JL, et al. Food-Specific IgG4 Is Elevated Throughout the Upper Gastrointestinal Tract in Eosinophilic Esophagitis. Dig Dis Sci 2023;68:2406–13. https://doi.org/10.1007/s10620-023-07924-2.

47. Kosaka S, Tanaka F, Nakata A, et al. Gastrointestinal IgG4 Deposition Is a New Histopathological Feature of Eosinophilic Gastroenteritis. Dig Dis Sci 2022;67:3639–48.

48. Chen X, Song X, Li K, et al. FcgammaR-Binding Is an Important Functional Attribute for Immune Checkpoint Antibodies in Cancer Immunotherapy. Front Immunol 2019;10:292.

49. Burton OT, Logsdon SL, Zhou JS, et al. Oral immunotherapy induces IgG antibodies that act through FcgammaRIIb to suppress IgE-mediated hypersensitivity. J Allergy Clin Immunol 2014;134:1310–1317 e1316.

50. Qin L, Tang LF, Cheng L, et al. The clinical significance of allergen-specific IgG4 in allergic diseases. Front Immunol 2022;13:1032909.

Role of Mast Cells in Eosinophilic Gastrointestinal Diseases

Paneez Khoury, MD, MHSc[a],*, Joshua B. Wechsler, MD, MSci[b]

KEYWORDS

- Mast cells • Eosinophils • Eosinophilic gastrointestinal disorders
- Eosinophilic esophagitis

KEY POINTS

- Mast cells are present in vascularized tissues and play an integral role in tissue homeostasis.
- Type 2 inflammation, including Eosinophilic Gastrointestinal Disorders (EGIDs), is associated with increases in mast cell density and/or activation.
- In EGIDs, mast cells regulate barrier integrity, nerve activation, smooth muscle hyperplasia, myofibroblast activation, and immune cell recruitment.
- Further studies are needed to define the role of mast cells in allergic inflammation.

INTRODUCTION

Unlike other granulocytes, mast cells are tissue resident cells that circulate as progenitors and mature in the tissue based on the microenvironment.[1–3] Mast cells survive for long periods and play a key role in maintaining homeostasis at the interface between the external environment and the host barrier and immune system.[1–3] Through a variety of stimuli, mast cells are capable of rapid activation (degranulation) with release of preformed contents from small molecules, such as histamine, to proteases, such as tryptase, chymase, and carboxypeptidase A3.[4–7] Mast cells can also synthesize and release leukotrienes, prostaglandins, and cytokines, such as interleukin-13 (IL-13) through late-phase activation.[8] Through their activation and cross talk with both structural and immune cells, mast cells contribute to a variety of pathologic conditions.[6]

Grant Support: J.B. Wechsler did not receive funding for this work. P. Khoury was funded, in part, by the Division of Intramural Research, United States, NIAID/NIH, United States.
[a] Human Eosinophil Section, National Institute of Allergy and Infectious Diseases, National Institutes of Health, 9000 Rockville Pike, Building 10, Room 12C103, Bethesda, MD 20892, USA;
[b] Simpson-Querrey 10-518, Stanley Manne Children's Research Institute, Ann & Robert H. Lurie Children's Hospital of Chicago, 225 E. Chicago Avenue, Box 65, Chicago, IL 60611, USA
* Corresponding author.
E-mail address: khouryp@nih.gov

Immunol Allergy Clin N Am 44 (2024) 311–327
https://doi.org/10.1016/j.iac.2024.01.004
0889-8561/24/Published by Elsevier Inc.

Eosinophilic Gastrointestinal Disorders (EGIDs) are characterized and currently diagnosed by demonstration of an increase in tissue eosinophils well above normal levels; however, several other immune cells increase in number and may be activated, including mast cells.[9] The role of mast cells in EGIDs is emerging with most research focused on Eosinophilic Esophagitis (EoE), a hallmark type 2 (T2) immune disease characterized by significant infiltration of eosinophils into the esophageal epithelium, loss of barrier integrity, and tissue remodeling, which results in symptoms such as dysphagia.[10] Along with an increase in density, mast cells become activated in EoE and release a variety of mediators that contribute to the loss of barrier integrity, nerve stimulation, fibroblast activation, and muscle contraction.[11] Although mast cell responses are intricately coordinated with other innate and adaptive cells in the tissues, this review focuses on the basic biology of mast cells, their role in the gastrointestinal (GI) tract, and most specifically, how mast cells may contribute to the pathogenesis in EGIDs. Potential future therapeutic considerations as well as clinical and research unmet needs are explored (**Table 1**).

Tissue Mast Cells Drive Type 2 Disorders

T2 immune diseases include EGIDs, such as EoE, as well as other atopic disorders, including asthma, atopic dermatitis, food allergy, and allergic rhinitis.[12] Together these disorders have a significant burden on quality of life frequently requiring controller medications and lifestyle modification for both patients and caretakers.[13,14] Although individual atopic conditions may develop early in life, accumulation or evolution of atopic disorders, referred to as the "atopic march," may occur and can include the development of EoE.[15] The pathogenesis of T2 disorders is multifactorial and complex with some heterogeneity; however, most disorders include mast cells as a component of either acute symptomatology, disease pathogenesis, or symptoms.

Mast cells play a critical role in maintaining homeostasis and driving inflammation through interaction with structural and immune cells.[16] Mast cells derive from a pluripotent hematopoietic progenitor that is $CD34^+$ and gives rise to other granulocytes.[2,17,18] Mast cell progenitors circulate in the bloodstream and mature locally in the tissue in response to the microenvironment.[2,18] Mast cells have prolonged survival in the tissue and are found in mucosa of the airway, skin, and GI tract where they facilitate interaction between the environment and the host immune system.[19] Mast cells are classified into 2 types based on the granule contents, which relate to their tissue localization.[20] This includes MC_T, which release tryptase, but not chymase, and are found in mucosal surfaces, and MC_{TC}, which secrete both tryptase and chymase, and are found in the submucosa and connective tissue.

Activation of mast cells is a key aspect of many T2 allergic diseases. Mast cells can be activated to release preformed contents as well as synthetize de novo mediators.[21] Rapid activation or degranulation is most well-described to occur through cross-linking of the high-affinity immunoglobulin E (IgE) receptor (FcεRI) after engagement of specific antigens to IgE bound to FcεRI.[21] In this manner, mast cells are poised to respond to foreign antigens to which they are sensitized, a hallmark of immediate hypersensitivity, such as occurs in food allergy. Degranulation can be triggered through non-IgE mechanisms, including mast-related G protein–coupled receptor X2 (MRGPRX2) receptors, toll-like receptors, and complement receptors.[6,21] Degranulation of mast cells leads to release of preformed proteases stored in granules, including tryptase (*TPSAB1/TPSB2*), chymase (*CMA1*), carboxypeptidase a3 (*CPA3*), and cathepsin-G (*CTSG*). Tryptase, chymase, and cathepsin-G are serine proteases that cleave N-terminus amino acids, whereas carboxypeptidase a3 cleaves C-terminus amino acids.[20] Tryptase and chymase are also known to interact with protease-activated receptor 2

Table 1
Unmet needs regarding mast cells in eosinophilic gastrointestinal disorders

Clinical	Research Question	Potential Studies
Therapies that limit mast cell activation	1. Do therapies that limit rapid mast cell activation (degranulation) improve histologic, endoscopic, and/or clinic parameters in EGIDs? 2. Are therapies that limit late-phase activation (prostaglandin, lipid mediator, cytokine release) effective in EGIDs?	1. Correlation of flow-based assessment of mast cell with clinical, histologic, and endoscopic outcome metrics 2. Clinical trial of agents that limit mast cells activation (BTK inhibitors, anti-Siglec6 antibodies, tyrosine kinase inhibitors, anti-KIT small molecule inhibitors) 3. Assess contribution of specific mast cell subtypes
Association of mast cells and chest pain	1. Are specific mast cell mediators responsible for EGID-associated chest pain?	1. Flow characterization and isolation of mast cells in EGID patients with and without chest pain for RNA-sequencing 2. Animal models of EoE that assess pain in mice lacking specific proteins in mast cells
Therapies that deplete mast cells	1. Do therapies that deplete mast cells improve histologic, endoscopic, and/or clinic parameters in EGIDs? 2. What is the optimal target/drug type to deplete esophageal mast cells?	1. Evaluation of mast cell-specific knockouts in ant gen-driven EoE and non-EoE EGID models 2. Clinical trials of anti-Siglec-6, anti-KIT biologics, and tyrosine kinase inhibitors
Lack of clinical remission with persistent esophageal mastocytosis	1. Effects on mast cell counts and the mast cell transcriptome following dupilumab therapy in EoE/EoG 2. Does adjunctive therapy in patients with low eosinophils lead to clinical remission 3. Is persistent mastocytosis a long-term phenomenon in EoE? 4. Are there specific food triggers of mast cells?	1. Quantification of mast cells and mast cell transcriptome in EGID patients before and after dupilumab 2. Clinical trial on patients with lack of clinical remission despite low eosinophils 3. Longitudinal studies of mast cells in patients with persistent lack of clinical remission 4. Studies of patients undergoing food reintroduction to assess mast cells changes
Blunting of fibrostenosis	1. Does mast cell-targeted therapy limit the development of fibrostenosis?	1. Correlation of mast cell immunohistochemistry and flow cytometric mast cell activation with EndoFLIP distensibility 2. Assessment of patients with long-term elevation in mast cells for development of fibrostenosis

(PAR2). Mast cell proteases have been implicated in a variety of functions relevant to T2 diseases, including loss of barrier integrity, nerve signaling, remodeling, muscle contraction, and cytokine release.[20,22,23] Degranulation of mast cells also releases bioactive small molecules, such as histamine, heparin, or serotonin. Mast cells are considered the largest source of histamine in the human body. Histamine signals via several histamine receptors and is well-described to play a key role in immediate hypersensitivity responses through vasodilation, increased vascular permeability, and smooth muscle contraction.[24–26] Histamine can act synergistically with other cytokines, such as IL-4, which together enhance expression of chemokines in macrophages.[27] Mast cell degranulation can occur chronically and is characterized by translocation of lysosomal-associated membrane proteins like Lysosomal Associated Membrane Protein-3 (LAMP3/CD63) to the cell surface, which has been adapted to in vitro assays to assess for evidence of functional IgE.[28]

Mast cells can further be activated to synthesize and release a variety of molecules, including leukotrienes, prostaglandins, and cytokines.[29] Mast cell involvement in the late phase response can have both proinflammatory and anti-inflammatory effects.[30–34] This has a key role in driving chronic inflammation in T2-driven disorders through interaction with and recruitment of other immune cells as well as interaction with structural cells to drive pathologic processes like mucous production and tissue remodeling, as described in the next section in more detail.[34–36] IL-13 is a key cytokine in many T2 disorders and can be released by mast cells in addition to other innate cell populations.[37] IL-13, in turn, can drive barrier dysfunction, tissue remodeling, smooth muscle contraction, and effector cell recruitment.[38,39] Thus, mast cells as tissue resident cells have significant cross talk with the local tissue environment and contribute to T2 diseases.

Biomarkers of mast cell activation remain a significant limitation in identifying localized tissue mast cell activation. This is due to the diversity in types of mast cells activation, the breadth of molecules that mast cells secrete, and the chronicity to which this occurs. Serum tryptase is broadly the best marker of mast cell activation, yet to some extent also measures mast cell burden. Other blood- and urine-based markers have been assessed, yet none have clear utility over tryptase.[40] However, these methods have limitation in analyzing tissue localized mast cell activation. Histologic analysis of pathology specimens for free granules or mast cells without an intact cell body has been performed[41] but has significant potential for subjectivity. One potentially useful methodology for assessing tissue mast cell activation is flow cytometry, which can be used to characterize the extent to which tissue mast cells have CD63 on their cell surface, which is externalized following rapid activation.[42]

Mast Cells in the Gastrointestinal Tract

The GI tract continuously interacts with the external environment. This includes interactions with the host microbiome, pathogens, ingested foods, and toxins. Mast cells can be found in all areas of the GI tract at homeostasis, although the density of mast cells varies in each location.[43] In the GI tract, mast cells are positioned within the mucosa, and near nerve cells, blood vessels, and smooth muscle.[16,44,45] This proximity facilitates a critical role for mast cells in the surveillance of foreign antigens or epithelial perturbations that may necessitate an immune response and tissue repair.[11] Mast cells are capable of increasing blood flow and propulsive motor activity through the release of histamine and other vasoactive molecules, such as bradykinin, or neuroactive molecules, such as serotonin.[25,26,46] Mast cells play a key role in the elimination of toxins through the release of proteases that can cleave key components of the toxins and facilitate tissue repair.[47] They participate in infection responses through detection of microbial ligands via pathogen-associated molecular pattern receptors that prime adaptive immune responses. Mast cells also participate in homeostatic functions, such as regulation of tight junctions and the epithelial barrier through proteolytic actions of chymase and tryptase with PAR2.[23]

A key obstacle to elucidating the role of mast cells in the gut is a limited understanding of normal homeostasis. Quantification of mast cells involves staining with either CD117 or tryptase. CD117 is a cell-surface receptor for stem cell factor and is also present on other immune cells, such as monocytes, so counts tend to be higher than with tryptase, an intracellular protease packed into granules. However, although tryptase is more specific, free granules can be stained that make counting difficult. Current knowledge regarding mast cells counts in the GI tract suggests some similarities to eosinophil density,[43] although a direct correlation is not found in many cases. In the esophagus, mast cells are sparse (0–8 per high-power field [HPF]) but are variably increased in the stomach (12–43), duodenum (18–33), jejunum (14–26), and colon (4–88).[43] The variability can, in part, be attributed to the different immunostains used, but may also be due to the lack of true healthy controls (HCs). During inflammatory states, mast cells can increase in density or be activated, although differentiating between these scenarios histopathologically is imperfect. Subtle increases have been found in other conditions, such as irritable bowel syndrome (IBS) and dyspepsia with increased mast cells near nerves.[48] There are also reports of increased mast cells in inflammatory bowel disease (IBD), Crohn's disease, and ulcerative colitis. Intestinal mastocytosis is associated with a dramatic increase in mast cells in clusters, with an increase in CD25 positivity. The increase in both mast cell density and activation is associated with nonspecific symptoms of abdominal pain or diarrhea, attributed to mediator release.[49] Mast cells have been implicated as contributing to a variety of non-T2 disorders and syndromes, including irritable bowel syndrome (IBS) and IBD.[50] In addition, bacterial infection and toxins can break oral tolerance leading to the production of local food-antigen–specific IgE in the tissue. Reexposure to the same food antigens triggers tissue mast cell activation and visceral pain in mice. Intramucosal injection of food antigens in human colonic tissue in human participants with IBS but not IgE-mediated food allergy elicited pain and immediate mucosal responses.[51] Stressful conditions can also increase gut permeability and are associated with mast cell activation, a potential mechanism of IBS. In murine models, mast cell–derived histamine and the histamine 4-receptor contribute to the severity of colitis through IL-6–mediated recruitment of neutrophils.[52] Patients with IBD have also been noted to have increased histamine metabolite levels in the urine, further supporting a role for mast cell activation.[53]

Mast Cell Interactions with Immune and Structural Cells

Mast cell interactions with various immune and structural cells contribute to disease pathogenesis in EoE (**Fig. 1**). As with other T2-high disorders, such as T2 asthma, mast cells and eosinophils often colocalize in affected tissues.[54] Some of the descriptions of cell-cell interactions originate from study of atopic disorders, wherein mast cells and eosinophils have been shown to modulate each other's actions via release of cellular products and direct interactions.[55] In mouse models and in vitro, eosinophil products, such as cytokines and extruded granule proteins, can stimulate mast cells. Similarly, mediators, such as cytokines (IL-5, IL-3, and granulocyte-macrophage colony-stimulating factor) known to be secreted by mast cells, can enhance eosinophil recruitment, activation, and survival, potentially synergizing and contributing to tissue inflammation. In a mouse model of EoE, blockade of stem cell factor (SCF) resulted in reduction of T-helper 2 (Th2) -mediated inflammation, reduction in eosinophils mast cells, and innate lymphoid cells (ILCs) as well as attenuation of T2 responses.[56] In c-kit–deficient "sash" mice, muscle layer thickness was found to be reduced without effects on eosinophils, suggesting that mast cells function independently from eosinophils to drive remodeling.[57] Furthermore, myofibroblasts are a likely source of SCF, a survival and maturation factor for mast cells; however, its role in other cell types, such as monocytes and T cells, makes conclusions about the role of mast cells difficult to discern.[56]

In the context of allergic and inflammatory diseases, mast cells are pivotal players in driving tissue remodeling and fibrosis through intricate interactions with fibroblasts. When activated, mast cell release of IL-13 directly influences fibroblasts to proliferate and triggers heightened collagen production—a hallmark of tissue fibrosis.[58,59] Simultaneously, as shown in decellularized intestinal scaffold models, tryptase and transforming growth factor-β1 (TGF-β1) directly activate fibroblasts, further promoting their proliferation and differentiation into a phenotype of fibrosis-promoting myofibroblast and augmenting collagen deposition.[60] The interplay between mast cells and fibroblasts underscores cellular interactions that may contribute to tissue remodeling in EGIDs.

At the epithelial barrier, dysregulated mast cells may contribute to loss of epithelial integrity and function (see **Fig. 1**). Mast cell–derived proteases can disrupt tight junctions within the epithelial layer, allowing antigen and microbial translocation, and tryptase release may activate PAR receptors on epithelial cells.[61] As a product of damaged epithelial cells as well as mast cells, thymic stromal lymphopoietin (TSLP) has been shown to be important for mast cell proliferation, and in concert with other inflammatory cytokines, a promoter of T2 cytokines released from mast cells.[62] Similar to TSLP, IL-33 can be produced by mast cells, in this case in response to IgE stimulation, as well as be a product of a damaged barrier and released by epithelial cells and keratinocytes,[63] potentially setting up a feedback loop between damaged epithelium and mast cells that contributes to disease persistence. Furthermore, in the lamina propria, mast cells play a central role in orchestrating extracellular matrix (ECM) remodeling, a process intimately associated with tissue fibrosis through release of tryptase and chymase and cleavage of ECM components fibronectin and collagen.[64,65]

Mast cell–derived tryptase, as well as pruritogenic cytokines IL-13, IL-33, and IL-31 (all produced by mast cells), have been implicated in the stimulation and dysregulation of sensory neurons.[66] These interactions have been better described in skin diseases, such as prurigo nodularis, atopic dermatitis, and T2-dominated inflammatory skin disorders, where sensitization of cutaneous sensory neurons has been demonstrated. In concert, both IL-4 and IL-13 have been identified as important for neuroimmune cross talk. Specifically, IL-13 effects on expression of TRPA1 channels on sensory neural cells in inflammatory conditions[67] bring attention to the possibility of these same pathways amplifying the perception of discomfort or pain, or visceral hypersensitivity in patients with EGID.[68,69] Mast cell activation and tryptase production also appear to drive neuron-evoked action potentials via a PAR2 activating peptide.[70] This direct link between mast cells and neural responses underscores their potential critical involvement in mediating the sensory aspects of EGID symptoms. Furthermore, it emphasizes the need to explore therapeutic strategies targeting mast cell–neuron interactions to alleviate pain associated with EGIDs.

Mast cells and leukocytes interact through coordinated regulation and counterbalance of cytokines and chemokines. For instance, mast cell–derived IL-13 has been implicated in recruiting and activating Th2 cells. Altered lipid metabolism and tissue resident pathogenic effector Th2 cell products, such as cytokines IL-5 and IL-13, attract both eosinophils and mast cells in EoE through shared receptor expression.[71] Chemokines released by mast cells contribute to the recruitment and activation of

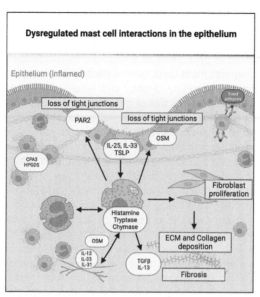

Fig. 1. Mast cell interactions with structural and immune cells in EGIDs. Mast cell interactions with eosinophils, nerves, fibroblasts, and the epithelial barrier are shown. Release of mast cell mediators (histamine, tryptase, chymase), cytokines (IL-13, IL-33, IL-31, OSM), and enzymes (Carboxypeptidase A3 [CPA3], hematopoietic prostaglandin D synthase [HGPDS]) contribute to loss of tight junctions, fibrosis, fibroblast proliferation, ECM and collagen deposition, activation of eosinophils, and stimulation and dysregulation of neurons. The G protein–coupled receptor PAR2 is expressed by mast cells and eosinophils as well as vascular endothelial cells and is activated when cleaved by proteases, such as tryptase, contributing to inflammatory processes. (Created with BioRender.com.)

other immune cells. For monocytes, mast cell–derived cytokines, such as IL-6 and tumor necrosis factor-alpha (TNF-α), have been shown to influence monocyte differentiation, promoting the development of proinflammatory subsets that contribute to disease pathogenesis, for example, in wound healing.[72] Furthermore, studies in IBD, a disease that shares some immune dysregulatory characteristics with EGIDs, highlight mast cell–mediated chemokine release, such as CCL2 (monocyte chemoattractant protein-1), directing monocyte recruitment and activation within the inflamed gut mucosa.[73] The immune responses shaped by cell-cell interactions further outline the coordinated and delicate balance required in the GI tract to maintain normal homeostasis.

Finally, mast cells have been implicated in promoting smooth muscle hypertrophy. In T2 asthma, mast cell–derived histamine and leukotrienes induce bronchoconstriction and airway hyperreactivity by promoting smooth muscle contraction. In addition, in the context of IBS, a condition that shares some clinical features with EGIDs, mast cell activation and the release of mediators have been associated with visceral hypersensitivity and alterations in GI motility,[74] further underscoring the role of mast cells in smooth muscle and potential interactions with motility.

Mast Cells in Eosinophilic Esophagitis

Mast cells are thought to play an important role in EoE, yet many questions remain, including signals for recruitment and activation, as well as the extent to which direct targeting could be useful as treatment. An increase in intraepithelial mast cells has been recognized in EoE since the early 1990s.[75] Subsequent studies have corroborated this observation, and more recent observations have demonstrated that the mast cell transcriptome is prominent in EoE biopsies, particularly in children.[76] Of these, *CPA3* is the highest mast cells gene detected in biopsy lysates.[41] However, mast cells do not always correlate directly with eosinophils and may vary by EoE phenotype.[77,78] Mast cells are effective at differentiating EoE from gastroesophageal reflux disease; however, no clear differences exist in mast cells between proton-pump inhibitor responsive and nonresponsive EoE.[78] Although many studies have shown a reduction in mast cells following treatment, this likely relates to the extent of response to treatment. One study demonstrated persistent mast cells in symptomatic children who had endoscopic furrows and histopathologic findings, such as basal zone hyperplasia, despite treatment suggesting a lack of response to treatment.[79] "Clinical remission" in this case was defined as the lack of endoscopic abnormalities and symptoms, which is in line with findings from other groups demonstrating that a composite histologic score for remission corresponded with low mast cell counts and gene expression among patients that met these criteria.[80] This observation raises key questions as to the duration of persistent esophageal mast cell proliferation, and the potential consequence on remodeling and symptoms. In addition, whether mast cell counts may be useful to assess treatment response requires further study especially in light of recent clinical trials demonstrating discordance between symptom resolution and targeted biologic therapies that deplete or reduce eosinophil counts in tissues.[81]

Although mast cell density appears to be a biomarker of tissue injury in EoE, mast cell counts are an unclear biomarker of symptoms with discordant findings in the available literature. One study reported a correlation between peak mast cell count and a nonvalidated symptom score,[82] whereas another group found no correlation between mast cell density and symptoms scores for dysphagia (measured by a visual analog scale), GERD (gastroesophageal reflux disease; measured by GERD-HRQL), and abdominal pain (measured by the SODA [Severity of Dyspepsia Assessment] score).[83] Several studies have evaluated the relationship of mast cell counts to symptoms in children with EoE. A correlation between dysphagia scores in children with EoE assessed by the Pediatric Eosinophilic Esophagitis Symptom Score and mast cell counts/gene levels was superior to eosinophils in one study.[84] The CEGIR (Consortium for Eosinophilic GastroIntestinal Research) group found increased *CPA3* and *HPGDS* (hematopoietic prostaglandin D2 synthase) in children and adults with EoE that reported pain; however, no relationship with dysphagia.[68] Although mucosal mast cells may be a biomarker to some extent, it is more likely that TGF-β expressing mast cells deeper in the esophageal tissue contributes to symptoms directly owing to smooth muscle–driven muscle contraction.[24]

The function of mast cells in EoE has been assessed using multiple methodologies, including single-cell transcriptomics, in both in vitro and in vivo models. Mast cells phenotypes as assessed by single-cell RNA sequencing include resident, transient, persistent, and proliferating within active and inactive EoE as compared with HCs.[37] Whereas HCs had very few mast cells and formed a single cluster of resident mast cells, patients with active EoE had diverse types of mast cells, including one cluster comprising mast cells with high expression of proliferative genes. One cluster comprising persistent mast cells was present in both active and inactive patients with EoE but absent in HCs. Importantly, patients with inactive EoE (<15 eosinophils per HPF) had a small number of persistent mast cells with a more activated transcriptional profile compared with resident mast cells, suggesting mast cells may remain poised for activation despite treatment. Alternatively, it may be the case that the type of treatment that these patients received failed to shut off this transcriptional activation; however, newer therapies, such as dupilumab, may help address this question. Furthermore, transient mast cells had high expression of ST2, the receptor for IL-33, whereas persistent mast cells had high protease expression of chymase and cathepsin G, recapitulating prior findings of increases in MC$_{TC}$ in EoE.

In vivo and in vitro studies have been crucial to facilitating an understanding of the role of mast cells in the esophagus and particularly in EoE. Many studies suggest a multifaceted role for mast cell activation to drive subepithelial fibrosis, muscle hypertrophy, afferent nerve stimulation, and epithelial barrier dysfunction. Several animal models have evidence of mast cell accumulation in the esophagus mimicking human EoE. Despite this, the specificity of mast cells in pain sensitization and food-antigen–driven EGIDs remains unclear. It is likely that use of mast cell–specific knockouts (eg, *CPA3*/Cre and m*CPT5*/Cre-DTA) in an antigen-driven model will be necessary to confirm the role of mast cells in EoE, including the presence of features of remodeling, such as basal cell hyperplasia. A role for mast cells in fibrosis using mice deficient in TRAIL (TNF-related apoptosis-inducing ligand) showed less muscularis externa thickening, collagen deposition, and mast cell accumulation independent of IL-13.[85] This finding should be validated in human EoE given the significant improvements seen in tissue inflammation with dupilumab. A reduction in mast cell accumulation, fibrosis, and Th2 cytokines after administration of disodium cromoglycate, a mast cell stabilizer, in murine EoE supports the notion that blocking mast cell activation instead of depletion could play an adjunctive, although not primary role in EoE.[86] A more recent study has supported a key role for mucosal mast cell activation driving epithelial barrier dysfunction using cocultures of IgE-activated mast cells with 2-dimensional epithelial cultures that contained both basal and stratified epithelium.[87] A key role for oncostatin M (OSM) released by IgE-activated mast cells was proposed to drive barrier dysfunction with a dose-dependent increase in OSM in cocultures resulting in reduced filaggrin and desmoglein-1 expression. OSM's role in prurigo nodularis, a chronic inflammatory skin disorder that is associated with fibrosis, hyperkeratosis, and pruritus, suggests that OSM's role in mast cell interactions in EoE may need further exploration (see **Table 1**).

Taken together, mast cell activation appears to play a key role in driving several key pathogenic aspects of EoE, including mucosal barrier disruption and tissue remodeling. It is therefore important to consider whether mast cell activation could be a target of therapy. Numerous drugs exist that could target mast cell activation (**Table 2**), including BTK inhibitors, tyrosine kinase inhibitors, and antibodies specific to c-kit. In addition, drugs that target intracellular mast cell signaling, such as JAK inhibitors, could be considered as well. A recent study examining the role of lirentelimab in patients with EoE failed to show improvement in symptoms,[81] suggesting that Siglec-8 may not be an ideal target in EoE; however, the specific effect of Siglec-8 on esophageal mast cells is not entirely clear. This negative finding should therefore not limit future clinical trials of other agents that target mast cells with a potential to benefit patients with EoE.

Mast Cells in Noneosinophilic Esophagitis Eosinophilic Gastrointestinal Disorders

Despite what is known about the role of mast cells in EoE, the role of mast cell activation in eosinophilic gastritis (EoG), eosinophilic duodenitis/enteritis (EoD/EoN), and eosinophilic colitis (EoC) is less clear. The normal gastric mucosa contains a small number of eosinophils as well as mast cells, typically found in the lamina propria. Similar to EoE, the mast cell transcriptome in EoG shows elevated *CPA3*, *TPSAB1/TPSB2*, and *HPGDS*.[88] CD117$^+$ cells are more numerous in EoG compared

Table 2
Therapies that target mast cells

Drug/Agent (Class)	Target	Mechanism of Action	Effect on Mast Cells	Potential Disorders	Refs.	Clinical Trial No.
Dupilumab (IL-4)	IL-4Rα subunit	Blocks IL-4 and IL-13 signaling	Reduces mast cell activation and survival	EoE, allergic conjunctivitis	Dellon et al,[97] 2022	NCT04296864
Glucocorticoids	Glucocorticoid receptor	Broadly anti-inflammatory by suppressing genes encoding inflammatory proteins	Indirectly suppresses mast cell degranulation and cytokine release	EoE, allergic conjunctivitis, others	Aceves et al,[24] 2010; Abonia et al,[41] 2010	
JAK inhibitors	Inhibition of combinations of JAK isoforms (JAK1-3)	Blocks downstream signaling of JAKs (JAK-STAT) pathway	Blocks signaling from JAKs and phosphorylation of STATs regulating mast cell growth, function, and survival	Under study for various allergic and autoimmune disorders; EoE	Morales et al,[98] 2010	
Bruton tyrosine kinase inhibitors	BTK protein	Inhibits the enzyme Bruton tyrosine kinase	May reduce activation and survival of mast cells	Under study for food allergy and prevention of anaphylaxis	Suresh et al,[99] 2023	
Barzolvolimab/tyrosine kinase inhibitor	KIT receptor	Inhibits KIT signaling pathway	Reduces mast cell proliferation and activation	ISM, CSU, and other mast cell disorders	Terhorst-Molawi et al,[100] 2023	
Lirentelimab (anti-Siglec 8)	Siglec-8 receptor	Binds to and promotes enhanced ADCC of eosinophils and inhibition of mast cell activation	Suppresses mast cell activation	Under study for CSU, AD, and other diseases where mast cells have been implicated	Dellon et al,[94] 2020	CSU: NCT055288 AD: NCT05155085

Abbreviations: AD, atopic dermatitis; ADCC, antibody-dependent cell-mediated cytotoxicity; CSU, chronic spontaneous urticaria; ISM, indolent systemic mastocytosis; JAK, Janus kinase; STAT, signal transducer and activator of transcription.

with controls (EoG 93.8 ± 33.1/HPF vs control 51.0 ± 3.8/HPF) and more frequently localized to the superficial lamina propria in EoG biopsies. In control biopsies, CD117+ cells were most numerous in the deep lamina propria but were also in the muscularis mucosa. Mast cells in the stomach of patients with EoG (44.2 ± 19.6 mast cells per HPF) are increased compared with controls (18.1 ± 7.2 mast cells per HPF)[89] and not correlated with eosinophils. In addition to numerical increases, degranulated mast cells have also been noted in the stomach of patients with EoG, characterized by high cell-surface expression of lysosomal-associated membrane proteins CD63 and CD107a.[90] In fact, the use of benralizumab in EoG, which depletes eosinophils, did not result in any change in the mast cells counts of patients with EGID, suggesting that mast cell recruitment or persistence is not dependent on eosinophils.[91] In EoD, there is an increased mast cell–related gene signature with high CPA3 similar to EoE and EoG.[92] Mast cells are also numerically increased in EoD (62.5 ± 38.8 mast cells per HPF) compared with HCs (23.6 ± 8.1 mast cells per HPF), with a weak correlation with eosinophils, as in EoG.[89] EoN with protein-losing enteropathy has significantly more mast cells despite comparable numbers of eosinophils.[93] Although anti-Siglec-8 antibody administration showed positive results in a phase 2 trial of EoG/EoD,[94] a phase 3 trial did not demonstrate clear symptomatic improvement. Whether study design aspects or heterogeneity in disease pathogenesis in EGIDs played a role in the discrepant findings is not clear. In EoC, mast cells appear to be increased as well with ~26 mast cells per HPF in EoC and 10/HPF in controls.[95]. Mast cell degranulation has been shown to be increased in patients with EoC (12/15) compared with that in patients with ulcerative colitis (1/10) and Crohn's disease (0/1) and can help differentiate IBD, which often contains an eosinophilic infiltrate, from EoC.[96] Interestingly, they found tryptase and IgE colocalize on enteric neurons in patients with allergic colitis but rarely in patients with IBD. Taken together, this supports an emerging role for mast cells in non-EoE EGIDs, although more research is clearly needed.

SUMMARY

In conclusion, mast cells play a significant role in the pathogenesis of EGIDs, including EoE. Their interactions with immune and structural cells, involvement in tissue remodeling, and contribution to symptoms make them attractive targets for therapeutic intervention. More is being discovered regarding the intricate interplay of mast cells and eosinophils. Recent studies demonstrating that depletion of eosinophils is insufficient to improve symptoms of EGIDs have raised the question of whether other cells may play a role in symptomatology and pathogenesis of EGIDs. The complexity of mast cell activation and the variability in EGID presentations necessitate further research to identify the specific role of mast cells. Whether mast cell–directed therapies can improve patient symptoms and outcomes is not yet known; however, future studies with more specific mast cell targets, such as KIT, are likely to help elucidate the role of mast cells in EGID pathogenesis.

CLINICS CARE POINTS

- The available data for contribution of mast cells in eosinophilic gastrointestinal disorders are evolving.
- Future guidelines on diagnosis of eosinophilic gastrointestinal disorders should include mast cells, as more data on the roles of mast cells in disease pathogenesis are clarified.

- Physicians should discuss the potential contribution of mast cells in eosinophilic gastrointestinal disorders with patients and consider adjunctive medications for mast cell release symptoms, if appropriate.
- Future studies using targeted mast cell therapeutics will address the impact of mast cell depletion on eosinophilic gastrointestinal disorders symptoms, disease progression, and outcomes.

DISCLOSURE

J.B. Wechsler provides medical advisory consulting for Regeneron/Sanofi, Allakos, Bristol-Myers Squibb, and Ellodi. J.B. Wechsler is a speaker for Regeneron/Sanofi. J.B. Wechsler received clinical trial funding from Regeneron, United States and Allakos. P. Khoury has nothing to disclose.

REFERENCES

1. Okayama Y, Kawakami T. Development, migration, and survival of mast cells. Immunol Res 2006;34:97–115.
2. Ribatti D. The development of human mast cells. An historical reappraisal. Exp Cell Res 2016;342:210–5.
3. Valent P, Akin C, Hartmann K, et al. Mast cells as a unique hematopoietic lineage and cell system: From Paul Ehrlich's visions to precision medicine concepts. Theranostics 2020;10:10743–68.
4. Burchett JR, Dailey JM, Kee SA, et al. Targeting Mast Cells in Allergic Disease: Current Therapies and Drug Repurposing. Cells 2022;11.
5. Kim HS, Kawakami Y, Kasakura K, et al. Recent advances in mast cell activation and regulation. F1000Res 2020;9.
6. Lyons DO, Pullen NA. Beyond IgE: Alternative Mast Cell Activation Across Different Disease States. Int J Mol Sci 2020;21.
7. Parente R, Giudice V, Cardamone C, et al. Secretory and Membrane-Associated Biomarkers of Mast Cell Activation and Proliferation. Int J Mol Sci 2023;24.
8. Banafea GH, Bakhashab S, Alshaibi HF, et al. The role of human mast cells in allergy and asthma. Bioengineered 2022;13:7049–64.
9. Gonsalves N. Eosinophilic Gastrointestinal Disorders. Clin Rev Allergy Immunol 2019;57:272–85.
10. Underwood B, Troutman TD, Schwartz JT. Breaking down the complex pathophysiology of eosinophilic esophagitis. Ann Allergy Asthma Immunol 2023;130:28–39.
11. Janarthanam R, Bolton SM, Wechsler JB. Role of mast cells in eosinophilic esophagitis. Curr Opin Gastroenterol 2022;38:541–8.
12. Hassoun D, Malard O, Barbarot S, et al. Type 2 immunity-driven diseases: Towards a multidisciplinary approach. Clin Exp Allergy 2021;51:1538–52.
13. Klinnert MD, Atkins D, Pan Z, et al. Symptom Burden and Quality of Life Over Time in Pediatric Eosinophilic Esophagitis. J Pediatr Gastroenterol Nutr 2019;69:682–9.
14. Roncada C, Medeiros TM, Strassburger MJ, et al. Comparison between the health-related quality of life of children/adolescents with asthma and that of their caregivers: a systematic review and meta-analysis. J Bras Pneumol 2020;46:e20190095.
15. Hill DA, Grundmeier RW, Ramos M, et al. Eosinophilic Esophagitis Is a Late Manifestation of the Allergic March. J Allergy Clin Immunol Pract 2018;6:1528–33.

16. Albert-Bayo M, Paracuellos I, Gonzalez-Castro AM, et al. Intestinal Mucosal Mast Cells: Key Modulators of Barrier Function and Homeostasis. Cells 2019;8.

17. Bian G, Gu Y, Xu C, et al. Early development and functional properties of tryptase/chymase double-positive mast cells from human pluripotent stem cells. J Mol Cell Biol 2021;13:104–15.

18. Ribatti D, d'Amati A. Hematopoiesis and Mast Cell Development. Int J Mol Sci 2023;24.

19. Ekoff M, Nilsson G. Mast cell apoptosis and survival. Adv Exp Med Biol 2011; 716:47–60.

20. Caughey GH. Mast cell tryptases and chymases in inflammation and host defense. Immunol Rev 2007;217:141–54.

21. Mukai K, Tsai M, Saito H, et al. Mast cells as sources of cytokines, chemokines, and growth factors. Immunol Rev 2018;282:121–50.

22. Groschwitz KR, Wu D, Osterfeld H, et al. Chymase-mediated intestinal epithelial permeability is regulated by a protease-activating receptor/matrix metalloproteinase-2-dependent mechanism. Am J Physiol Gastrointest Liver Physiol 2013;304:G479–89.

23. Jacob C, Yang PC, Darmoul D, et al. Mast cell tryptase controls paracellular permeability of the intestine. Role of protease-activated receptor 2 and beta-arrestins. J Biol Chem 2005;280:31936–48.

24. Aceves SS, Chen D, Newbury RO, et al. Mast cells infiltrate the esophageal smooth muscle in patients with eosinophilic esophagitis, express TGF-beta1, and increase esophageal smooth muscle contraction. J Allergy Clin Immunol 2010;126:1198–11204 e4.

25. Greaves MW, Sabroe RA. Histamine: the quintessential mediator. J Dermatol 1996;23:735–40.

26. Thangam EB, Jemima EA, Singh H, et al. The Role of Histamine and Histamine Receptors in Mast Cell-Mediated Allergy and Inflammation: The Hunt for New Therapeutic Targets. Front Immunol 2018;9:1873.

27. Mommert S, Schaper JT, Schaper-Gerhardt K, et al. Histamine Increases Th2 Cytokine-Induced CCL18 Expression in Human M2 Macrophages. Int J Mol Sci 2021;22:11648.

28. Bahri R, Bulfone-Paus S. Mast Cell Activation Test (MAT). Methods Mol Biol 2020;2163:227–38.

29. Castells M. Mast cell mediators in allergic inflammation and mastocytosis. Immunol Allergy Clin North Am 2006;26:465–85.

30. Alim MA, Peterson M, Pejler G. Do Mast Cells Have a Role in Tendon Healing and Inflammation? Cells 2020;9:1134.

31. Dileepan KN, Raveendran VV, Sharma R, et al. Mast cell-mediated immune regulation in health and disease. Front Med 2023;10:1213320.

32. Loucks A, Maerz T, Hankenson K, et al. The multifaceted role of mast cells in joint inflammation and arthritis. Osteoarthritis Cartilage 2023;31:567–75.

33. Tete G, D'Orto B, Ferrante L, et al. Role of mast cells in oral inflammation. J Biol Regul Homeost Agents 2021;35:65–70.

34. Wozniak E, Owczarczyk-Saczonek A, Lange M, et al. The Role of Mast Cells in the Induction and Maintenance of Inflammation in Selected Skin Diseases. Int J Mol Sci 2023;24.

35. Amin K. The role of mast cells in allergic inflammation. Respir Med 2012; 106:9–14.

36. Kwon SY, Kim JH. Role of Leukotriene B(4) Receptor-2 in Mast Cells in Allergic Airway Inflammation. Int J Mol Sci 2019;20:2897.

37. Ben-Baruch Morgenstern N, Ballaban AY, Wen T, et al. Single-cell RNA sequencing of mast cells in eosinophilic esophagitis reveals heterogeneity, local proliferation, and activation that persists in remission. J Allergy Clin Immunol 2022;149(6):2062–77.

38. Khokhar D, Marella S, Idelman G, et al. Eosinophilic esophagitis: Immune mechanisms and therapeutic targets. Clin Exp Allergy 2022;52(10):1142–56.

39. Zhernov YV, Vysochanskaya SO, Sukhov VA, et al. Molecular Mechanisms of Eosinophilic Esophagitis. Int J Mol Sci 2021;22.

40. Butterfield JH. Increased Excretion of Mast Cell Mediator Metabolites During Mast Cell Activation Syndrome. J Allergy Clin Immunol Pract 2023;11:2542–6.

41. Abonia JP, Blanchard C, Butz BB, et al. Involvement of mast cells in eosinophilic esophagitis. J Allergy Clin Immunol 2010;126:140–9.

42. Kritikou E, Depuydt MAC, de Vries MR, et al. Flow Cytometry-Based Characterization of Mast Cells in Human Atherosclerosis. Cells 2019;8:334.

43. Genta RM, Turner KO, Collins MH, et al. Quantification of Mucosal Mast Cells in the Gastrointestinal Tract: A Primer for Practicing Pathologists. Arch Pathol Lab Med 2023. https://doi.org/10.5858/arpa.2023-0070-OA.

44. Nakano N, Kitaura J. Mucosal Mast Cells as Key Effector Cells in Food Allergies. Cells 2022;11.

45. Ravanbakhsh N, Kesavan A. The role of mast cells in pediatric gastrointestinal disease. Ann Gastroenterol 2019;32:338–45.

46. Lavich TR, Cordeiro RS, Calixto JB, et al. Combined action of vasoactive amines and bradykinin mediates allergen-evoked thermal hyperalgesia in rats. Eur J Pharmacol 2003;462:185–92.

47. Dudeck A, Koberle M, Goldmann O, et al. Mast cells as protectors of health. J Allergy Clin Immunol 2019;144:S4–18.

48. Hasler WL, Grabauskas G, Singh P, et al. Mast cell mediation of visceral sensation and permeability in irritable bowel syndrome. Neuro Gastroenterol Motil 2022;34:e14339.

49. Elvevi A, Elli EM, Luca M, et al. Clinical challenge for gastroenterologists-Gastrointestinal manifestations of systemic mastocytosis: A comprehensive review. World J Gastroenterol 2022;28:3767–79.

50. Hamilton MJ, Frei SM, Stevens RL. The multifaceted mast cell in inflammatory bowel disease. Inflamm Bowel Dis 2014;20:2364–78.

51. Aguilera-Lizarraga J, Florens MV, Viola MF, et al. Local immune response to food antigens drives meal-induced abdominal pain. Nature 2021;590:151–6.

52. Wechsler JB, Szabo A, Hsu CL, et al. Histamine drives severity of innate inflammation via histamine 4 receptor in murine experimental colitis. Mucosal Immunol 2018;11:861–70.

53. Marakova K, Piestansky J, Zelinkova Z, et al. Simultaneous determination of twelve biogenic amines in human urine as potential biomarkers of inflammatory bowel diseases by capillary electrophoresis - tandem mass spectrometry. J Pharm Biomed Anal 2020;186:113294.

54. Dougherty RH, Sidhu SS, Raman K, et al. Accumulation of intraepithelial mast cells with a unique protease phenotype in T(H)2-high asthma. J Allergy Clin Immunol 2010;125:1046–1053 e8.

55. Elishmereni M, Alenius HT, Bradding P, et al. Physical interactions between mast cells and eosinophils: a novel mechanism enhancing eosinophil survival in vitro. Allergy 2011;66:376–85.

56. Ptaschinski C, Zhu D, Fonseca W, et al. Stem cell factor inhibition reduces Th2 inflammation and cellular infiltration in a mouse model of eosinophilic esophagitis. Mucosal Immunol 2023;16:727–39.

57. Niranjan R, Mavi P, Rayapudi M, et al. Pathogenic role of mast cells in experimental eosinophilic esophagitis. Am J Physiol Gastrointest Liver Physiol 2013; 304:G1087–94.

58. Firszt R, Francisco D, Church TD, et al. Interleukin-13 induces collagen type-1 expression through matrix metalloproteinase-2 and transforming growth factor-beta1 in airway fibroblasts in asthma. Eur Respir J 2014;43:464–73.

59. Garbuzenko E, Nagler A, Pickholtz D, et al. Human mast cells stimulate fibroblast proliferation, collagen synthesis and lattice contraction: a direct role for mast cells in skin fibrosis. Clin Exp Allergy 2002;32:237–46.

60. Wan J, Wu T, Liu Y, et al. Mast Cells Tryptase Promotes Intestinal Fibrosis in Natural Decellularized Intestinal Scaffolds. Tissue Eng Regen Med 2022;19:717–26.

61. Wang Z, Hao M, Wu L, et al. Mast cells disrupt the duodenal mucosal integrity: Implications for the mechanisms of barrier dysfunction in functional dyspepsia. Scand J Gastroenterol 2023;58:460–70.

62. Allakhverdi Z, Comeau MR, Jessup HK, et al. Thymic stromal lymphopoietin is released by human epithelial cells in response to microbes, trauma, or inflammation and potently activates mast cells. J Exp Med 2007;204:253–8.

63. Hsu CL, Neilsen CV, Bryce PJ. IL-33 is produced by mast cells and regulates IgE-dependent inflammation. PLoS One 2010;5:e11944.

64. St John AL, Rathore APS, Ginhoux F. New perspectives on the origins and heterogeneity of mast cells. Nat Rev Immunol 2023;23:55–68.

65. Bradding P, Pejler G. The controversial role of mast cells in fibrosis. Immunol Rev 2018;282:198–231.

66. Green DP, Limjunyawong N, Gour N, et al. A Mast-Cell-Specific Receptor Mediates Neurogenic Inflammation and Pain. Neuron 2019;101:412–420 e3.

67. Oh MH, Oh SY, Lu J, et al. TRPA1-dependent pruritus in IL-13-induced chronic atopic dermatitis. J Immunol 2013;191:5371–82.

68. Zhang S, Shoda T, Aceves SS, et al. Mast cell-pain connection in eosinophilic esophagitis. Allergy 2022;77(6):1895–9.

69. Matthews PJ, Aziz Q, Facer P, et al. Increased capsaicin receptor TRPV1 nerve fibres in the inflamed human oesophagus. Eur J Gastroenterol Hepatol 2004;16:897–902.

70. Yu S, Gao G, Peterson BZ, et al. TRPA1 in mast cell activation-induced long-lasting mechanical hypersensitivity of vagal afferent C-fibers in guinea pig esophagus. Am J Physiol Gastrointest Liver Physiol 2009;297:G34–42.

71. Morgan DM, Ruiter B, Smith NP, et al. Clonally expanded, GPR15-expressing pathogenic effector TH2 cells are associated with eosinophilic esophagitis. Sci Immunol 2021;6.

72. Komi DEA, Khomtchouk K, Santa Maria PL. A Review of the Contribution of Mast Cells in Wound Healing: Involved Molecular and Cellular Mechanisms. Clin Rev Allergy Immunol 2020;58:298–312.

73. Jones GR, Bain CC, Fenton TM, et al. Dynamics of Colon Monocyte and Macrophage Activation During Colitis. Front Immunol 2018;9:2764.

74. Barbara G, Wang B, Stanghellini V, et al. Mast cell-dependent excitation of visceral-nociceptive sensory neurons in irritable bowel syndrome. Gastroenterology 2007;132:26–37.

75. Attwood SE, Smyrk TC, Demeester TR, et al. Esophageal eosinophilia with dysphagia. A distinct clinicopathologic syndrome. Dig Dis Sci 1993;38:109–16.

76. Jacobse J, Brown R, Revetta F, et al. A synthesis and subgroup analysis of the Eosinophilic Esophagitis tissue transcriptome. J Allergy Clin Immunol 2023. https://doi.org/10.1016/j.jaci.2023.10.002.

77. Sallis BF, Acar U, Hawthorne K, et al. A Distinct Esophageal mRNA Pattern Identifies Eosinophilic Esophagitis Patients With Food Impactions. Front Immunol 2018;9:2059.

78. Wen T, Dellon ES, Moawad FJ, et al. Transcriptome analysis of proton pump inhibitor-responsive esophageal eosinophilia reveals proton pump inhibitor-reversible allergic inflammation. J Allergy Clin Immunol 2015;135:187–97.

79. Bolton SM, Kagalwalla AF, Arva NC, et al. Mast Cell Infiltration Is Associated With Persistent Symptoms and Endoscopic Abnormalities Despite Resolution of Eosinophilia in Pediatric Eosinophilic Esophagitis. Am J Gastroenterol 2020; 115:224–33.

80. Collins MH, Martin LJ, Wen T, et al. Eosinophilic Esophagitis Histology Remission Score: Significant Relations to Measures of Disease Activity and Symptoms. J Pediatr Gastroenterol Nutr 2020;70:598–603.

81. Dellon ES, Spergel JM. Biologics in eosinophilic gastrointestinal diseases. Ann Allergy Asthma Immunol 2023;130:21–7.

82. Arias A, Lucendo AJ, Martinez-Fernandez P, et al. Dietary treatment modulates mast cell phenotype, density, and activity in adult eosinophilic oesophagitis. Clin Exp Allergy 2016;46:78–91.

83. Tappata M, Eluri S, Perjar I, et al. Association of mast cells with clinical, endoscopic, and histologic findings in adults with eosinophilic esophagitis. Allergy 2018;73:2088–92.

84. Martin LJ, Franciosi JP, Collins MH, et al. Pediatric Eosinophilic Esophagitis Symptom Scores (PEESS v2.0) identify histologic and molecular correlates of the key clinical features of disease. J Allergy Clin Immunol 2015;135:1519–15128 e8.

85. Collison AM, Sokulsky LA, Sherrill JD, et al. TNF-related apoptosis-inducing ligand (TRAIL) regulates midline-1, thymic stromal lymphopoietin, inflammation, and remodeling in experimental eosinophilic esophagitis. J Allergy Clin Immunol 2015;136:971–82.

86. Silva F, de Oliveira EE, Ambrosio MGE, et al. Disodium cromoglycate treatment reduces TH2 immune response and immunohistopathological features in a murine model of Eosinophilic Esophagitis. Int Immunopharmacol 2020;83:106422.

87. Kleuskens MTA, Bek MK, Al Halabi Y, et al. Mast cells disrupt the function of the esophageal epithelial barrier. Mucosal Immunol 2023;16(5):567–77.

88. Caldwell JM, Collins MH, Stucke EM, et al. Histologic eosinophilic gastritis is a systemic disorder associated with blood and extragastric eosinophilia, TH2 immunity, and a unique gastric transcriptome. J Allergy Clin Immunol 2014;134: 1114–24.

89. Reed CC, Genta RM, Youngblood BA, et al. Mast Cell and Eosinophil Counts in Gastric and Duodenal Biopsy Specimens From Patients With and Without Eosinophilic Gastroenteritis. Clin Gastroenterol Hepatol 2021;19:2102–11.

90. Youngblood BA, Brock EC, Leung J, et al. Siglec-8 antibody reduces eosinophils and mast cells in a transgenic mouse model of eosinophilic gastroenteritis. JCI Insight 2019;4.

91. Kuang FL, Legrand F, Makiya M, et al. Benralizumab for PDGFRA-Negative Hypereosinophilic Syndrome. N Engl J Med 2019;380:1336–46.

92. Shoda T, Rochman M, Collins MH, et al. Molecular analysis of duodenal eosinophilia. J Allergy Clin Immunol 2023;151:1027–39.

93. Chehade M, Magid MS, Mofidi S, et al. Allergic eosinophilic gastroenteritis with protein-losing enteropathy: intestinal pathology, clinical course, and long-term follow-up. J Pediatr Gastroenterol Nutr 2006;42:516–21.

94. Dellon ES, Peterson KA, Murray JA, et al. Anti-Siglec-8 Antibody for Eosinophilic Gastritis and Duodenitis. N Engl J Med 2020;383:1624–34.

95. Awad H, Sfaira A, Abu Osba Y, et al. Mast Cell Numbers in Primary Eosinophilic Colitis are Significantly Higher than in Secondary Tissue Eosinophilia and Normal Control: a Possible Link to Pathogenesis. Iran J Immunol 2021;18:220–9.

96. Torrente F, Barabino A, Bellini T, et al. Intraepithelial lymphocyte eotaxin-2 expression and perineural mast cell degranulation differentiate allergic/eosinophilic colitis from classic IBD. J Pediatr Gastroenterol Nutr 2014;59:300–7.

97. Dellon ES, Rothenberg ME, Collins MH, et al. Dupilumab in Adults and Adolescents with Eosinophilic Esophagitis. N Engl J Med 2022;387:2317–30.

98. Morales JK, Falanga YT, Depcrynski A, et al. Mast cell homeostasis and the JAK-STAT pathway. Genes Immun 2010;11:599–608.

99. Suresh RV, Dunnam C, Vaidya D, et al. A phase II study of Bruton's tyrosine kinase inhibition for the prevention of anaphylaxis. J Clin Invest 2023;133.

100. Terhorst-Molawi D, Hawro T, Grekowitz E, et al. Anti-KIT antibody, barzolvolimab, reduces skin mast cells and disease activity in chronic inducible urticaria. Allergy 2023;78:1269–79.

Associations of Eosinophilic Gastrointestinal Disorders with Other Gastrointestinal and Allergic Diseases

Salvatore Oliva, MD, PhD[a],*, Emily Clarke McGowan, MD, PhD[b]

KEYWORDS

- Eosinophilic esophagitis • Eosinophilic gastrointestinal diseases • Allergy
- Inflammatory bowel disease • Celiac disease

KEY POINTS

- Eosinophilic gastrointestinal disorders (EGIDs) are characterized by allergic inflammation, and the prevalence of other allergic conditions in EGIDs patients is high.
- The presentation and management of eosinophilic esophagitis (EoE) may be influenced by other allergic conditions, in particular food allergy and allergic rhinitis.
- Although EGIDs are defined by the exclusion of other causes of gastrointestinal (GI) eosinophilia, these conditions may also coexist with inflammatory bowel disease, celiac disease, gastroesophageal reflux disease, and motility disorders.
- The exact prevalence of coexisting GI conditions with EoE and non-EoE EGIDs remains unclear, posing a challenge in determining whether these associations are genuine or if there is an overlap in clinical presentation complicating the diagnostic process.
- Ongoing research is essential to better understand the relationships between these allergic and GI conditions, providing insights into their interplay and implications for diagnosis and treatment.

INTRODUCTION

Eosinophilic gastrointestinal disorders (EGIDs) constitute a diverse group of conditions marked by substantial eosinophilic inflammation affecting various segments of the digestive tract. These disorders manifest in the absence of secondary factors such as infections or drug reactions.[1,2] Eosinophils typically exhibit an activated state,

[a] Department of Maternal and Child Health, Pediatric Gastroenterology and Liver Unit, Sapienza University of Rome, Viale Regina Elena 324, Rome 00161, Italy; [b] Division of Allergy and Immunology, Departments of Internal Medicine and Pediatrics, University of Virginia School of Medicine, P.O. Box 801355, Charlottesville, VA 22908, USA
* Corresponding author.
E-mail address: salvatore.oliva@uniroma1.it

Immunol Allergy Clin N Am 44 (2024) 329–348
https://doi.org/10.1016/j.iac.2024.01.005
0889-8561/24/© 2024 Elsevier Inc. All rights reserved.
immunology.theclinics.com

leading to symptoms stemming from organ dysfunction. EGIDs encompass distinct entities based on the specific site of inflammation, including eosinophilic esophagitis (EoE), eosinophilic gastritis/enteritis (EoG/EoN), and eosinophilic colitis (EoC).[3] Although these conditions can affect both pediatric and adult populations, their clinical presentations differ by age.[4]

Recognition of these disorders is on the rise, although their true prevalence has likely been underestimated due to limited awareness and a lack of standardized diagnostic criteria.[5,6] Moreover, because definitive diagnosis often hinges on endoscopic procedures, recent data suggest that these conditions may be underdiagnosed. Of note, EoE is the most prevalent EGID (0.5–1 per 1000 individuals in the general population), making it the most extensively researched.[7] In contrast, the prevalence of EoG, EoN, and EoC may only reach as high as 6.3 per 100,000, 8.4 per 100,000, and 3.3 per 100,000, respectively.[8]

Since the time of their initial description, EGIDs have been considered to be an allergic disease. EoE is characterized by epithelial barrier dysfunction,[9] epithelial cell production of thymic stromal lymphopoietin, tissue infiltration of eosinophils, mast cells, and T cells, and increased levels of Th2 cytokines.[10–13] Similarly, genome-wide transcript profiles in EoG demonstrate increased interleukin (IL)-4, IL-5, IL-13, and mast cell-specific transcripts, which are characteristic of allergic inflammation.[14] In addition, EoE and non-EoE EGIDs are known to be triggered by food in the majority of individuals, as patients achieve both histologic and clinical remission on elemental and empirical elimination diets.[15–20] Finally, the vast majority of patients with EGIDs have other allergic diseases such as food allergy, asthma, eczema, or allergic rhinitis,[21–24] and two recent screening studies suggest that the prevalence of EoE may be markedly higher in patients with allergic disease than previous estimates.[5]

The objective of this review is to present a summary of the association between EGIDs and other allergic conditions both in adults and children. Concurrently, we have explored potential associations between EGIDs and other GI ailments that frequently exhibit overlapping symptoms or are considered in the differential diagnosis process, such as gastroesophageal reflux disease (GERD), celiac disease, motility disorders, achalasia, and inflammatory bowel disease (IBD). The aim of this review is to improve the diagnosis and management of allergic and gastrointestinal (GI) comorbidities in patients with EGIDs and identify areas for future research.

ALLERGY AND EOSINOPHILIC GASTROINTESTINAL DISORDERS

Epidemiologic data strongly suggest an association between EGIDs and allergic disease, as the vast majority of patients with these conditions have allergic comorbidities, including IgE-mediated food allergy, allergic rhinitis, asthma, and eczema.[21–24] In addition, many studies have shown that EGIDs may be influenced by other allergic conditions, in particular food allergy and allergic rhinitis, which has led some to suggest that EGIDs (in particular EoE) may be part of the atopic march.[25,26] The association between allergic disease and EGIDs has been best studied in EoE—given the higher overall prevalence of this condition—but recent studies have also demonstrated similar trends in EoG and EoN. It has been suggested that EoC may not have as strong of an association with allergic disease, as gene expression profiling demonstrated minimal evidence of underlying Th2 mechanisms in this condition.[27] The authors summarize the existing data for an association between EGID and food allergy, allergic rhinitis, asthma, and atopic dermatitis (AD), with considerations for both EoE and non-EoE EGIDs.

Immunoglobulin E-Mediated Food Allergy

Eosinophilic esophagitis

Although EoE, EoG, and EoN have been shown to be driven by food allergens, the inflammatory response is distinct from that seen in "classic" immunoglobulin E (IgE)-mediated food allergy, in which a systemic response happens immediately on ingestion of a relevant food allergen due to IgE cross-linking on mast cells and basophils. Recent data, however, suggest that there is a close association between EoE and IgE-mediated food allergy. Epidemiologically, approximately 25% to 70% of patients with EoE have concomitant IgE-mediated food allergy.[28,29] Conversely, among patients with IgE-mediated food allergy, Hill and colleagues reported an EoE prevalence of 4.7%, which is approximately 100-fold higher than in the general population.[30] This observation was recently confirmed in a registry study of patients with IgE-mediated food allergy, where 5% (309/6074) of subjects with food allergy reported a diagnosis of EoE. Furthermore, the risk of EoE was higher in those with a greater number of food allergies, more food allergy reactions, and higher measures of reaction severity,[31] suggesting coexistence in a more severe food allergy phenotype.

Because the symptoms of EoE are gradually progressive, the diagnosis requires an upper endoscopy, and there have not been any large-scale screening studies, it is possible that the prevalence of EoE among patients with food allergy is higher than current estimates. When performing upper endoscopies in children with a history of anaphylaxis to cow's milk, Barbosa and colleagues found that 38% had esophageal eosinophilia (>15 eosinophils per high-powered field), and many did not report chronic GI or esophageal symptoms.[32] Similarly, 14% of adults with peanut allergy who had screening endoscopies before initiation of oral immunotherapy (OIT) were found to have subclinical esophageal eosinophilia at baseline.[33] Given the lack of large-scale screening studies, the true prevalence of EoE and asymptomatic esophageal eosinophilia among patients with food allergy—and whether asymptomatic disease requires therapy—is currently unknown and warrants further study.

The relationship between EoE and IgE-mediated food allergy is further complicated in the setting of OIT, a treatment for food allergy in which a patient receives increasing doses of the relevant food allergen to achieve desensitization and/or sustained unresponsiveness. The most common cause for discontinuing this therapy is the development of GI symptoms, specifically abdominal pain.[34] Recent studies have demonstrated that patients on OIT may develop EoE, which is estimated to occur in 2.7% to 5.1% of patients based on a retrospective review and meta-analysis.[34,35] However, these estimates are based on endoscopic evaluation, which does not occur in all patients, so this is likely an underestimate of the true prevalence. Whether EoE develops de novo, or previously existed as subclinical disease that was unmasked during OIT, is currently unknown.

Non-eosinophilic esophagitis eosinophilic gastrointestinal disorders

Early case studies and single-center retrospective studies have similarly demonstrated an association between food allergy and non-EoE EGIDs.[36,37] This was then extended in 2017 using a population-based database of more than 75 million individuals enrolled in commercial insurance from 2009 to 2011. In this study, Jensen and colleagues found that the prevalence of food allergy was higher in the EoG, EoN, and EoC populations than the source controls (1.2%, 3.4%, 2.0%, and 0.2%, respectively).[22] These results were then confirmed in population-based study of more than 35 million individuals in the United States from 2012 to 2017, where those with EoG/EoN and EoC were more likely to be diagnosed with food allergy than controls (EoG/EoN OR 12.20; $P<.0001$; EoC OR 8.25, $P < .0001$).[23] Finally, in a retrospective study of

373 patients with non-EoE EGIDs seen at six tertiary care centers in the United States between 2005 and 2016, 117 (31%) had a history of food allergy (EoG 29%, EoN 46%, EoC 19%),[24] confirming the association between these two conditions.[38]

Owing to the lack of a noninvasive biomarker or diagnostic test for non-EoE EGIDs, the prevalence of these conditions among patients with food allergy is currently unknown. However, there are emerging data to suggest that the prevalence of non-EoE EGIDs among patients with food allergy may be higher than in other populations. In the same screening study of adults with food allergy presenting for peanut OIT described above, the investigators also assessed for gastric and duodenal eosinophilia before initiating therapy.[33] They found that 42% of subjects had gastric (>12 eos/hpf) and duodenal (>26 eos/hpf) eosinophilia at baseline.[33] Furthermore, during OIT, all patients were found to have either gastric or duodenal eosinophilia, and 29% exceeded the thresholds for EoG and EoN (>30 eos in 5 and 2 hpf, respectively).[39] Further study on the prevalence and predictors of non-EoE EGIDs in patients with food allergy, as well as the development of a noninvasive biomarker or screening tool, is clearly needed.

Allergic Rhinitis

Eosinophilic esophagitis

It is now well established that there is a strong association between allergic rhinitis—or hay fever—and EoE. A large systematic review and meta-analysis of 12 studies found that allergic rhinitis was significantly more common in patients with EoE than healthy controls (OR 5.09; 95% CI 2.91–8.90), and this was seen in both children and adults.[28] More recently, large-scale cohort studies have demonstrated that approximately 60% of patients with EoE have comorbid allergic rhinitis.[21,40] Conversely, a recent study using administrative coding across six academic institutions in the US suggests that the prevalence of EoE among patients with chronic rhinosinusitis may be eightfold higher than in the general population.[41]

In addition to this epidemiologic association, it is increasingly recognized that aeroallergen exposure may contribute to EoE symptoms in some individuals. Several studies have now demonstrated an increase in the diagnosis of EoE during spring, summer, and fall months.[42–44] Similarly, esophageal food impactions due to EoE have been shown to occur more frequently in the summer and fall.[45] Furthermore, among children and adults with established EoE, a subset had biopsy-confirmed variation in their esophageal eosinophil counts with aeroallergen exposure.[46,47] Using a national pathology database, Jensen and colleagues further demonstrated that the odds of having a biopsy with esophageal eosinophilia was higher in the late spring and summer months (OR 1.13; 95% CI 1.03–1.24).[48] These data suggest that aeroallergen exposure may contribute to disease exacerbation in select patients.

There are also data to suggest that pollen exposure may affect treatment response in patients with aeroallergen sensitization (ie, positive skin prick test or serum IgE > 0.35 kU/L). A recent study examined the efficacy of the six-food elimination diet (SFED) by pollen season among adults with EoE. They found that those sensitized to aeroallergens (ie, IgE to birch and/or grass pollen) had a lower response to the SFED during the pollen season (21.4%) compared with the same individuals outside the pollen season (77.3%). Among patients without sensitization, however, 77.8% achieved remission with the SFED during the pollen season.[49] Similar findings were observed in children with EoE, in which those who were sensitized to perennial and mold allergens were less likely to respond to proton pump inhibitor (PPI) therapy.[50] Case reports have suggested that subcutaneous immunotherapy as treatment for allergic rhinitis may benefit a subset of EoE patients, but these data are currently limited.[51,52] These observations suggest that treatment response may vary by season in select individuals, and optimizing treatment of allergic rhinitis in patients with EoE is essential.

Non-eosinophilic esophagitis eosinophilic gastrointestinal disorders

Previous studies have consistently demonstrated an association between allergic rhinitis and non-EoE EGIDs, but with less convincing evidence than for EoE. In the cross-sectional study of commercially insured individuals in the United States mentioned above, Jensen and colleagues found a higher prevalence of allergic rhinitis in the EoG, EoN, and EoC populations than controls (EoG: 27.7%; EoN: 30.2%; EoC: 30.0%; and controls: 13.3%, respectively). In comparison, the prevalence of allergic rhinitis in the EoE population in this study was 48.1%.[22] Mansoor and colleagues similarly found that individuals with EoG and EoN were more likely to have allergic rhinitis than controls (EoG: 33.5%; EoN: 27.3%; controls: 8.9%).[23] This high prevalence of allergic rhinitis was subsequently confirmed in a cohort of EGIDs patients seen at six tertiary care centers in the United States (EoG: 24%; EoN: 31%; EoC: 14%).[38] To date, no studies have identified seasonal variation in non-EoE EGIDs symptoms or complications, and whether aeroallergens play a role in the pathophysiology of these conditions is unclear.

Asthma

Eosinophilic esophagitis

As with the other allergic conditions discussed in this review, there is a strong association between asthma and EoE. Most of the existing literature on coexisting disease is derived from studies examining the prevalence of asthma among patients with EoE. Retrospective studies have demonstrated that 12% to 68% of adults with EoE have a diagnosis of asthma[21,53–56] and studies using administrative databases have identified a prevalence of 23% to 29%.[57–59] Among children with EoE, there is similarly a high prevalence, with an estimate of 22% to 70%.[21,60,61] In the systematic review and meta-analysis described above, 16 studies examined the frequency of asthma in patients with EoE and were included in the analysis. The investigators found that asthma is more common in individuals with EoE than controls (OR 3.01; 95% CI 1.96–4.62), and this is true for both children and adults.[28]

A few studies to date have examined whether the presence of asthma impacts the clinical presentation or treatment of EoE. One recent case report described an adult with previously controlled asthma who had recurrent asthma exacerbations in the setting of newly diagnosed EoE, which improved with treatment of her EoE.[62] In a prospective study of esophageal remodeling in children with EoE, Rajan and colleagues found that children who had concomitant asthma had higher esophageal eosinophil levels at baseline than those without asthma. They further found that more children with asthma did not respond to topical steroid treatment of their EoE than those without asthma.[63] In an exploratory analysis of 33 children with EoE, Krupp and colleagues further found that children who had EoE and asthma had higher levels of fibroblast growth factor-2 than EoE patients without asthma. Finally, when comparing 156 adults with asthma and EoE to 276 adults with only asthma, Harer and colleagues found that those with asthma and EoE were more likely to be younger, male, have allergic asthma and have peripheral eosinophilia.[64]

Non-eosinophilic esophagitis eosinophilic gastrointestinal disorders

Similar to EoE, individuals with non-EoE EGIDs have a higher prevalence of asthma than the general population. In cross-sectional studies of administrative databases in the United States, the prevalence of asthma is 16% to 33% among patients with

EoG/EoN and 15% to 23% among patients with EoC.[22,38] This is significantly higher than the prevalence of asthma in the study control populations (8%–9%; $P < .01$). There are no studies to our knowledge demonstrating differences in clinical presentation or treatment outcomes among patients with non-EoE EGIDs and asthma. However, there are case reports of patients who have improvement in their EoG/EoN with anti-IL5 therapy for severe asthma[65,66] suggesting shared underlying mechanisms.

Atopic Dermatitis

Eosinophilic esophagitis

EoE and AD are both characterized by T2 inflammation and a disrupted epithelial barrier,[67,68] and recent studies have shown that AD and EoE share a common set of disease-specific ribonucleic acid (RNA) transcripts centered around the IL-13 pathway.[69] Similar to the other allergic conditions discussed in this review, patients with EoE are at higher risk for AD, with an estimated prevalence of 6% to 28% in adults and 17% to 61% in children.[21,54,58,61] A recent systematic review and meta-analysis compiled data from 10 studies and found that AD is more common in patients with EoE than controls (OR 2.85; 95% CI 1.87–4.34), and this risk is higher in both children and adults.[28] Conversely, the prevalence of EoE among patients with AD was recently explored in the All of Us Research Program, a National Institutes of Health research program in which recruitment is prioritized from groups that are historically underrepresented in clinical research. In this cross-sectional study of 240,635 subjects, the prevalence of EoE among those with AD was 0.8%, which was significantly higher than in the non-AD population (0.3%), for an odds ratio of 1.82 (95% CI 1.43–2.30; $P < .01$).[70]

One study to date has examined whether EoE disease severity is modified by the presence of AD. In a single-center retrospective study of 76 children with EoE, Daley and colleagues found that subjects with EoE and AD had a higher level of esophageal eosinophilia at the time of diagnosis, but there was no association with esophageal fibrosis, strictures, or food impactions. This study was limited, however, by the small sample size and the limited number of fibrostenotic complications in the study population.[71] Sessions and colleagues examined whether the presence of AD modifies treatment outcomes in children with EoE. In a single-center retrospective review of 137 children with EoE, the investigators found that children with AD achieved histologic remission faster than those with asthma, food allergies, or allergic rhinitis.[72] Whether this finding is true in the adult population, and whether the presence of AD confers a milder EoE phenotype is unclear and warrants further investigation.

Non-eosinophilic esophagitis eosinophilic gastrointestinal disorders

Atopic dermatitis is estimated to affect 5% to 20% of patients with EoG/EoN and 6% to 18% of patients with EoC, compared with 3% to 6% in the general population.[22,38] To our knowledge, whether the presence of AD impacts the clinical presentation or treatment outcomes in patients with non-EoE EGIDs has not yet been examined but warrants future investigation.

OTHER GASTROINTESTINAL CONDITIONS AND EOSINOPHILIC GASTROINTESTINAL DISORDERS
Inflammatory Bowel Disease

Eosinophilic esophagitis

IBD and EoE exhibit numerous similarities, encompassing shared etiologic mechanisms, such as environmental exposure in genetically predisposed individuals. Both conditions demonstrate parallel epidemiologic trends, with an increasing incidence, more prevalence in developed nations, and a higher occurrence among young patients.[73,74] In addition, there are overlapping features such as potential inflammatory and fibrotic phenotypes, and, to some extent, shared therapeutic interventions.[75] Key treatment modalities for both diseases involve anti-inflammatory measures and dietary interventions, forming the cornerstone of induction and maintenance therapy. Of note, a recent research has proposed common pathogenetic pathways linking these conditions, particularly involving abnormalities in intestinal epithelial barrier function.[76] For instance, Crohn's disease is marked by heightened mucosal expression of IL-5 and eosinophilic infiltrate, akin to the increased presence of eotaxin in ulcerative colitis (UC), a protein facilitating eosinophil recruitment. The Predicting Response to Standardized Pediatric Colitis Therapy study has further suggested that UC patients with eosinophilic infiltrates in rectal biopsies exhibit less aggressive disease.[77]

Although the diagnosis of EoE requires the exclusion of other causes of esophageal eosinophilia, including IBD, EoE and IBD have been reported to coexist in children and adults. A recent paper revealed that the overall prevalence of EoE within the pediatric IBD population is 0.35%, showing a modest, though statistically nonsignificant, increase over the past 6 years compared with the preceding period (0.45% vs 0.2%).[78] These results align with previous reports, although the limited existing literature on this subject in children presents divergent findings. Of note, another study by Moore and colleagues reported a higher prevalence of EoE within the pediatric IBD population (1.5%), whereas earlier small-scale studies yielded lower prevalence.[79] In the realm of adults, epidemiologic data exhibit considerable heterogeneity. For instance, Limketkai and colleagues, in a population-based cohort comprising 376,822 patients with Crohn's, reported a prevalence of 594.2 per 100,000, with rates significantly higher in Crohn's patients compared with the non-IBD population.[80] Conversely, Fan and colleagues observed a lower prevalence (0.1%) in their cohort of adults with IBD.[81] These variations underscore the complexity and variability in the prevalence of EoE and IBD comorbidity across different populations and studies. Nonetheless, numerous pieces of evidence indicate a notable surge in the incidence and prevalence of both EoE and IBD over recent decades, particularly in industrialized nations.[82–87] Currently, the impact of a concurrent diagnosis on the phenotype, natural history, and specific clinical implications for each disease remains uncertain and warrants further study.

These findings strongly suggest the existence of potential common pathogenetic mechanisms and shared environmental factors underpinning EoE and IBD.[88] Of note, both conditions are linked to family clusters and specific predisposition genes, exhibiting an overexpression of pro-eosinophilic cytokines and increased toll-like receptor activity.[89–91] Furthermore, a recent research highlights an augmented mucosal expression of IL-13, a cytokine implicated in the compromised functionality of the GI barrier. This may lead to possible aberrant responses to the microbiota inhabiting the digestive tract.[92]

Recently, a pediatric paper also investigated the clinical trajectory of IBD in individuals concurrently diagnosed with EoE. This study strongly suggests that the coexistence of both disorders is linked to a milder disease course when compared with individuals with IBD alone. Specifically, they revealed that patients diagnosed with only IBD exhibited a significantly higher risk of escalating treatment and experiencing hospitalizations at the 2-year follow-up, in contrast to those with the dual diagnosis of EoE-IBD.[78] Conversely, other studies did not reveal substantial differences in the natural progression and phenotype between IBD-only and cases associated with EoE.[93] Further prospective studies will elucidate potential pathogenetic mechanisms common to both conditions and provide additional support for the epidemiologic and phenotypic distinctions between the two groups.

Non-eosinophilic esophagitis eosinophilic gastrointestinal disorders

Although the precise nature of the relationship remains to be fully elucidated, it has been noted that EGIDs have been reported in conjunction with IBD.[8,94] Early studies describing mucosal biopsies of patients with IBD revealed mucosal eosinophilia compared with healthy controls. Unlike the esophagus, eosinophils are resident cells of the small and large intestines, and the normal number of eosinophils is not well-defined, making interpretation of pathologic intestinal eosinophilia difficult. Clinical implications of mucosal eosinophils in IBD are unknown, especially because mucosal eosinophilia is increased in IBD compared with irritable bowel syndrome.[95,96] Of note, gastric eosinophil counts, encompassing both the gastric antrum and gastric body, were significantly elevated in children diagnosed with celiac disease (CD) compared with children with functional abdominal pain disorders or individuals with no GI issues. However, when comparing eosinophil counts between the latter two groups, it is important to note that eosinophil counts were higher at all levels of the GI tract, spanning from the stomach to the rectum.[97] Some studies found that the severity of eosinophilic inflammation in patients with UC was the most significant predictor of lack of response to therapy.[98] Given the infrequency of EGIDs and the potential presence of eosinophils in mucosal inflammatory infiltration associated with IBD, it is crucial to ascertain whether the coexistence of these two conditions is genuine or if it simply reflects IBD with unconventional mucosal alterations involving eosinophils. To navigate this distinction, it may be beneficial to consider the histologic thresholds recommended by the recent ESPGHAN/NASPGHAN guidelines for EGIDs.[8]

Celiac Disease

Eosinophilic esophagitis

Both celiac disease and EoE are immune-mediated disorders triggered by dietary antigens. Symptom resolution and histologic improvements in both CD and EoE can be achieved through the avoidance of these dietary triggers.[99] The etiology of both diseases involves an imbalance in the Th1/Th2 pathway. Despite sharing similarities in symptoms, immune-mediated origins, and the management approach involving allergen avoidance, it is crucial to recognize that CD and EoE are distinct entities. Numerous studies, both in adults and children, have explored the potential association between CD and EoE.[100,101] However, the findings have been inconsistent, with varying degrees of association or dissociation between these two conditions. Consequently, recommendations regarding the necessity of routine esophageal biopsies during CD evaluations have been inconsistent as well.[102]

The exploration of the association between CD and EoE gained momentum following Verzegnassi and colleagues' description of their co-occurrence.[103] Subsequent studies have reported varying degrees of co-occurrence, reaching as high as 35.2%.[104] In cases where patients underwent both esophageal and duodenal biopsies simultaneously, the prevalence of CD and EoE coexistence was lower than initially reported but still significantly higher than their individual prevalence in the general population.[105]

The incidence and prevalence of both CD and EoE are on the rise.[83] However, whether this signifies a genuine surge in incidence or is attributed to heightened awareness, improved diagnostic tests, or an increased number of endoscopic procedures in children is unclear. Children with either condition often exhibit similar GI symptoms, with abdominal pain and vomiting being the most commonly reported.[100]

Consequently, the simultaneous presence of both conditions should be anticipated, particularly in children presenting with suggestive GI symptoms seeking medical attention.

Non-eosinophilic esophagitis eosinophilic gastrointestinal disorders

Celiac disease and non-EoE EGIDs are distinct conditions, but there is ongoing research exploring potential associations and connections between them. Celiac disease and EGIDs can share some GI symptoms, such as abdominal pain, diarrhea, and nausea. This overlap in clinical presentation might lead to misdiagnosis or delayed diagnosis, highlighting the importance of considering both conditions in patients with persistent GI issues.[106]

As celiac disease and some EGIDs involve autoimmune responses, there may be a complex interplay between the immune mechanisms responsible for each condition. Understanding how these autoimmune pathways interact could provide valuable insights into their potential association.[107]

It is crucial to note that the current understanding of the relationship between celiac disease and non-EoE EGIDs is still evolving, and more research is needed to establish a clear connection. Clinicians should remain vigilant in considering the possibility of coexisting conditions in patients with GI symptoms and pursue thorough diagnostic evaluations to ensure accurate and timely management.

Gastroesophageal Reflux Disease

Eosinophilic esophagitis

GERD and EoE have evolved as distinct disorders, each presenting with unique clinical features. Although GERD commonly manifests with heartburn and regurgitation, EoE presents with dysphagia and food impaction. However, symptom overlap made it challenging to differentiate the two initially, leading to the misconception that eosinophils in the esophagus were solely indicative of GERD. The diagnostic landscape shifted with the recognition of PPI-responsive esophageal eosinophilia (PPI-REE), blurring the lines between GERD and EoE. The 2018 AGREE conference redefined PPIs as a treatment rather than a diagnostic criterion for EoE, acknowledging the substantial overlap between PPI-REE and EoE.[108] Importantly, the use of PPIs in infancy has been linked to an increased risk of developing EoE.[109] The interplay between GERD and EoE involves complex mechanisms, with GERD potentially increasing esophageal mucosal permeability, allowing food antigens to incite allergic responses and contribute to EoE. Conversely, EoE may influence GERD by altering lower esophageal sphincter (LES) function and esophageal motility. Research priorities aim to unravel the fundamental pathophysiology of EoE, striving to understand why this allergic disorder has become increasingly prevalent over the past two decades and how it is pathologically distinct from GERD.

Non-eosinophilic esophagitis eosinophilic gastrointestinal disorders

Given that non-EoE EGIDs primarily impact areas other than the esophagus, the simultaneous presence of GERD may not necessarily be linked to the underlying condition. Nevertheless, inflammation in the upper GI tract can induce GERD-like symptoms. Many non-EoE EGIDs patients often require PPIs for symptom management. Although the direct use of PPIs in treating non-EoE EGIDs remains uncertain, some reports suggest a connection to their conventional use in comorbid peptic disease. Of note, case reports mention PPI use in patients with EoG. In a recent retrospective multicenter study involving children with EoC and EoG, PPIs were used in 30% of patients alongside various treatments such as elimination diets, combination therapies involving diet and medication, systemic steroids, topical steroids/crushed enteric budesonide, and 5-aminosalicylates (5-ASA).[110] Consequently, the coexistence of GERD with EGIDs is plausible, emphasizing the importance of tailored treatment based on symptomatology.

Motility Disorders

Eosinophilic esophagitis

The functional pathophysiology of symptoms in EoE is often overshadowed, with a primary focus on histology and endoscopic appearances. Although fibrosis-related strictures and narrowing can occur in EoE, there are instances where patients remain symptomatic despite achieving histologic remission and showing no signs of fibrostenotic disease during endoscopy.[111] In this scenario, it is helpful to suspect a possible association with a motility disorder. Indeed, high-resolution manometry (HRM) becomes a reasonable next step in the assessment of patients who continue to experience esophageal symptoms even after seemingly adequate treatment for EoE.

Studies investigating esophageal motility patterns in EoE reveal a spectrum of patterns, ranging from nonspecific and normal to hypotensive and ineffective motility, and even obstructive features resembling achalasia. Using HRM, several alterations in esophageal motility were found in patients with EoE, such as esophagogastric junction outflow obstruction, ineffective esophageal motility, distal esophageal spasm, hypercontractile esophagus, and many of these alterations often resolved after surgical or drug therapy.[112] Dysmotility seems to correlate with disease severity, duration, and symptoms, especially in cases of obstruction. Esophageal wall thickness also seems to relate to contractile vigor and, consequently, symptoms.[113,114]

Achalasia, a severe esophageal motility disorder characterized by the absence of esophageal peristalsis and LES relaxation, has traditionally been regarded as rare but has shown a substantial increase in incidence and prevalence in recent years.[115,116] This surge parallels the rising frequency of allergic disorders, including EoE. Eosinophils, key effector cells in allergies, are not typically found in the esophagus but have been observed in achalasia patients.[117] Numerous reports document cases of individuals with both achalasia and EoE, and achalasia-like motility abnormalities have been known to resolve with steroid treatment for EoE. A retrospective cohort study from the United Kingdom found a significant association between achalasia and atopic disorders in patients less than 40 years.[118] The accumulation of eosinophils and mast cells in the EoE esophagus produces substances that can affect esophageal smooth muscle and potentially cause motility disturbances characteristic of achalasia. The strong association between achalasia and EoE suggests the possibility of an allergic etiology for some cases of achalasia.[119] As there are documented cases of achalasia-like motility abnormalities resolving with EoE treatment, careful evaluation for EoE in achalasia patients before initiating invasive achalasia therapies is recommended, as treating underlying allergic pathology may restore normal esophageal function in some achalasia cases.[120]

Esophageal planimetry, such as endoluminal functional lumen imaging probe (EndoFLIP), offers a potential means of assessing esophageal compliance. Although currently experimental, it may find its way into routine clinical practice in the future.[114] One potential limitation in these studies is that HRM assessments are often conducted using small volume water swallows, which may not accurately replicate the symptoms experienced by EoE patients when consuming solid food. In addition, it may not reflect normal eating behavior. The correlation of HRM metrics with symptoms in patients is not yet fully established. Given that EoE frequently involves solid food dysphagia, relying solely on small volume water swallows during HRM might explain the variability in manometry patterns documented in the literature. Studies have shown an increased diagnostic yield of motility disorders by including solid swallows during HRM, especially in patients with functional obstruction, leading to its incorporation as a standard in the latest iteration of the Chicago Classification of motility disorders.[119]

To address persistent, refractory dysphagia in EoE patients with seemingly normal endoscopic findings, the British guideline recommends a comprehensive evaluation, incorporating esophageal physiologic testing and, where appropriate, barium swallow studies.[120] Moreover, the inclusion of solid swallows during HRM is suggested to better replicate the symptoms associated with EoE.

Non-eosinophilic esophagitis eosinophilic gastrointestinal disorders

The link between non-EoE EGIDs and motility disorders underscores the varied clinical expressions of these conditions. EoG manifests with persistent nonspecific GI symptoms that can mimic gastroparesis, whereas the clinical presentation of EoC varies based on mucosal, transmural, or serosal involvement.[121] Despite the potential similarity in clinical presentation to chronic intestinal pseudo-obstruction,[122] the investigation into motility alterations in these disorders remains limited. However, it is crucial to consistently explore the exclusion of motility disorders before arriving at a conclusive diagnosis of non-EoE EGIDs.[8]

A significant challenge in diagnosing the coexistence of these conditions arises from their rarity, and measurements of enteric nervous system involvement often rely on surgical samples obtained when complications, such as bowel obstructions and prompt intervention. As both conditions are infrequent, there is a critical need for more in-depth research into their shared motility aspects to enhance diagnostic accuracy and refine treatment strategies.

SUMMARY

In summary, there is an intricate connection between EGIDs, allergic conditions, and other GI conditions. Shared etiologic mechanisms and epidemiologic trends exist, prompting exploration into common pathogenetic pathways. Many individuals diagnosed with EoE and non-EoE EGIDs often concurrently experience other allergic conditions, including but not limited to food allergies, allergic rhinitis, asthma, and eczema. Recent data suggest that the presence of these coexisting conditions may impact the manifestation and treatment of EoE. Although this connection is being explored, further investigation is required to discern whether these factors similarly influence the diagnosis and management of non-EoE EGIDs. In addition, both EoE and non-EGIDs are frequently linked with other GI conditions such as IBD, celiac disease, GERD, and motility disorders. The precise prevalence of these coexisting conditions with EoE and non-EoE EGIDs remains unknown. Determining whether there is a genuine association or if the observed overlap in clinical presentation complicates the diagnostic process is often a challenging task. The overlap between IBD, celiac disease, and EoE, both immune-mediated and influenced by dietary triggers, underscores the necessity of considering these conditions concurrently, given the simultaneous increase in their incidence and prevalence. The evolving landscape of GERD and EoE relationships highlights dynamic diagnostic criteria and complex mechanisms, necessitating ongoing research to unravel their fundamental pathophysiology. Motility disorders, especially in the context of EoE, add complexity, emphasizing the importance of considering motility assessments in patients with persistent symptoms. The intricate relationships between non-EoE EGIDs and various GI conditions reinforce the need for a holistic diagnostic approach. In conclusion, this review enhances our understanding of allergy-GI relationships, emphasizing the imperative for ongoing research to elucidate mechanisms and improve diagnostic precision. The complexities unveiled pave the way for future investigations, contributing to more effective management approaches and improved patient outcomes in allergy-associated GI disorders.

CLINICS CARE POINTS

- Interconnection betwenn EGIDs, Allergy, and GI conditions
- Overlap Between Celiac Disease and EoE
- Dynamic GERD and EoE relationship
- Significance of Motility Disoders
- Holistic Diagnostic Approach for Non-EoE EGIDs
- Ongoing Research and Improved Precision
- Future Directions

DISCLOSURE

S. Oliva serves as a consultant and speaker and has received grants from Medtronic, Regeneron/Sanofi, Bristol Myers Squibb. E.C. McGowan has received grant support from the National Institutes of Health, the American College of Gastroenterology and Regeneron/Sanofi (all funds to the University of Virginia) and has served as a consultant to Regeneron/Sanofi. No honorarium, grant, or other form of payment was given to anyone to write or produce the article.

REFERENCES

1. Cianferoni A, Spergel JM. Eosinophilic Esophagitis and Gastroenteritis. Curr Allergy Asthma Rep 2015;15(9):58. https://doi.org/10.1007/s11882-015-0558-5.
2. Spergel JM, Brown-Whitehorn TA, Muir A, et al. Medical algorithm: Diagnosis and treatment of eosinophilic esophagitis in children. Allergy 2020;75(6):1522–4. https://doi.org/10.1111/all.14188.
3. Dellon ES, Gonsalves N, Abonia JP, et al. International Consensus Recommendations for Eosinophilic Gastrointestinal Disease Nomenclature. Clin Gastroenterol Hepatol 2022;20(11):2474–2484 e3. https://doi.org/10.1016/j.cgh.2022.02.017.
4. Oliva S, Dias JA, Rea F, et al. Characterization of Eosinophilic Esophagitis From the European Pediatric Eosinophilic Esophagitis Registry (pEEr) of ESPGHAN. J Pediatr Gastroenterol Nutr 2022;75(3):325–33. https://doi.org/10.1097/MPG.0000000000003530.
5. Eid R, Noonan E, Borish L, et al. High prevalence of gastrointestinal symptoms and undiagnosed eosino-philic esophagitis among allergic adults. J Allergy Clin Immunol Pract 2022;10(12):3325–3327 e1. https://doi.org/10.1016/j.jaip.2022.09.028.
6. Allin KH, Poulsen G, Melgaard D, et al. Eosinophilic oesophagitis in Denmark: Population-based incidence and prevalence in a nationwide study from 2008 to 2018. United European Gastroenterol J 2022;10(7):640–50. https://doi.org/10.1002/ueg2.12273.
7. Lam AY, Lee JK, Coward S, et al. Epidemiologic Burden and Projections for Eosinophilic Esophagitis-Associated Emergency Department Visits in the United States: 2009-2030. Clin Gastroenterol Hepatol 2023;21(12):3041–50, e3.

8. Papadopoulou A, Amil-Dias J, Auth MK, et al. Joint ESPGHAN/NASPG! Guidelines on Childhood Eosinophilic Gastrointestinal Disorders beyond Eos ophilic Esophagitis. J Pediatr Gastroenterol Nutr 2023. https://doi.org/10.1097/ MPG.0000000000003877.

9. O'Shea KM, Aceves SS, Dellon ES, et al. Pathophysiology of Eosinophilic Esophagitis. Gastroenterology 2018;154(2):333–45. https://doi.org/10.1053/j. gastro.2017.06.065.

10. Rothenberg ME, Spergel JM, Sherrill JD, et al. Common variants at 5q22 associate with pediatric eosinophilic esophagitis. Nat Genet 2010;42(4):289–91. https://doi.org/10.1038/ng.547.

11. Chandramouleeswaran PM, Shen D, Lee AJ, et al. Preferential Secretion of Thymic Stromal Lymphopoietin (TSLP) by Terminally Differentiated Esophageal Epithelial Cells: Relevance to Eosinophilic Esophagitis (EoE). PLoS One 2016; 11(3):e0150968. https://doi.org/10.1371/journal.pone.0150968.

12. Wen T, Aronow BJ, Rochman Y, et al. Single-cell RNA sequencing identifies inflammatory tissue T cells in eosinophilic esophagitis. J Clin Invest 2019;129(5): 2014–28. https://doi.org/10.1172/JCI125917.

13. Morgan DM, Ruiter B, Smith NP, et al. Clonally expanded, GPR15-expressing pathogenic effector T(H)2 cells are associated with eosinophilic esophagitis. Sci Immunol 2021;(62):6. https://doi.org/10.1126/sciimmunol.abi5586.

14. Caldwell JM, Collins MH, Stucke EM, et al. Histologic eosinophilic gastritis is a systemic disorder associated with blood and extragastric eosinophilia, TH2 immunity, and a unique gastric transcriptome. J Allergy Clin Immunol 2014;134(5): 1114–24. https://doi.org/10.1016/j.jaci.2014.07.026.

15. Younes M, Schueler SA, Borum M. Histologic Evaluation of Eosinophilic Esophagitis as Part of the Recently Proposed Clinical Severity Index. Gastroenterology 2022;163(6):1719–20. https://doi.org/10.1053/j.gastro.2022.07.025.

16. Kagalwalla AF, Sentongo TA, Ritz S, et al. Effect of six-food elimination diet on clinical and histologic outcomes in eosinophilic esophagitis. Clin Gastroenterol Hepatol 2006;4(9):1097–102. https://doi.org/10.1016/j.cgh.2006.05.026.

17. Molina-Infante J, Arias A, Barrio J, et al. Four-food group elimination diet for adult eosinophilic esophagitis: A prospective multicenter study. J Allergy Clin Immunol 2014;134(5):1093–1099 e1. https://doi.org/10.1016/j.jaci.2014.07.023.

18. Molina-Infante J, Arias A, Alcedo J, et al. Step-up empiric elimination diet for pediatric and adult eosinophilic esophagitis: The 2-4-6 study. J Allergy Clin Immunol 2018;141(4):1365–72. https://doi.org/10.1016/j.jaci.2017.08.038.

19. Wechsler JB, Schwartz S, Arva NC, et al. A Single-Food Milk Elimination Diet Is Effective for Treatment of Eosinophilic Esophagitis in Children. Clin Gastroenterol Hepatol 2022;20(8):1748–56, e11.

20. Gonsalves N, Doerfler B, Zalewski A, et al. Prospective study of an amino acid-based elemental diet in an eosinophilic gastritis and gastroenteritis nutrition trial. J Allergy Clin Immunol 2023;152(3):676–88. https://doi.org/10.1016/j.jaci.2023. 05.024.

21. Chehade M, Jones SM, Pesek RD, et al. Phenotypic Characterization of Eosinophilic Esophagitis in a Large Multicenter Patient Population from the Consortium for Food Allergy Research. J Allergy Clin Immunol Pract 2018;6(5): 1534–1544 e5. https://doi.org/10.1016/j.jaip.2018.05.038.

22. Jensen ET, Martin CF, Kappelman MD, et al. Prevalence of Eosinophilic Gastritis, Gastroenteritis, and Colitis: Estimates From a National Administrative Database. J Pediatr Gastroenterol Nutr 2016;62(1):36–42. https://doi.org/10.1097/MPG. 0000000000000865.

23. Mansoor E, Saleh MA, Cooper GS. Prevalence of Eosinophilic Gastroenteritis and Colitis in a Population-Based Study, From 2012 to 2017. Clin Gastroenterol Hepatol 2017;15(11):1733–41. https://doi.org/10.1016/j.cgh.2017.05.050.

24. Pesek RD, Reed CC, Muir AB, et al. Increasing Rates of Diagnosis, Substantial Co-Occurrence, and Variable Treatment Patterns of Eosinophilic Gastritis, Gastroenteritis, and Colitis Based on 10-Year Data Across a Multicenter Consortium. Am J Gastroenterol 2019;114(6):984–94. https://doi.org/10.14309/ajg.0000000000000228.

25. Hill DA, Grundmeier RW, Ramos M, et al. Eosinophilic Esophagitis Is a Late Manifestation of the Allergic March. J Allergy Clin Immunol Pract 2018;6(5):1528–33. https://doi.org/10.1016/j.jaip.2018.05.010.

26. Hill DA, Spergel JM. Is eosinophilic esophagitis a member of the atopic march? Ann Allergy Asthma Immunol 2018;120(2):113–4. https://doi.org/10.1016/j.anai.2017.10.003.

27. Shoda T, Collins MH, Rochman M, et al. Evaluating Eosinophilic Colitis as a Unique Disease Using Colonic Molecular Profiles: A Multi-Site Study. Gastroenterology 2022;162(6):1635–49. https://doi.org/10.1053/j.gastro.2022.01.022.

28. Gonzalez-Cervera J, Arias A, Redondo-Gonzalez O, et al. Association between atopic manifestations and eosinophilic esophagitis: A systematic review and meta-analysis. Ann Allergy Asthma Immunol 2017;118(5):582–590 e2. https://doi.org/10.1016/j.anai.2017.02.006.

29. Capucilli P, Hill DA. Allergic Comorbidity in Eosinophilic Esophagitis: Mechanistic Relevance and Clinical Implications. Clin Rev Allergy Immunol 2019;57(1):111–27. https://doi.org/10.1007/s12016-019-08733-0.

30. Hill DA, Dudley JW, Spergel JM. The Prevalence of Eosinophilic Esophagitis in Pediatric Patients with IgE-Mediated Food Allergy. J Allergy Clin Immunol Pract 2017;5(2):369–75. https://doi.org/10.1016/j.jaip.2016.11.020.

31. Guarnieri KM, Saba NK, Schwartz JT, et al. Food Allergy Characteristics Associated With Coexisting Eosinophilic Esophagitis in FARE Registry Participants. J Allergy Clin Immunol Pract 2023;11(5):1509–1521 e6. https://doi.org/10.1016/j.jaip.2023.02.008.

32. Barbosa AC, Castro FM, Meireles PR, et al. Eosinophilic Esophagitis: Latent Disease in Patients with Anaphylactic Reaction to Cow's Milk. J Allergy Clin Immunol Pract 2018;6(2):451–456 e1. https://doi.org/10.1016/j.jaip.2017.04.037.

33. Wright BL, Fernandez-Becker NQ, Kambham N, et al. Baseline Gastrointestinal Eosinophilia Is Common in Oral Immunotherapy Subjects With IgE-Mediated Peanut Allergy. Front Immunol 2018;9:2624. https://doi.org/10.3389/fimmu.2018.02624.

34. Petroni D, Spergel JM. Eosinophilic esophagitis and symptoms possibly related to eosinophilic esophagitis in oral immunotherapy. Ann Allergy Asthma Immunol 2018;120(3):237–40, e4.

35. Lucendo AJ, Arias A, Tenias JM. Relation between eosinophilic esophagitis and oral immunotherapy for food allergy: a systematic review with meta-analysis. Ann Allergy Asthma Immunol 2014;113(6):624–9. https://doi.org/10.1016/j.anai.2014.08.004.

36. Ko HM, Morotti RA, Yershov O, et al. Eosinophilic gastritis in children: clinicopathological correlation, disease course, and response to therapy. Am J Gastroenterol 2014;109(8):1277–85. https://doi.org/10.1038/ajg.2014.166.

37. Reed C, Woosley JT, Dellon ES. Clinical characteristics, treatment outcomes, and resource utilization in children and adults with eosinophilic gastroenteritis. Dig Liver Dis 2015;47(3):197–201. https://doi.org/10.1016/j.dld.2014.11.009.

38. Pesek RD, Reed CC, Collins MH, et al. Association Between Endoscopic and Histologic Findings in a Multicenter Retrospective Cohort of Patients with Non-esophageal Eosinophilic Gastrointestinal Disorders. Dig Dis Sci 2020;65(7): 2024–35. https://doi.org/10.1007/s10620-019-05961-4.

39. Wright BL, Fernandez-Becker NQ, Kambham N, et al. Gastrointestinal Eosinophil Responses in a Longitudinal, Randomized Trial of Peanut Oral Immunotherapy. Clin Gastroenterol Hepatol 2021;19(6):1151–1159 e14. https://doi.org/10.1016/j.cgh.2020.05.019.

40. Capucilli P, Cianferoni A, Grundmeier RW, et al. Comparison of comorbid diagnoses in children with and without eosinophilic esophagitis in a large population. Ann Allergy Asthma Immunol 2018;121(6):711–6. https://doi.org/10.1016/j.anai.2018.08.022.

41. Simmons JK, Leiman DA, Patil SU, et al. Increased Prevalence of Eosinophilic Esophagitis in Patients With Chronic Rhinosinusitis. Am J Rhinol Allergy 2022; 36(6):804–7. https://doi.org/10.1177/19458924221116162.

42. Fahey L, Robinson G, Weinberger K, et al. Correlation Between Aeroallergen Levels and New Diagnosis of Eosinophilic Esophagitis in New York City. J Pediatr Gastroenterol Nutr 2017;64(1):22–5. https://doi.org/10.1097/MPG.0000000000001245.

43. Iwanczak B, Janczyk W, Ryzko J, et al. Eosinophilic esophagitis in children: frequency, clinical manifestations, endoscopic findings, and seasonal distribution. Adv Med Sci 2011;56(2):151–7. https://doi.org/10.2478/v10039-011-0038-7.

44. Almansa C, Krishna M, Buchner AM, et al. Seasonal distribution in newly diagnosed cases of eosinophilic esophagitis in adults. Am J Gastroenterol 2009; 104(4):828–33. https://doi.org/10.1038/ajg.2008.169.

45. Ekre M, Tytor J, Bove M, et al. Retrospective chart review: seasonal variation in incidence of bolus impaction is maintained and statistically significant in subgroups with atopy and eosinophilic esophagitis. Dis Esophagus 2020;33(6). https://doi.org/10.1093/dote/doaa013.

46. Ram G, Lee J, Ott M, et al. Seasonal exacerbation of esophageal eosinophilia in children with eosinophilic esophagitis and allergic rhinitis. Ann Allergy Asthma Immunol 2015;115(3):224–228 e1. https://doi.org/10.1016/j.anai.2015.07.004.

47. Reed CC, Iglesia EGA, Commins SP, et al. Seasonal exacerbation of eosinophilic esophagitis histologic activity in adults and children implicates role of aeroallergens. Ann Allergy Asthma Immunol 2019;122(3):296–301. https://doi.org/10.1016/j.anai.2018.12.013.

48. Jensen ET, Shah ND, Hoffman K, et al. Seasonal variation in detection of oesophageal eosinophilia and eosinophilic oesophagitis. Aliment Pharmacol Ther 2015;42(4):461–9. https://doi.org/10.1111/apt.13273.

49. Visaggi P, Savarino E, Del Corso G, et al. Six-Food Elimination Diet Is Less Effective During Pollen Season in Adults With Eosinophilic Esophagitis Sensitized to Pollens. Am J Gastroenterol 2023;118(11):1957–62. https://doi.org/10.14309/ajg.0000000000002357.

50. Pesek RD, Rettiganti M, O'Brien E, et al. Effects of allergen sensitization on response to therapy in children with eosinophilic esophagitis. Ann Allergy Asthma Immunol 2017;119(2):177–83. https://doi.org/10.1016/j.anai.2017.06.006.

51. Iglesia EGA, Commins SP, Dellon ES. Complete remission of eosinophilic esophagitis with multi-aeroallergen subcutaneous immunotherapy: A case report. J Allergy Clin Immunol Pract 2021;9(6):2517–2519 e2. https://doi.org/10.1016/j.jaip.2021.01.045.

52. Robey BS, Eluri S, Reed CC, et al. Subcutaneous immunotherapy in patients with eosinophilic esophagitis. Ann Allergy Asthma Immunol 2019;122(5): 532–3, e3.

53. Hruz P, Straumann A, Bussmann C, et al. Escalating incidence of eosinophilic esophagitis: a 20-year prospective, population-based study in Olten County, Switzerland. J Allergy Clin Immunol 2011;128(6):1349–1350 e5. https://doi. org/10.1016/j.jaci.2011.09.013.

54. Leigh LY, Spergel JM. An in-depth characterization of a large cohort of adult patients with eosinophilic esophagitis. Ann Allergy Asthma Immunol 2019;122(1): 65–72 e1. https://doi.org/10.1016/j.anai.2018.09.452.

55. Prasad GA, Alexander JA, Schleck CD, et al. Epidemiology of eosinophilic esophagitis over three decades in Olmsted County, Minnesota. Clin Gastroenterol Hepatol 2009;7(10):1055–61. https://doi.org/10.1016/j.cgh.2009.06.023.

56. Simon D, Marti H, Heer P, et al. Eosinophilic esophagitis is frequently associated with IgE-mediated allergic airway diseases. J Allergy Clin Immunol 2005;115(5): 1090–2. https://doi.org/10.1016/j.jaci.2005.01.017.

57. Mansoor E, Cooper GS. The 2010-2015 Prevalence of Eosinophilic Esophagitis in the USA: A Population-Based Study. Dig Dis Sci 2016;61(10):2928–34. https:// doi.org/10.1007/s10620-016-4204-4.

58. Dellon ES, Jensen ET, Martin CF, et al. Prevalence of eosinophilic esophagitis in the United States. Clin Gastroenterol Hepatol 2014;12(4):589–596 e1. https:// doi.org/10.1016/j.cgh.2013.09.008.

59. Maradey-Romero C, Prakash R, Lewis S, et al. The 2011-2014 prevalence of eosinophilic oesophagitis in the elderly amongst 10 million patients in the United States. Aliment Pharmacol Ther 2015;41(10):1016–22. https://doi.org/10.1111/ apt.13171.

60. Krupp NL, Sehra S, Slaven JE, et al. Increased prevalence of airway reactivity in children with eosinophilic esophagitis. Pediatr Pulmonol 2016;51(5):478–83. https://doi.org/10.1002/ppul.23327.

61. Sorser SA, Barawi M, Hagglund K, et al. Eosinophilic esophagitis in children and adolescents: epidemiology, clinical presentation and seasonal variation. J Gastroenterol 2013;48(1):81–5. https://doi.org/10.1007/s00535-012-0608-x.

62. Bova M, Petraroli A, Loffredo S, et al. A Unique Case of Angioedema With Anti-C1 Inhibitor Antibodies and Normal C1 Inhibitor Levels. J Investig Allergol Clin Immunol 2016;26(2):111–2. https://doi.org/10.18176/jiaci.0021.

63. Rajan J, Newbury RO, Anilkumar A, et al. Long-term assessment of esophageal remodeling in patients with pediatric eosinophilic esophagitis treated with topical corticosteroids. J Allergy Clin Immunol 2016;137(1):147–156 e8. https://doi.org/10.1016/j.jaci.2015.05.045.

64. Harer KN, Enders FT, Lim KG, et al. An allergic phenotype and the use of steroid inhalers predict eosinophilic oesophagitis in patients with asthma. Aliment Pharmacol Ther 2013;37(1):107–13. https://doi.org/10.1111/apt.12131.

65. Caruso C, Colantuono S, Pugliese D, et al. Severe eosinophilic asthma and aspirin-exacerbated respiratory disease associated to eosinophilic gastroenteritis treated with mepolizumab: a case report. Allergy Asthma Clin Immunol 2020; 16:27. https://doi.org/10.1186/s13223-020-00423-3.

66. Han D, Lee JK. Severe asthma with eosinophilic gastroenteritis effectively managed by mepolizumab and omalizumab. Ann Allergy Asthma Immunol 2018;121(6):742–3. https://doi.org/10.1016/j.anai.2018.07.030.

67. Straumann A, Bauer M, Fischer B, et al. Idiopathic eosinophilic esophagitis is associated with a T(H)2-type allergic inflammatory response. J Allergy Clin Immunol 2001;108(6):954–61. https://doi.org/10.1067/mai.2001.119917.

68. Simon D, Simon HU. Relationship of skin barrier breakdown and eosinophilic esophagitis. J Allergy Clin Immunol 2020;145(1):90–92 e1. https://doi.org/10.1016/j.jaci.2019.11.005.

69. Doucet-Ladeveze R, Holvoet S, Raymond F, et al. Transcriptomic Analysis Links Eosinophilic Esophagitis and Atopic Dermatitis. Front Pediatr 2019;7:467. https://doi.org/10.3389/fped.2019.00467.

70. Chen G, Cohen J, Haven C. Association between atopic dermatitis and eosinophilic esophagitis: a cross-sectional study in the All of Us Research Program. PLoS One 2022;17(6):e0265531.

71. Aparna Daley EL, Pooja Jhaveri MS. Association of initial esophageal eosinophil counts with atopic dermatitis in patients with eosinophilic esophagitis. Allergy 2021;76(11):3307–13.

72. Sessions J, Purington N, Wang Y, et al. Pediatric eosinophilic esophagitis outcomes vary with co-morbid eczema and pollen food syndrome. Front Allergy 2022;3:981961. https://doi.org/10.3389/falgy.2022.981961.

73. Buie MJ, Quan J, Windsor JW, et al. Global Hospitalization Trends for Crohn's Disease and Ulcerative Colitis in the 21st Century: A Systematic Review With Temporal Analyses. Clin Gastroenterol Hepatol 2023;21(9):2211–21.

74. Navarro P, Arias A, Arias-Gonzalez L, et al. Systematic review with meta-analysis: the growing incidence and prevalence of eosinophilic oesophagitis in children and adults in population-based studies. Aliment Pharmacol Ther 2019;49(9):1116–25. https://doi.org/10.1111/apt.15231.

75. Lucendo AJ, Molina-Infante J, Arias A, et al. Guidelines on eosinophilic esophagitis: evidence-based statements and recommendations for diagnosis and management in children and adults. United European Gastroenterol J 2017;5(3):335–58. https://doi.org/10.1177/2050640616689525.

76. Akdis CA. Does the epithelial barrier hypothesis explain the increase in allergy, autoimmunity and other chronic conditions? Nat Rev Immunol 2021;21(11):739–51. https://doi.org/10.1038/s41577-021-00538-7.

77. Hyams JS, Davis Thomas S, Gotman N, et al. Clinical and biological predictors of response to standardised paediatric colitis therapy (PROTECT): a multicentre inception cohort study. Lancet 2019;393(10182):1708–20. https://doi.org/10.1016/S0140-6736(18)32592-3.

78. Aloi M, D'Arcangelo G, Rossetti D, et al. Occurrence and Clinical Impact of Eosinophilic Esophagitis in a Large Cohort of Children With Inflammatory Bowel Disease. Inflamm Bowel Dis 2023;29(7):1057–64. https://doi.org/10.1093/ibd/izac172.

79. Moore H, Wechsler J, Frost C, et al. Comorbid Diagnosis of Eosinophilic Esophagitis and Inflammatory Bowel Disease in the Pediatric Population. J Pediatr Gastroenterol Nutr 2021;72(3):398–403. https://doi.org/10.1097/MPG.0000000000003002.

80. Limketkai BN, Shah SC, Hirano I, et al. Epidemiology and implications of concurrent diagnosis of eosinophilic oesophagitis and IBD based on a prospective population-based analysis. Gut 2019;68(12):2152–60. https://doi.org/10.1136/gutjnl-2018-318074.

81. Fan YC, Steele D, Kochar B, et al. Increased Prevalence of Esophageal Eosinophilia in Patients with Inflammatory Bowel Disease. Inflamm Intest Dis 2019;3(4):180–6. https://doi.org/10.1159/000497236.

82. Shah MZ, Polk BI. Eosinophilic Esophagitis: The Role of Environmental Expo-
    sures. Immunol Allergy Clin North Am 2022;42(4):761–70. https://doi.org/10.
    1016/j.iac.2022.05.006.

83. Soon IS, Butzner JD, Kaplan GG, et al. Incidence and prevalence of eosinophilic
    esophagitis in children. J Pediatr Gastroenterol Nutr 2013;57(1):72–80. https://
    doi.org/10.1097/MPG.0b013e318291fee2.

84. Robson J, O'Gorman M, McClain A, et al. Incidence and Prevalence of Pediatric
    Eosinophilic Esophagitis in Utah Based on a 5-Year Population-Based Study.
    Clin Gastroenterol Hepatol 2019;17(1):107–114 e1. https://doi.org/10.1016/j.
    cgh.2018.06.028.

85. Ye Y, Manne S, Treem WR, et al. Prevalence of Inflammatory Bowel Disease in
    Pediatric and Adult Populations: Recent Estimates From Large National Data-
    bases in the United States, 2007-2016. Inflamm Bowel Dis 2020;26(4):619–25.
    https://doi.org/10.1093/ibd/izz182.

86. Alvisi P, Labriola F, Scarallo L, et al. Epidemiological trends of pediatric IBD in
    Italy: A 10-year analysis of the Italian society of pediatric gastroenterology, hep-
    atology and nutrition registry. Dig Liver Dis 2022;54(4):469–76. https://doi.org/
    10.1016/j.dld.2021.12.018.

87. Kuenzig ME, Fung SG, Marderfeld L, et al. Twenty-first Century Trends in the
    Global Epidemiology of Pediatric-Onset Inflammatory Bowel Disease: System-
    atic Review. Gastroenterology 2022;162(4):1147–59, e4.

88. Muir A, Falk GW. Eosinophilic Esophagitis: A Review. JAMA 2021;326(13):
    1310–8. https://doi.org/10.1001/jama.2021.14920.

89. Strober W, Fuss IJ. Proinflammatory cytokines in the pathogenesis of inflamma-
    tory bowel diseases. Gastroenterology 2011;140(6):1756–67. https://doi.org/10.
    1053/j.gastro.2011.02.016.

90. Arias A, Vicario M, Bernardo D, et al. Toll-like receptors-mediated pathways acti-
    vate inflammatory responses in the esophageal mucosa of adult eosinophilic
    esophagitis. Clin Transl Gastroenterol 2018;9(4):147. https://doi.org/10.1038/
    s41424-018-0017-4.

91. Hausmann M, Kiessling S, Mestermann S, et al. Toll-like receptors 2 and 4 are
    up-regulated during intestinal inflammation. Gastroenterology 2002;122(7):
    1987–2000. https://doi.org/10.1053/gast.2002.33662.

92. Sartor RB, Wu GD. Roles for Intestinal Bacteria, Viruses, and Fungi in Pathogen-
    esis of Inflammatory Bowel Diseases and Therapeutic Approaches. Gastroen-
    terology 2017;152(2):327–39, e4.

93. Mintz MJ, Ananthakrishnan AN. Phenotype and Natural History of Inflammatory
    Bowel Disease in Patients With Concomitant Eosinophilic Esophagitis. Inflamm
    Bowel Dis 2021;27(4):469–75. https://doi.org/10.1093/ibd/izaa094.

94. Dellon ES. Eosinophilic Gastrointestinal Diseases Beyond Eosinophilic Esopha-
    gitis. Am J Gastroenterol 2022;117(5):697–700. https://doi.org/10.14309/ajg.
    0000000000001658.

95. Hoofien A, Oliva S, Karl-Heinz Auth M, et al. A Quantitative Assessment of
    Mucosal Eosinophils in the Gastrointestinal Tract of Children Without Detectable
    Organic Disease. Pediatr Dev Pathol 2022;25(2):99–106. https://doi.org/10.
    1177/10935266211039474.

96. Koutri E, Patereli A, Noni M, et al. Distribution of eosinophils in the gastrointes-
    tinal tract of children with no organic disease. Ann Gastroenterol 2020;33(5):
    508–15. https://doi.org/10.20524/aog.2020.0518.

97. Mehta P, Furuta GT. Eosinophils in Gastrointestinal Disorders: Eosinophilic
    Gastrointestinal Diseases, Celiac Disease, Inflammatory Bowel Diseases, and

Parasitic Infections. Immunol Allergy Clin North Am 2015;35(3):413–37. https://doi.org/10.1016/j.iac.2015.04.003.

98. Nguyen N, Burger C, Skirka S, et al. One Year Into Dupilumab: Physician and Patient Experiences In Initiating Dupilumab for Pediatric Eosinophilic Esophagitis. J Pediatr Gastroenterol Nutr 2023;77(4):536–9. https://doi.org/10.1097/MPG.0000000000003901.

99. Coburn S, Germone M, McGarva J, et al. Psychological Considerations for Food Intolerances: Celiac Sprue, Eosinophilic Esophagitis, and Non-Celiac Gluten Sensitivity. Gastroenterol Clin North Am 2022;51(4):753–64. https://doi.org/10.1016/j.gtc.2022.07.003.

100. Hommeida S, Alsawas M, Murad MH, et al. The Association Between Celiac Disease and Eosinophilic Esophagitis: Mayo Experience and Meta-analysis of the Literature. J Pediatr Gastroenterol Nutr 2017;65(1):58–63. https://doi.org/10.1097/MPG.0000000000001499.

101. Castrodad-Rodriguez CA, Cheng J, Westerhoff M, et al. Clinical and Pathological Correlation in Concomitant Celiac Disease and Eosinophilic Esophagitis Suggests Separate Etiologies. Int J Surg Pathol 2023. https://doi.org/10.1177/10668969231167526. 10668969231167526.

102. Cristofori F, D'Abramo FS, Rutigliano V, et al. Esophageal Eosinophilia and Eosinophilic Esophagitis in Celiac Children: A Ten Year Prospective Observational Study. Nutrients 2021;(11):13. https://doi.org/10.3390/nu13113755.

103. Verzegnassi F JB. Eosinophilic oesophagitis and coeliac disease: is it just a casual association? Gut 2007;56(7):1028–9. https://doi.org/10.1136/gut.2006.118380.

104. Thompson J, Lebwohl B, Green P. Increased incidence of eosinophilic esophagitis in children and adults with celiac disease. J Clin Gastroenterol Hepatol 2012;46:e6–11.

105. Stewart M, Shaffer E, Storr M. The association between celiac disease and eosinophilic esophagitis in children and adults. BMC Gastroenterol 2013;13.

106. Votto M, Lenti MV, De Silvestri A, et al. Evaluation of diagnostic time in pediatric patients with eosinophilic gastrointestinal disorders according to their clinical features. Ital J Pediatr 2023;49(1):9. https://doi.org/10.1186/s13052-023-01410-1.

107. Xue Z, Miller TL, Abramson L, et al. Association of eosinophilic esophagitis with autoimmune and connective tissue disorders, and the impact on treatment response. Dis Esophagus 2022;36(1). https://doi.org/10.1093/dote/doac043.

108. Franciosi JP, Mougey EB, Dellon ES, et al. Proton Pump Inhibitor Therapy for Eosinophilic Esophagitis: History, Mechanisms, Efficacy, and Future Directions. J Asthma Allergy 2022;15:281–302. https://doi.org/10.2147/JAA.S274524.

109. Jensen ET, Svane HM, Erichsen R, et al. Maternal and Infant Antibiotic and Acid Suppressant Use and Risk of Eosinophilic Esophagitis. JAMA Pediatr 2023. https://doi.org/10.1001/jamapediatrics.2023.4609.

110. Visaggi P, Ghisa M, Barberio B, et al. Treatment Trends for Eosinophilic Esophagitis and the Other Eosinophilic Gastrointestinal Diseases: Systematic Review of Clinical Trials. Dig Liver Dis 2023;55(2):208–22. https://doi.org/10.1016/j.dld.2022.05.004.

111. Underwood B, Troutman TD, Schwartz JT. Breaking down the complex pathophysiology of eosinophilic esophagitis. Ann Allergy Asthma Immunol 2023;130(1):28–39. https://doi.org/10.1016/j.anai.2022.10.026.

112. van Rhijn BD, Oors JM, Smout AJ, et al. Prevalence of esophageal motility abnormalities increases with longer disease duration in adult patients with

eosinophilic esophagitis. Neurogastroenterol Motil 2014;26(9):1349–55. https://doi.org/10.1111/nmo.12400.

113. Pasman EA, Rubin Z, Hooper AR, et al. Quantitative Analysis of Tug Sign: An Endoscopic Finding of Eosinophilic Esophagitis. Clin Gastroenterol Hepatol 2023;21(4):1108–1110 e1. https://doi.org/10.1016/j.cgh.2022.02.042.

114. Hoffmann NV, Keeley K, Wechsler JB. Esophageal Distensibility Defines Fibrostenotic Severity in Pediatric Eosinophilic Esophagitis. Clin Gastroenterol Hepatol 2023;21(5):1188–1197 e4. https://doi.org/10.1016/j.cgh.2022.08.044.

115. Lanzoni G, Sembenini C, Gastaldo S, et al. Esophageal Dysphagia in Children: State of the Art and Proposal for a Symptom-Based Diagnostic Approach. Front Pediatr 2022;10:885308. https://doi.org/10.3389/fped.2022.885308.

116. Zaninotto G, Bennett C, Boeckxstaens G, et al. The 2018 ISDE achalasia guidelines. Dis Esophagus 2018;(9):31. https://doi.org/10.1093/dote/doy071.

117. Zhao W, Wang B, Zhang L, et al. Eosinophils Infiltration in Esophageal Muscularis Propria Induces Achalasia-like Esophageal Motility Disorder in Mice. Biomolecules 2022;(12):12. https://doi.org/10.3390/biom12121865.

118. Reddy CA, Allen-Brady K, Uchida AM, et al. Achalasia is Strongly Associated with Eosinophilic Esophagitis and Other Allergic Disorders. Clin Gastroenterol Hepatol 2023. https://doi.org/10.1016/j.cgh.2023.06.013.

119. Reddy SB, Ketchem CJ, Dougherty MK, et al. Association between eosinophilic esophagitis and esophageal dysmotility: A systematic review and meta-analysis. Neurogastroenterol Motil 2023;35(2):e14475. https://doi.org/10.1111/nmo.14475.

120. Dhar A, Haboubi HN, Attwood SE, et al. British Society of Gastroenterology (BSG) and British Society of Paediatric Gastroenterology, Hepatology and Nutrition (BSPGHAN) joint consensus guidelines on the diagnosis and management of eosinophilic oesophagitis in children and adults. Gut 2022;71(8):1459–87. https://doi.org/10.1136/gutjnl-2022-327326.

121. Walker MM, Potter MD, Talley NJ. Eosinophilic colitis and colonic eosinophilia. Curr Opin Gastroenterol 2019;35(1):42–50. https://doi.org/10.1097/MOG.0000000000000492.

122. Walker MM, Potter M, Talley NJ. Eosinophilic gastroenteritis and other eosinophilic gut diseases distal to the oesophagus. Lancet Gastroenterol Hepatol 2018;3(4):271–80. https://doi.org/10.1016/S2468-1253(18)30005-0.

Clinical Presentation of Patients with Eosinophilic Gastrointestinal Diseases beyond Eosinophilic Esophagitis

Alexandra Papadopoulou, MD[a],*, Noam Zevit, MD[b]

KEYWORDS

- Eosinophilic gastrointestinal diseases • Eosinophilic gastritis • Eosinophilic enteritis
- Eosinophilic colitis

KEY POINTS

- The vast majority of *eosinophilic gastrointestinal diseases beyond eosinophilic esophagitis (non-EoE EGIDs)* are of the mucosal subtype in which the main component of eosinophilic involvement is localized to the mucosa of the affected GI region.
- Symptoms of mucosal *non-EoE EGIDs* are wide ranged and non-specific.
- They may mimic many other organic diseases (eg, inflammatory bowel disease, peptic ulcer disease) and functional gastrointestinal disorders (eg, irritable bowel syndrome, functional dyspepsia, functional abdominal pain, functional constipation), and therefore *non-EoE EGIDs* may remain undiagnosed or misdiagnosed for long periods of time.

CLINICAL PRESENTATION OF MUCOSAL SUBTYPE OF *EOSINOPHILIC GASTROINTESTINAL DISEASES BEYOND EOSINOPHILIC ESOPHAGITIS*

The vast majority of *eosinophilic gastrointestinal diseases beyond eosinophilic esophagitis (non-EoE EGIDs)* are of the mucosal subtype in which the main component of eosinophilic involvement is localized to the mucosa of the affected GI region (**Fig. 1**). Symptoms of mucosal *non-EoE EGIDs* are wide ranged and non-specific. They may mimic many other organic (eg, inflammatory bowel disease, peptic ulcer disease) and functional gastrointestinal disorders (eg, irritable bowel syndrome, functional dyspepsia, functional abdominal pain, functional constipation), and therefore *non-EoE EGIDs* may remain undiagnosed or misdiagnosed for long periods of time.[1]

[a] Division of Gastroenterology and Hepatology, First Department of Pediatrics, University of Athens, Children's Hospital Agia Sophia, Thivon and Papadiamantopoulou, Athens 11527, Greece; [b] Institute of Gastroenterology, Nutrition, and Liver Diseases, Schneider Children's Medical Center of Israel, Tel-Aviv University, 14 Kaplan Street, PO Box 559, Petach Tikvah 4920235, Israel
* Corresponding author.
E-mail address: office.alexandra.papadopoulou@gmail.com

Immunol Allergy Clin N Am 44 (2024) 349–355
https://doi.org/10.1016/j.iac.2024.01.006
0889-8561/24/© 2024 Elsevier Inc. All rights reserved.

immunology.theclinics.com

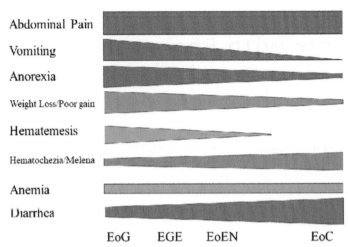

Abdominal Pain

Vomiting

Anorexia

Weight Loss/Poor gain

Hematemesis

Hematochezia/Melena

Anemia

Diarrhea

EoG   EGE   EoEN   EoC

Fig. 1. Schematic representation of symptoms of eosinophilic gastrointestinal diseases beyond eosinophilic esophagitis by region of eosinophilic involvement.

Signs and symptoms of mucosal *non-EoE EGIDs* may result from disruption of the epithelium (ulcers, erosions), effects of the inflammation on gut neurosensory modulation[2] (pain, dyspepsia), or may be secondary to blood loss (acute or chronic) associated with the tissue damage. For a number of years, the lack of uniform definitions for these conditions hampered the ability to perform collaborative studies, and therefore research and clinical practice was based on small case series and case reports that used a wide range of diagnostic criteria for the *non-EoE EGIDs*. Recently, the first international guideline defined clinical and histologic criteria of *non-EoE EGIDs*.[3]

The specific signs and symptoms associated with *non-EoE EGIDs* depend in part on the specific segment of the GI tract involved as well as the depth of tissue involvement; however, significant overlap in symptoms exists between different regions involved. In many case series, clinical symptoms of patients with *non-EoE EGIDs* remained broad and non-descript thus making organ-specific symptomology challenging to define. In addition, the rarity of *non-EoE EGIDs* created a need for a high index of suspicion when approaching a patient with symptoms possibly attributable to *non-EoE EGIDs* as well as a wide range of mucosal biopsies involving multiple segments of the GI tract. In general, according to the available data, with the exclusion of allergic proctocolitis of infancy, which is considered an entity separate from the primary *non-EoE EGIDs* and specifically from eosinophilic colitis, the *non-EoE EGIDs* present in a similar manner in adult and pediatric disease. An exception to this generalization is that infants and younger children may fail to gain weight and thrive, while teenagers and adults often lose weight.

In the largest retrospective case series of *non-EoE EGIDs*, the Consortium of Eosinophilic Gastrointestinal Disease Researchers retrospectively recorded the symptoms of 373 adult and pediatric patients.[4] While symptoms were reported according to site of involvement, the authors did not report exclusivity of the segment involved and noted that 154/373 (41%) had more than one GI region with eosinophilic inflammation. Of the whole cohort, 142 had eosinophilic gastritis (EoG). The diagnosis of EoG in these patients was based on the presence of symptoms and >30eos/HPF in gastric biopsies. The predominant symptoms were abdominal pain (48%), nausea/vomiting (54%), regurgitation (18%), and early satiety (13%) as well as food aversion (13%).

However, diarrhea and constipation were present in up to one-fifth of patients, and symptoms such as irritability, weight loss, bloating, bloody stool, and chest pain were also infrequently reported, indicating potential involvement of other sites besides the stomach. Eosinophilio gastroenteritis (EoN; n – 123) was defined based on symptoms and the histological finding in GI biopsies of ≥50eos/HPF, in the absence of alternative causes for tissue eosinophilia. The main symptom was nausea/vomiting (52%), followed by abdominal pain (50%), diarrhea (32%), regurgitation (12%), and more rarely weight loss, chest pain, irritability, early satiety, dysphagia, and food aversion. Isolated EoN was not reported in the cohort; however, eosinophilic colitis (EoC) was present in 108 patients who most frequently reported abdominal pain (60%), diarrhea (52%), nausea/vomiting (38%), and bloody stools (24%) followed by constipation, dysphagia, early satiety, weight loss, and bloating. Raffaele and colleagues, using strict histologic criteria, reported that children with EoC (n = 50) presented most commonly with abdominal pain (66%) and diarrhea (64%) while 8% had chronic constipation and 4% rectal bleeding.[5] In contrast, abdominal pain was present in 27% and abdominal pain in 38% of a large adult cohort (n = 194) of patients with colonic eosinophilia without evidence of secondary causes. Hematochezia was present in 10%.

In a case series of adults from Switzerland, Grandinetti and colleagues reported 22 patients with *non-EoE EGIDs* in whom gastric involvement was observed in 3, duodenal in 7, terminal ileal in 5, and 15 had colonic with 77% having overlapping involvement.[6] All 22 patients in the cohort reported abdominal pain, while other symptoms included diarrhea (59%), nausea/vomiting (36%), bloating (27%), loss of appetite/weight loss (18%), fatigue (18%), and reflux (14%). Similarly, in a largely pediatric cohort of 44 patients diagnosed with EoG and/or EoN as defined by symptoms attributable to the GI tract and ≥20eos/HPF in the biopsies taken from the stomach or duodenum, Reed and colleagues reported pooled symptoms of patients.[7] Of note, 30% of the cohort had concomitant eosinophilic esophagitis (EoE). Interestingly, while the vast majority of adult patients had abdominal pain (91%), this symptom was only reported by 53% of the children. Other common symptoms included vomiting, nausea, diarrhea, constipation, bloating, and dysphagia. A small prospective trial of amino acid– based formula in adults (n = 15) with EoG and EoN reported baseline symptoms that included abdominal pain (73%), dysphagia (73%), diarrhea (47%), and nausea or vomiting in 33% and 27%, respectively.[8] Similar results have been reported by others.[1,9,10]

Peripheral blood eosinophilia is common as is iron deficiency which may explain fatigue in patients with *non-EoE EGIDs*.[3,6–8] Protein losing enteropathy[7] with hypoalbuminemia may also be found at diagnosis; however, elevated inflammatory markers should raise concern for alternative diagnoses prior to diagnosing a primary *non-EoE EGIDs*,[3,6] although this too has been described. Elevated total blood immunoglobulin (Ig)E may also be found.[11]

CLINICAL PRESENTATION OF MUSCULAR SUBTYPE OF *NON-EoE EGIDs*

In muscular disease, eosinophilic infiltration of the muscular layer of the GI tract may lead to thickening of the gastric and/or intestinal wall, resulting in symptoms such as nausea, vomiting, and abdominal distention, which are indicative of obstruction. In addition, eosinophilic infiltration of the myenteric plexus may cause secondary pseudoobstruction of the intestine, while severe eosinophilic infiltration of the muscular layer may even lead to perforation of the small intestine and rarely the colon. Imaging studies of the gastrointestinal tract, such as abdominal ultrasonography, barium studies, abdominal computed tomography, or MRI, may show irregular narrowing of the lumen, especially in the distal antrum and proximal small intestine. However, the afore-mentioned findings are not specific for *non-EoE EGIDs*, and GI endoscopy and full-thickness biopsy, if necessary, are required to confirm the diagnosis after ruling out other causes.

Choi and colleagues[12] described a 1-month-old baby who presented with persistent vomiting since birth and failure to thrive and who showed segmental concentric wall thickening in the gastric antrum and an intact pylorus and duodenal bulb on ultrasound, whereas the upper GI series showed severe gastric outlet obstruction and poor passage of contrast to the duodenum on a 6-h delayed image. Peripheral eosinophil count and serum IgE levels were not elevated. Esophagogastroduodenoscopy showed marked antral swelling with pyloric narrowing, while gastric biopsies showed dense eosinophil infiltration in the antrum and pylorus. Barium passage gradually improved with a short course of corticosteroids in combination with amino acid formula given via a transpyloric feeding tube, which was removed after 3 months. Kellermayer and colleagues[13] described a previously healthy girl who presented with a 3-month history of worsening postprandial vomiting that resulted in inability to tolerate food. She had mild peripheral eosinophilia (740 × 106/L) but normal IgE and no history of atopy. Upper GI follow through showed marked pyloric narrowing, upper GI endoscopy showed antral edema and severe pyloric stenosis, while mucosal biopsies showed dense eosinophilic inflammation confirming the diagnosis of EoG. The patient was placed on intravenous steroids (methylprednisolone 2 mg/kg/day) and within 2 days she began to tolerate liquid food. Five days later, repeat upper endoscopy and biopsies showed resolution of eosinophilic infiltrate, and the patient was gradually switched to oral prednisolone (0.5 mg/kg per day). Oral steroids were discontinued after 8 weeks, while the patient remained asymptomatic 6 months after steroid discontinuation. Furthermore, a rare case of invagination of the thickened duodenal wall due to severe eosinophilic inflammation into the common bile duct causing jaundice was described by Hamamoto and colleagues[14] in an adult patient with EoG and eosinophilic duodenitis (EoD). Duodenal wall thickening was revealed with abdominal contrast-enhanced computed tomography, while upper GI endoscopy and duodenal biopsies showed dense eosinophilic infiltration of the gastroduodenal mucosa. Symptoms and findings in imaging studies and histology resolved after steroid therapy.

In the small intestine, eosinophilic infiltration of the muscular layer may cause wall thickening or narrowing of the intestinal lumen as a mechanical phenomenon, but may also affect neuronal ganglia causing eosinophilic ganglionitis and secondary pseudo-obstruction. Schäppi and colleagues[15] described 3 children (aged 1 month to 15 years) with severe functional intestinal obstruction due to inflammation of the lamina propria of the colon and myenteric plexus. The inflammatory infiltrate in the myenteric plexus was predominantly eosinophilic and had none of the immunologic features of lymphocytic ganglionitis. Neurons in the myenteric ganglia expressed the potent eosinophilic chemoattractant interleukin 5. None of the patients responded to dietary exclusion but all 3 responded to immunosuppressive/anti-inflammatory drugs. The authors claimed that eosinophilic ganglionitis associated with a pseudo-obstructive syndrome responded well to anti-inflammatory treatment.

Intususeption and perforation have also been reported in children with muscular involvement in the context of *non-EoE EGIDs*. Bramuso and colleagues[16] reported multiple ileoileal intussusceptions in a 6-year-old patient with EoN who presented with a 1-month history of diarrhea without blood or mucus, weight loss, and abdominal distension. Abdominal radiography showed air-fluid levels, while abdominal ultrasound revealed multiple ileoileal intussusceptions. Surgical reduction without bowel resection was performed. Due to persistent abdominal pain and diarrhea, ileocolono-scopy was performed, which revealed diffuse mucosal inflammation and patchy aph-thoid mucosal lesions in the proximal and distal ileum and colon, while histology of biopsies from the terminal ileum and colon showed massive eosinophilic infiltrates without architectural distortion. The patient had no history of allergy or peripheral eosinophilia. The stool was negative for bacterial enteropathogens, ova, and para-sites. EoN was diagnosed, and the child was treated with oral budesonide, with symp-toms resolving after few weeks of treatment. Siahanidou and colleagues[17] reported gastric perforation and ileoileal intussusception in a 1-month-old infant with EoG and EoN. Intussusception was manually reduced and the gastric perforation was sur-gically closed, while biopsy specimens from the area of the perforated gastric wall showed eosinophilic infiltration of the mucosa, submucosa, and muscularis of the stomach. The infant was placed on amino acid formula and was still asymptomatic af-ter 18 months. Huang and colleagues[18] described an 8-month-old boy who presented with periodic irritability for 4 days followed by bilious vomiting. Abdominal ultrasonog-raphy revealed a discrete mass with dense central echoes and hypoechoic periphery. Barium enema was subsequently performed, but persistent obstruction of retrograde barium flow at the proximal ascending colon was noted. A laparotomy was performed, which revealed an inflammatory mass in the ileocecal region with perforation and adhesion to the adjacent intestinal loops and mesentery. The mass was resected and an end-to-end ileocolic anastomosis was performed. Histologic examination revealed transmural eosinophilic inflammation of the ileum.

CLINICAL PRESENTATION OF SUBSEROSAL SUBTYPE OF *NON-EoE EGIDs*

If the inflammatory process is deep within the colon wall and involves the subserosal level, ascites and abdominal distension may occur. Menon and colleagues[19] described an 11-year-old girl who presented with colicky abdominal pain and massive eosinophilic ascites with peripheral eosinophilia, elevated IgE levels, and positive skin prick tests. Abdominal ultrasonography showed thickening of the muscular layer of both the stomach and small intestine and massive ascites. Ascitic fluid analysis revealed 8000/mm^3 cells, 90% of which were eosinophilic. Upper and lower GI endos-copy was macroscopically normal as was the mucosal histology. The authors reported a dramatic response to prednisolone with complete resolution of ascites within 1 week. Steroid treatment was reduced and discontinued over 3 months after normal sonography, eosinophil count, and IgE levels were documented. The authors reported that the patient subsequently relapsed twice with identical symptoms and elevated eosinophil and IgE levels 1 and 2 years later, citing seafood and yeast as the main possible triggers. The relapses were diagnosed by endoscopic ultrasound, which confirmed thickening of the muscle layer in the antro-pyloric region, duodenum, and jejunum. The first relapse was treated with prednisolone, which was continued at a low dose for 1 year; the second relapse occurred 1 month after discontinuation of ste-roids. Because she had developed a cushingoid habitus, montelukast was recom-mended in addition to lower doses of prednisolone (5 mg), with strict avoidance of dietary triggers. In contrast to the afore-mentioned case report in which there was muscular but not mucosal involvement, Ming and colleagues[20] reported an 11-year-old boy who presented with abdominal pain and ascites associated with peripheral blood eosinophilia and elevated serum IgE levels, and histologic finding of dense eosinophilic infiltration of the gastric antrum. The authors reported improvement of symptoms and clinical findings after 2 weeks of corticosteroid and anti-allergy treatment.

SUMMARY

Non-EoE EGIDs pose a clinical challenge to physicians treating patients with non-specific gastrointestinal symptoms, mandating a high index of suspicion to avoid delaying diagnoses and prolonging patient suffering. Many of the symptoms of *non-EoE EGIDs* in different regions of the GI tract are shared, and therefore, in the appropriate clinical setting endoscopy with multiple tissue biopsies both from well and ill-appearing mucosa should be sampled to avoid missing the diagnosis. In the correct context, full thickness biopsies or diagnostic paracentesis may be necessary to diagnose the rarer subtypes of *non-EoE EGIDs*.

CLINICS CARE POINTS

- Children suspected of having *non-EoE EGIDs* may present with vague or non-specific symptoms including diarrhea, abdominal pain, vomiting, and bleeding.
- If other etiologies have been addressed for common place symptoms, an endoscopic assessment with mucosal biopsy may be indicated even if findings associated with *non-EoE EGIDs*, including peripheral eosinophilia or atopic history, are not present

DISCLOSURE

None.

REFERENCES

1. Chehade M, Kamboj AP, Atkins D, et al. Diagnostic Delay in Patients with Eosinophilic Gastritis and/or Duodenitis: A Population-Based Study. J Allergy Clin Immunol Pract 2021;9(5):2050–9.e20.
2. Walker M, Warwick A, Ung C, et al. The role of eosinophils and mast cells in intestinal functional disease. Curr Gastroenterol Rep 2011;13(4):323–30.
3. Papadopoulou A, Amil-Dias J, Auth MK, et al. Joint ESPGHAN/NASPGHAN Guidelines on Childhood Eosinophilic Gastrointestinal Disorders Beyond Eosinophilic Esophagitis. J Pediatr Gastroenterol Nutr 2024;78(1):122–52.
4. Pesek RD, Reed CC, Muir AB, et al. increasing rates of diagnosis, substantial co-occurrence, and variable treatment patterns of eosinophilic gastritis, gastroenteritis, and colitis based on 10-year data across a multicenter consortium. Am J Gastroenterol 2019;114(6):984–94.
5. Raffaele A, Vatta F, Votto M, et al. Eosinophilic colitis in children: a new and elusive enemy? Pediatr Surg Int 2021;37(4):485–90.
6. Grandinetti TB L, Bussmann C, Straumann A, et al. eosinophilic gastroenteritis: clinical manifestation, natural course, and evaluation of treatment with corticosteroids and vedolizumab. Dig Dis Sci 2019;64(8):2231–41.
7. Reed C, Woosley JT, Dellon ES. Clinical characteristics, treatment outcomes, and resource utilization in children and adults with eosinophilic gastroenteritis. Dig Liver Dis 2015;47(3):197–201.
8. Gonsalves N, Doerfler B, Zalewski A, et al. Prospective study of an amino acid-based elemental diet in an eosinophilic gastritis and gastroenteritis nutrition trial. J Allergy Clin Immunol 2023;152(3):676–88.
9. Kobayashi S, Tsunoda T, Umetsu S, et al. Clinical features of pediatric eosinophilic gastroenteritis. Pediatr Int 2022;64(1):e15322.

10. Bagheri M, Ashrafi M, Mohamadnejad M, et al. Eosinophilic gastroenteritis: a case series from iran. Middle East J Dig Dis 2011;3(2):115–8.
11. Turner KS, Neumann WL, Genta RM, et al. primary colonic eosinophilia and eosinophilic colitis in adults. Am J Surg Pathol 2017;41(2):225–33.
12. Choi S-JJ, Yun-Jin, Choe Byung-Ho, et al. Eosinophilic gastritis with gastric outlet obstruction mimicking infantile hypertrophic pyloric stenosis. J Pediatr Gastroenterol Nutr 2014;59(1):e9–11.
13. Kellermayer RT N, Klish W, Shulman RJ, et al. Steroid responsive eosinophilic gastric outlet obstruction in a child. World J Gastroenterol 2008;14(14):2270–1.
14. Hamamoto HH, Taguchi H, Kojima I, et al. A eosinophilic gastroenteritis in which obstructive jaundice developed due to invagination of the duodenal wall. Intern Med 2018;57(13):1841–7.
15. Schäppi MS, Milla VV, Lindley PJ, et al. Eosinophilic myenteric ganglionitis is associated with functional intestinal obstruction. Gut 2003;52(5):752–5.
16. Bramuzzo MM, Stefano, Villanacci Vincenzo, et al. Ileoileal intussusceptions caused by eosinophilic enteropathy. J Pediatr Gastroenterol Nutr 2016;62(e60).
17. Siahanidou TM, Dimitriadis H, Van-Vliet D, et al. Eosinophilic gastroenteritis complicated with perforation and intussusception in a neonate. J Pediatr Gastroenterol Nutr 2001;32(3):335–7.
18. Huang FK SF, Huang SC, Lee SY, et al. Eosinophilic gastroenteritis with perforation mimicking intussusception. J Pediatr Gastroenterol Nutr 2001;33(5):613–5.
19. Menon JV V, Bhatia A, Rana SS, et al. an unusual presentation of eosinophilic gastroenteritis in a child. Trop Doct 2020;50(3):277–9.
20. Ming GB, Li-Ping Y. Eosinophilic gastroenteritis with ascites in a child. Indian Pediatr 2015;52(8):707–8.

Endoscopic Features of Eosinophilic Gastrointestinal Diseases

Thomas Greuter, MD[a,b,c],*, David Katzka, MD[d]

KEYWORDS

- Eosinophilic gastrointestinal diseases • Biopsies • Eosinophilic esophagitis
- Eosinophilic gastritis • Endoscopy

KEY POINTS

- Eosinophilic esophagitis (EoE) is a chronic inflammatory disease of the esophagus, defined clinically by the presence of symptoms of esophageal dysfunction and histologically by an eosinophil predominant infiltration of the esophageal mucosa.
- In analogy, eosinophilic gastrointestinal diseases (EGIDs) beyond the esophagus are defined by the presence of gastrointestinal symptoms and an eosinophil infiltration of various gastrointestinal segments (such as the stomach, duodenum, or the colon).
- Although not a diagnostic criterion, endoscopic changes have long been appreciated as key features of EoE and EGIDs, which have culminated in the development of 2 standardized endoscopic reference scores: the Endoscopic REFerence Score for EoE and the EG-REFS for eosinophilic gastritis.

INTRODUCTION

Eosinophilic esophagitis (EoE) is a chronic inflammatory disease of the esophagus, defined clinically by the presence of symptoms of esophageal dysfunction and histologically by an eosinophil predominant infiltration of the esophageal mucosa.[1] In analogy, eosinophilic gastrointestinal diseases (EGIDs) beyond the esophagus are defined by the presence of gastrointestinal symptoms and an eosinophil infiltration of various gastrointestinal segments (such as the stomach, duodenum, or the colon). Although not a diagnostic criterion, endoscopic changes have long been appreciated as key features of EoE and EGIDs, which have culminated in the development of 2 standardized endoscopic reference scores, the Endoscopic REFerence Score (EREFS) for

[a] Division of Gastroenterology and Hepatology, University Hospital Lausanne - CHUV, Lausanne Switzerland; [b] Department of Gastroenterology and Hepatology, University Hospital Zurich, Zurich, Switzerland; [c] Department of Internal Medicine, GZO – Zurich Regional Health Center, Spitalstrassse 66, Wetzikon 8610, Switzerland; [d] Division of Digestive and Liver Diseases, Presbyterian Hospital, 622 West 168th Street, New York, NY 10032, USA
* Corresponding author.
E-mail address: thomas.greuter@gzo.ch

Immunol Allergy Clin N Am 44 (2024) 357–368
https://doi.org/10.1016/j.iac.2024.01.007
0889-8561/24/© 2024 Elsevier Inc. All rights reserved.
immunology.theclinics.com

EoE,[2] and the Eosinophilic Gastritis Endoscopic Reference System (EG-REFS) for eosinophilic gastritis.[3] For less-prevalent EGIDs, such as eosinophilic colitis or enteritis, such classification systems are lacking. In contrast to other chronic gastrointestinal diseases, where diagnosis and disease monitoring rely heavily on endoscopic appearance with histology being less important (such as in ulcerative colitis and Crohn disease), the diagnosis and follow-up of EGIDs focus on eosinophil infiltration in biopsies, although assessment of disease severity by gross endoscopic features is emerging in importance.[4,5] Indeed, endoscopic assessment of severity seems to be on the verge of complementing and in some cases replacing histology. In the following article, we will discuss the most commonly used endoscopic scores in EGIDs, their validity for the diagnosis and follow-up of disease activity, as well as endoscopic interventions and areas of uncertainty.

ENDOSCOPIC SCORES IN EOSINOPHILIC ESOPHAGITIS

In its early years, endoscopic disease severity was graded semiquantitatively and generally (remission, mild, moderate, and severe) or based on a visual analog scale ranging from 0 to 10, both at the treating physician's discretion (global assessment).[6–8] This changed with the development of the EREFS score in the seminal publication of Hirano and colleagues in 2013.[2] The EREFS score considers both inflammatory and fibrotic changes in the esophagus. Depending on how the edema subscore is counted, the score ranges from 0 (no activity) to 8 to 9 (most severe endoscopic activity). The following inflammatory features are included in the score: edema, exudates, and furrows; whereas, rings and strictures are fibrotic readouts (conveniently, also, EREFS—Edema, Rings, Exudates, Furrows, Stricture). **Table 1** summarizes the EREFS score with its individual components.

Although the initial score also accounted for other features such as a feline esophagus or a narrow caliber, these components were eliminated due to poor interobserver agreement. As described by Hirano and colleagues, the 4 major components rings, furrows, exudates, and edema and the additional feature stricture demonstrated good interobserver agreement (71%–81%).[2] Although crepe paper esophagus reached good agreement as well (92%), this feature usually is less frequently reported

Table 1		
EREFS classification for grading of the endoscopic disease activity in EoE		
EREFS	**Characteristics**	**Subscores**
Edema	Swelling of the esophageal mucosa resulting in a decreased (absent) visibility of blood vessels	0: no edema 1: edema 2: severe edema
Rings	Presence of rings within the esophagus resembling the trachea, also referred to as trachealization	0: no rings 1: mild 2: moderate 3: severe
Exudates	White spots (purulent), also referred to as plaques	0: none 1: mild, <10% of the surface area 2: severe, >10% of the surface area
Furrows	Vertical lines running down the esophagus ("tram-lines," "train tracks")	0: absent 1: present
Strictures	Narrowing of the opening of the esophagus	0: absent 1: present

in clinical practice.[2] The EREFS score has been validated in both the United States and Europe.[9,10]

Despite its dramatic impact on the endoscopic assessment of EoE, the EREFS score has several drawbacks, among which are as follows: (1) the extent of inflammation is not considered; (2) strictures as a severe complication are probably underestimated (with 1 point only); (3) endoscopic signs do not account for transmural changes; and (4) it is unclear if an average or worst score of esophageal involvement is most important. Furthermore, there is no consensus about clear definitions of disease severity based on the EREFS score. In other words, it remains unclear, what grade should reflect mild, moderate, or severe disease based on the available EREFS scoring. Although some authors consider an EREFS score of 0 as remission, others include patients with an EREFS of 1 and some an EREFS of 1 if it is due to mild rings.

ENDOSCOPIC SCORES IN NON-EoE EOSINOPHILIC GASTROINTESTINAL DISEASES

Non-EoE EGIDs are characterized by the presence of chronic gastrointestinal symptoms and an eosinophil infiltration in gastrointestinal segments other than the esophagus.[11] However, the esophagus can exhibit eosinophilic inflammation in combination with another EGID. Whether this represents a continuum of disease from more distal organs or an association of EoE with EGIDs is debated. Until last year, endoscopic changes in Non-EoE EGIDs have been appreciated only as nonspecific. However, this has changed lately with the development of the first endoscopic grading system for eosinophilic gastritis, the EG-REFS.[3] The EG-REFS has been developed and prospectively evaluated by a collaborative approach of researchers involved in the Consortium of Eosinophilic GastroIntestinal disease Researchers (CEGIR).[3] Similarly to the EREFS in EoE, the EG-REFS takes into account inflammatory and fibrotic features of the disease. Those are erosions/ulcerations, granularity, raised lesions/nodules, erythema, friability/bleeding, thickened folds and pyloric stenosis. The EG-REFS ranges from 0 (no activity) to 46 (most severe endoscopic disease activity). Except for pyloric stenosis (which is scored as yes or no), scoring is done for each of the three regions of the stomach separately (fundus, body and antrum) and subscores are then summed up to a total score.[3] **Table 2** summarizes the EG-REFS score with its individual components.

The EG-REFS score has been demonstrated to strongly correlate with physician global assessment (r = 0.84), with most features being described in the antrum rather than the fundus or body.[3] Most importantly, the EG-REFS correlated with eosinophil infiltration of the gastric mucosa (defined by a threshold of 30 eosinophils per high power field [hpf]) although up to 50% of patients with active gastritis may have a normal appearing stomach on endoscopy. This is in contrast to EoE where a normal appearance is seen in only 5% to 10% of patients despite active disease.[3]

As a recently implemented endoscopic score, the EG-REFS has its limitations: Because eosinophilic gastritis is a rare disease, EG-REFS was based on expert opinion and literature review but is not a validated instrument. It was mainly described in patients already diagnosed and under medical/dietary treatment, with most of the patients being children. In the absence of a prior scoring system, however, EG-REFS serves at least as a start in more accurately staging endoscopic activity in eosinophilic gastritis.

Although no endoscopic score has been developed for EGIDs beyond the stomach, various endoscopic features have been described in the small intestinal tract and the colon. Among those are mucosal edema, erythema, flattening of the villi in the small

Table 2
EG-REFS classification for grading of the endoscopic disease activity in eosinophilic gastritis

EG-REFS	Characteristics	Subscores
Erosion/Ulceration	Erosions (mild) or ulcerations (severe) of the gastric mucosa	0: none 1: <5 erosions 2: ≥5 erosions 3: shallow/superficial ulceration(s) 4: deep/excavated ulceration <25% of the surface area of specified location 5: deep/excavated ulceration 25%–50% of the surface area of specified location 6: deep/excavated ulceration >50% of the surface area of specified location
Granularity	Gastric mucosa looks granular	0: none 1: fine 2: coarse
Raised lesions/ nodularity	Raised lesions of the gastric mucosa appearing as nodular surface	0: none 1: mild (width greater than height) 2: severe (height greater than width)
Erythema	Redness of the mucosa	0: none 1: mild (pink) 2: severe (red/hemorrhagic)
Friability/Bleeding	Mucosa is friable, bleeds on contact or spontaneously	0: none 1: mild (contact bleeding) 2: severe (spontaneous bleeding)
Folds	Gastric folds seem thickened	0: none 1: thickened folds
Pyloric stenosis	Stenosis of the pylorus not passable with a diagnostic gastroscope of 8–10 mm	0: none 1: present

intestine, ulcerations and nodularity of the mucosa. Many of the patients with eosinophilic colitis, however, have a normal-appearing endoscopy.[12] Similar to eosinophilic gastritis, suspicion of an EGID warrants biopsies in the presence of normal-appearing gastrointestinal mucosa.

THE ROLE OF ENDOSCOPIC FEATURES IN DIAGNOSIS AND FOLLOW-UP OF EOSINOPHILIC GASTROINTESTINAL DISEASES
Endoscopic Features in Eosinophilic Esophagitis

Although EoE can present in a sizable proportion of patients with a normal-appearing esophagus (up to 25%, particularly in children),[13,14] endoscopic features are increasingly recognized for the diagnosis and treatment monitoring of EoE. The EREFS score has been shown to be an accurate tool for both, diagnosis and determining response to treatment. Dellon and colleagues prospectively evaluated 67 adult patients and compared them to 144 subjects without EoE, showing an AUC for an accurate identification of EoE of 0.934.[15] A significant reduction in the EREFS was observed after treatment, particularly in patients with a histologic response. The responsiveness of the total EREFS score was maximized when subscores for exudates, rings, and edema were doubled.[15] Thus, endoscopic assessment was able to accurately diagnose EoE vs healthy controls, and assess treatment response. Disease activity and treatment effects have also been accurately identified by EREFS scoring in children, both older and younger.[16,17] However, some drawbacks remain: a subset of patients would be missed if endoscopic assessment is solely relied on; (2) It remains to be determined how well the EREFS can diagnostically discriminate between EoE and other esophageal diseases, particularly gastro-esophageal reflux disease (GERD); and (3) some endoscopic features might be overestimated or underestimated when it comes to therapeutic response. A second study in 69 patients demonstrated a modest correlation of the EREFS with peak eosinophil counts but an insufficient predictive value for disease activity.[18] Of note, lower peak eosinophil counts were not associated with a decrease in EREFS in the follow-up of 35 patients.[18] The latter further underscores that mechanisms beyond simple eosinophil infiltration might contribute to disease activity in EoE. However, these data also emphasize the complementary nature of EREFS to peak eosinophil count in assessing EoE activity and response to therapy.

Fibrostenosis is a common complication of EoE.[19] The EREFS score assesses fibrotic features by measuring both rings and strictures. However, endoscopy has its limitations: particularly in the proximal tier, stenosis can be easily missed.[20] Moreover, the pathophysiology behind the fibrotic endoscopic features remains largely unknown. Whether increased lamina propria fibrosis leads to rings and strictures is a valid hypothesis but still speculative. In addition, endoscopy fails to differentiate the transmural components of edema and fibrosis in EoE, which causes ongoing clinical symptoms in otherwise well-controlled and treated disease.[21–24] The functional luminal imaging probe (EndoFLIP) is an established technology that evaluates hollow organ distention by using high-resolution impedance planimetry.[25] Thus, this technique could potentially overcome the drawbacks of an isolated endoscopic assessment. EndoFLIP is an increasingly used tool in the context of EoE to assess esophageal distensibility.[26,27] In fact, it is well known that patients with EoE have a less-distensible esophagus compared with control patients without EoE.[25] Of note, patients with lower distensibility seem to have an increased risk for food bolus impactions.[28,29] Thus, EndoFLIP seems to be a surrogate marker for tissue remodeling. Nevertheless, the EREFS still has its value in the assessment of fibrotic changes. Studies have shown correlation between the severity of endoscopically identified rings and a reduction in esophageal distensibility measured by EndoFLIP.[30]

Although uniformly applied in all prospective clinical EoE studies now (and used at least as a secondary treatment outcome) and encouraged to use in clinical practice,[31] the role of the EREFS has been questioned lately. In fact, assessments of endoscopic activity vary among endoscopists and a simple scoring system (VAS 0–3) seems to not be any worse in detecting endoscopic changes.[32] Therefore, not surprisingly, the newly developed and proposed clinical severity index in EoE considers only the presence versus absence of inflammatory endoscopic features (and whether they are localized or diffuse), and the presence of fibrostenotic features (and whether or not a standard endoscope can pass) instead of including all EREFS components individually.[33] At the very least, a standardized endoscopic scoring system of some type should be used.

Endoscopic Features in Non-EoE Eosinophilic Gastrointestinal Diseases

In contrast to EoE, endoscopic scoring remains in the preliminary stages when it comes to EGIDs beyond the esophagus. Although standardized, the recently developed EG-REFS has not been validated and its value for the diagnosis and monitoring of disease activity remains completely unknown. One key value of the new scoring system, however, lies in the possibility to educate endoscopists and raise awareness of the subtle endoscopic changes that can be found in eosinophilic gastritis. Despite being novel, the role of the EG-REFS has already been questioned. A recent analysis from a randomized controlled phase II trial[34] with the anti-Siglec 8 antibody, Lirentelimab, revealed that most patients with eosinophilic gastritis have normal gastric mucosa or only mild endoscopic changes (mainly mild mucosal erythema and mild granularity).[35] In fact, 91% of the included patients had an EG-REFS score of 15 or lesser. Furthermore, no correlation was found between the EG-REFS and clinical or histologic severity of the disease (based on peak eosinophil or mast cell counts in gastric biopsies). Finally, the EG-REFS score was not different in eosinophilic gastritis versus controls. Thus, at the current stage, endoscopic assessment alone is not reliable for the diagnosis of eosinophilic gastritis. Nevertheless, the availability of the EG-REFS allows for standardized assessment of endoscopic disease severity, which is now used as secondary outcome and a means of assessing response to therapy in many prospective phase II and III trials in eosinophilic gastritis.[36]

ENDOSCOPIC INTERVENTIONS

Long diagnostic delay is a considerable concern in the management of patients with EoE and despite increasing disease awareness, the duration of this diagnostic delay has not changed in recent years.[37] This is a particular problem given well-documented findings demonstrating that a longer diagnostic delay is associated with increased rates of stricture formation.[19] The efficacy of current EoE treatment options for fibrosis and strictures is not well investigated. Therefore, for patients with severe and/or persistently symptomatic fibrostenotic features endoscopic dilation is needed.[38] It has to be kept in mind that endoscopic dilation should never be the sole treatment because it does not target ongoing inflammation.[39] Dilation should rather be considered as an add-on therapy. One of the great advantages of endoscopy in EoE is the possibility of combining assessment of disease activity and direct endoscopic interventions. Inflammatory changes are not a contraindication to endoscopic dilation and do not increase the risk of complications.[40,41] Such dilation can be performed by different techniques based on the endoscopist's preferences. There are 3 techniques available: balloon dilation, bougie dilation over a Savary guidewire, and dilation using a BougieCap.[42] Current guidelines do not prefer one dilation modality over the other.[40,41] A target diameter of 15 to 18 mm should be achieved, often through multiple sessions, in order to follow the rule of 3.[39] If performed gently by experienced hands, the risk of perforation is very low (0.3%).[43] Although perforation can occur, most of these complications can be treated conservatively with observation or stenting. Fatal outcomes are extremely rare.

Endoscopic features of the EREFS score help in the assessment before versus after endoscopic dilation. Patients with severe fibrostenotic signs, such as high-grade rings and strictures, particularly those with a narrow-caliber esophagus, and patients with ongoing symptoms despite control of inflammation, are ideal candidates for dilation therapy. After dilation, immediate endoscopic assessment ideally shows mucosal laceration, which is not regarded as a complication but rather an intended outcome.[4,14] A major drawback of endoscopic dilations is that the improvement in dysphagia leads to a greater discrepancy between esophageal eosinophilic inflammation and symptoms.[44] This is why, in most studies, patients with a recent dilation (and therefore a severe fibrostenotic phenotype) are excluded so as to optimize the performance of symptom scores in response to medical therapy. This also explains why data regarding the effect of antieosinophil treatment on tissue remodeling and eventual reversal of stricture formation are scarce.

THE ROLE OF ENDOSCOPY IN EOSINOPHILIC ESOPHAGITIS-LIKE DISEASES

EoE-like disease was first described by Straumann and colleagues in 2016 with the description of 5 patients from 4 EoE families.[45] These patients presented with a typical history for EoE (mainly solid-food dysphagia) but without eosinophilic infiltration of the esophageal epithelium. The entity has been further defined in a recent multicenter study, where the term EoE variants has been used to describe inflammatory conditions of the esophagus resembling EoE but not fulfilling diagnostic criteria (in the absence of an antieosinophil treatment).[46] The umbrella term EoE variants was further divided into EoE-like esophagitis,[45] nonspecific esophagitis, and lymphocytic esophagitis.[47] These patients had clinically active disease without a considerable eosinophil infiltration of the esophagus. More than 50% of these patients showed endoscopic abnormalities that were captured by the EREFS score, with both inflammatory (mainly edema) and fibrostenotic features (rings and strictures). In fact, more than 25% of the patients had an EREFS score of 3 or greater indicating at least moderately severe disease. In addition to features captured by the EREFS scoring system, a granular mucosa and plaques have been described in the esophagus.[45] These findings highlight that endoscopic changes can be observed regardless of the eosinophil count in the esophagus, similarly to what has been recently shown in eosinophilic gastritis.[35] Furthermore, they define EoE-like disease in the presence of unremarkable histology. Careful endoscopic assessment is warranted in all patients presenting with solid-food dysphagia but the presence of EoE typical endoscopic changes does not necessarily imply the diagnosis of EoE. EoE variants need to be considered as an important differential diagnosis, particularly when other (motility) disorders of the esophagus are excluded.

AREA OF UNCERTAINTY

Despite the implementation of the EREFS score in EoE, its frequent use in clinical practice and its universal use for research purposes, several uncertainties and open questions remain. One obvious and looming question—particularly when comparing EoE with other chronic intestinal diseases such as Crohn disease or ulcerative colitis—is whether endoscopy can replace the need for biopsies. This is particularly noteworthy in the context of increasing uncertainty about the role of eosinophils. In fact, the role of eosinophils as the culprit cell in EoE pathophysiology has been questioned lately.[48–51] Accurate endoscopic assessment would omit the reliance on peak eosinophil counts, and such strategy would be even cost-saving. However, the EREFS is far from being perfect and data on the need of esophageal biopsies are just emerging.[52] Furthermore, inflammatory bowel disease (IBD) and now EoE investigators have put forth the concept of deep remission, that is, resolution of symptoms, endoscopic abnormalities, and histopathology. As a result, although endoscopic evaluation may gain refinement and importance, it will likely remain one of several combined measured parameters for EoE diagnosis and response to therapy. Other areas of uncertainty include the relative importance of inflammatory versus fibrostenotic features and the accuracy with which they predict transmural disease activity, the dominant contributor to esophageal narrowing. If an endoscopic and/or pathologic finding, such as lamina propria fibrosis for the latter, could be reliably associated with esophageal wall fibrosis, more invasive testing such as endoscopic ultrasound could be avoided. Finally, it remains to be determined whether EREFS should be used to assess the esophagus as a whole or by segment, for example, proximal and distal esophagus. Longitudinal prospective studies will be needed to correlate these different means of calculating EREFS score with other measures and clinical outcome.

In non-EoE EGIDs, the role of endoscopic assessment is in its infancy. The EG-REFS is a start but needs in-depth validation. A major question in EGIDs will be how to assess the extent of inflammation. It is still unknown, whether patients with eosinophilic gastritis and duodenitis should undergo further endoscopic and/or capsule imaging of the small intestine and eventually colonoscopy (in the absence of symptoms warranting such further examination). Another area of uncertainty is the role of tissue remodeling in EGIDs. In EoE, the EREFS accounts for 2 features (rings and strictures), while the EG-REFS only assesses one fibrotic sign (pyloric stenosis). Although appealing, the role of EndoFLIP of the pylorus has not been evaluated in EGIDs. For both EoE and eosinophilic gastritis, the role of nonstandardized endoscopic signs, such as a granular mucosa or plaques (other than exudates) in the esophagus remains to be determined and correlated to histology and other objective measures. It is also possible there are endoscopic features that will be recognized in the future that are not apparent now due to the relative rarity but now increased recognition of these diseases. This and other novel findings may emerge from application of more accurate means of endoscopic imaging or application of artificial intelligence to image recognition in eosinophilic gastrointestinal diseases.

With regards to endoscopic interventions, several questions remain unanswered, such as the optimal timepoint of the first endoscopic dilation and the optimal interval between repetitive dilations in EoE. Further studies are also needed to determine whether effective medical treatment with control of esophageal inflammation can delay or obviate dilation. Studies comparing different endoscopic dilation techniques are urgently needed (bougie vs balloon dilation vs BougieCap). It seems that for some cases, one technique might be preferred over the other (such as for long vs short strictures) but data are lacking. Whether endoscopic dilations are beneficial for nondysphagia symptoms related to EoE is unknown, as it is for dilations beyond 16 to 18 mm.

FUTURE PERSPECTIVE

Endoscopic recognition and assessment of EoE and EGIDs is in the preliminary stages but already great progress has been made during past decades. At the very least, these scoring systems yield a common language for gastroenterologists to consider. As the fine points of optimal imaging and recognition of key findings are investigated, endoscopy may play a greater role in diagnosis and monitoring disease. Additionally, further correlation of these findings with other objective tools such as histology and impedance planimetry may help us gain further understanding of the pathophysiology and course of these diseases. This is particularly true with the increasing use of EndoFLIP as the best available means of detecting physiologic abnormalities of the esophageal wall reflected in a perturbation of distensibility. However, for now, endoscopy (and EndoFLIP) remains an important but additional outcome with the primary outcomes still being clinical and histologic response and remission.

DISCLOSURE

T. Greuter has consulting contracts with Sanofi-Regeneron, Janssen, BMS, Takeda, Abbvie and Falk Pharma GmbH, received travel grants from Falk Pharma GmbH and Vifor, speaker's fee from Norgine and an unrestricted research grant from Novartis, Switzerland. D. Katzka received research funding from Shire, a Takeda company, and consulting fees from Receptos, Celgene and Bristol Myers Squibb. No company representative was involved in conception, writing, or financing of this study.

This study was supported by a grant from the Swiss National Science Foundation, United States to T. Greuter (grant no. P2ZHP3_168561). This study was further supported by a young investigator award from the Swiss Society of Gastroenterology to T. Greuter, a research grant from the Novartis Foundation for Medical-Biological Research, Switzerland to T. Greuter, a research award from the Swiss IBDnet to T. Greuter, a project grant from the EoE Foundation, United States to T. Greuter, and a training grant from the CEGIR to T. Greuter. CEGIR (U54 AI117804) is part of the Rare Disease Clinical Research Network (RDCRN), an initiative of the Office of Rare Diseases Research, National Center for Advancing Translational Sciences (NCATS), and is funded through collaboration between the National Institute of Allergy and Infectious Diseases, United States, National Institute of Diabetes and Digestive and Kidney Diseases, United States, and NCATS, United States. CEGIR is also supported by patient advocacy groups including the American Partnership for Eosinophilic Disorders, United States, Campaign Urging Research for Eosinophilic Disease, United States, and Eosinophilic Family Coalition, United States. As a member of the RDCRN, CEGIR is also supported by its Data Management and Coordinating Center (U2CTR002818).

REFERENCES

1. Liacouras CA, Furuta GT, Hirano I, et al. Eosinophilic esophagitis: updated consensus recommendations for children and adults. J Allergy Clin Immunol 2011;128(1):3–20, e6; quiz 1-2.
2. Hirano I, Moy N, Heckman MG, et al. Endoscopic assessment of the oesophageal features of eosinophilic oesophagitis: validation of a novel classification and grading system. Gut 2013;62(4):489–95.
3. Hirano I, Collins MH, King E, et al, CEGIR investigators. Prospective endoscopic activity assessment for eosinophilic gastritis in a multisite cohort. Am J Gastroenterol 2022;117(3):413–23.
4. Lucendo AJ, Molina-Infante J, Arias Á, et al. Guidelines on eosinophilic esophagitis: evidence-based statements and recommendations for diagnosis and management in children and adults. United European Gastroenterol J 2017;5(3): 335–58.
5. Arnim UV, Biedermann L, Aceves SS, et al, EUREOS and TIGERs. Monitoring patients with eosinophilic esophagitis in routine clinical practice - international expert recommendations. Clin Gastroenterol Hepatol 2023;21(10):2526–33.
6. Warners MJ, Hindryckx P, Levesque BG, et al. Systematic review: disease activity indices in eosinophilic esophagitis. Am J Gastroenterol 2017;112(11):1658–69.
7. Straumann A, Conus S, Degen L, et al. Budesonide is effective in adolescent and adult patients with active eosinophilic esophagitis. Gastroenterology 2010; 139(5):1526–37, 37.e1.
8. Straumann A, Conus S, Degen L, et al. Long-term budesonide maintenance treatment is partially effective for patients with eosinophilic esophagitis. Clin Gastroenterol Hepatol 2011;9(5):400–9.e1.
9. van Rhijn BD, Warners MJ, Curvers WL, et al. Evaluating the endoscopic reference score for eosinophilic esophagitis: moderate to substantial intra- and interobserver reliability. Endoscopy 2014;46(12):1049–55.
10. Kochar B, Dellon ES. Endoscopic findings in eosinophilic esophagitis and esophageal distensibility: a proxy for transmural modeling? Gastroenterology 2017; 152(1):298–9.
11. Dellon ES, Gonsalves N, Abonia JP, et al. International consensus recommendations for eosinophilic gastrointestinal disease nomenclature. Clin Gastroenterol Hepatol 2022;20(11):2474–84.e3.

12. Grandinetti T, Biedermann L, Bussmann C, et al. Eosinophilic gastroenteritis: clinical manifestation, natural course, and evaluation of treatment with corticosteroids and vedolizumab. Dig Dis Sci 2019;64(8):2231–41.

13. Prasad GA, Alexander JA, Schleck CD, et al. Epidemiology of eosinophilic esophagitis over three decades in Olmsted County, Minnesota. Clin Gastroenterol Hepatol 2009;7(10):1055–61.

14. Visaggi P, Savarino E, Sciume G, et al. Eosinophilic esophagitis: clinical, endoscopic, histologic and therapeutic differences and similarities between children and adults. Therap Adv Gastroenterol 2021;14. 1756284820980860.

15. Dellon ES, Cotton CC, Gebhart JH, et al. Accuracy of the eosinophilic esophagitis endoscopic reference score in diagnosis and determining response to treatment. Clin Gastroenterol Hepatol 2016;14(1):31–9.

16. Wechsler JB, Bolton SM, Amsden K, et al. Eosinophilic esophagitis reference score accurately identifies disease activity and treatment effects in children. Clin Gastroenterol Hepatol 2018;16(7):1056–63.

17. Ahuja N, Weedon J, Schwarz SM, et al. Applying the eosinophilic esophagitis endoscopic reference scores (EREFS) to different aged children. J Pediatr Gastroenterol Nutr 2020;71(3):328–32.

18. van Rhijn BD, Verheij J, Smout AJ, et al. The endoscopic reference score shows modest accuracy to predict histologic remission in adult patients with eosinophilic esophagitis. Neuro Gastroenterol Motil 2016;28(11):1714–22.

19. Schoepfer AM, Safroneeva E, Bussmann C, et al. Delay in diagnosis of eosinophilic esophagitis increases risk for stricture formation in a time-dependent manner. Gastroenterology 2013;145(6):1230–6, e1-2.

20. Gentile N, Katzka D, Ravi K, et al. Oesophageal narrowing is common and frequently under-appreciated at endoscopy in patients with oesophageal eosinophilia. Aliment Pharmacol Ther 2014;40(11–12):1333–40.

21. Hirano I, Aceves SS. Clinical implications and pathogenesis of esophageal remodeling in eosinophilic esophagitis. Gastroenterol Clin North Am 2014;43(2):297–316.

22. Saffari H, Peterson KA, Fang JC, et al. Patchy eosinophil distributions in an esophagectomy specimen from a patient with eosinophilic esophagitis: Implications for endoscopic biopsy. J Allergy Clin Immunol 2012;130(3):798–800.

23. Rieder F, Nonevski I, Ma J, et al. T-helper 2 cytokines, transforming growth factor β1, and eosinophil products induce fibrogenesis and alter muscle motility in patients with eosinophilic esophagitis. Gastroenterology 2014;146(5):1266–77, e1-9.

24. Fox VL, Nurko S, Teitelbaum JE, et al. High-resolution EUS in children with eosinophilic "allergic" esophagitis. Gastrointest Endosc 2003;57(1):30–6.

25. Kwiatek MA, Hirano I, Kahrilas PJ, et al. Mechanical properties of the esophagus in eosinophilic esophagitis. Gastroenterology 2011;140(1):82–90.

26. Hirano I, Pandolfino JE, Boeckxstaens GE. Functional lumen imaging probe for the management of esophageal disorders: expert review from the clinical practice updates committee of the AGA institute. Clin Gastroenterol Hepatol 2017;15(3):325–34.

27. Donnan EN, Pandolfino JE. EndoFLIP in the esophagus: assessing sphincter function, wall stiffness, and motility to guide treatment. Gastroenterol Clin North Am 2020;49(3):427–35.

28. Nicodème F, Hirano I, Chen J, et al. Esophageal distensibility as a measure of disease severity in patients with eosinophilic esophagitis. Clin Gastroenterol Hepatol 2013;11(9):1101–7.e1.

29. Read AJ, Pandolfino JE. Biomechanics of esophageal function in eosinophilic esophagitis. J Neurogastroenterol Motil 2012;18(4):357–64.

30. Chen JW, Pandolfino JE, Lin Z, et al. Severity of endoscopically identified esophagoal rings correlates with reduced esophageal distensibility in eosinophilic esophagitis. Endoscopy 2016;48(9):794–801.

31. Dellon ES. Do you see what I see? Towards standardized reporting of endoscopic findings in eosinophilic esophagitis. Endoscopy 2014;46(12):1043–5.

32. Schoepfer AM, Hirano I, Coslovsky M, et al, International EEsAI Study Group. variation in endoscopic activity assessment and endoscopy score validation in adults with eosinophilic esophagitis. Clin Gastroenterol Hepatol 2019;17(8): 1477–88.e10.

33. Dellon ES, Khoury P, Muir AB, et al. A clinical severity index for eosinophilic esophagitis: development, consensus, and future directions. Gastroenterology 2022;163(1):59–76.

34. Dellon ES, Peterson KA, Murray JA, et al. Anti-siglec-8 antibody for eosinophilic gastritis and duodenitis. N Engl J Med 2020;383(17):1624–34.

35. Dellon ES, Gonsalves N, Rothenberg ME, et al. Determination of biopsy yield that optimally detects eosinophilic gastritis and/or duodenitis in a randomized trial of lirentelimab. Clin Gastroenterol Hepatol 2022;20(3):535–45.e15.

36. Kliewer KL, Murray-Petzold C, Collins MH, et al. Benralizumab for eosinophilic gastritis: a single-site, randomised, double-blind, placebo-controlled, phase 2 trial. Lancet Gastroenterol Hepatol 2023;8(9):803–15.

37. Murray FR, Kreienbuehl AS, Greuter T, et al. Diagnostic delay in patients with eosinophilic esophagitis has not changed since the first description 30 years ago: diagnostic delay in eosinophilic esophagitis. Am J Gastroenterol 2022; 117(11):1772–9.

38. Moawad FJ, Molina-Infante J, Lucendo AJ, et al. Systematic review with meta-analysis: endoscopic dilation is highly effective and safe in children and adults with eosinophilic oesophagitis. Aliment Pharmacol Ther 2017;46(2):96–105.

39. Greuter T, Straumann A. Medical algorithm: diagnosis and treatment of eosinophilic esophagitis in adults. Allergy 2020;75(3):727–30.

40. Aceves SS, Alexander JA, Baron TH, et al. Endoscopic approach to eosinophilic esophagitis: american society for gastrointestinal endoscopy consensus conference. Gastrointest Endosc 2022;96(4):576–92.e1.

41. Pouw RE, Barret M, Biermann K, et al. Endoscopic tissue sampling - Part 1: Upper gastrointestinal and hepatopancreatobiliary tracts. European Society of Gastrointestinal Endoscopy (ESGE) Guideline. Endoscopy 2021;53(11):1174–88.

42. Schoepfer AM, Henchoz S, Biedermann L, et al. Technical feasibility, clinical effectiveness, and safety of esophageal stricture dilation using a novel endoscopic attachment cap in adults with eosinophilic esophagitis. Gastrointest Endosc 2021;94(5):912–9.e2.

43. Moawad FJ, Cheatham JG, DeZee KJ. Meta-analysis: the safety and efficacy of dilation in eosinophilic oesophagitis. Aliment Pharmacol Ther 2013;38(7):713–20.

44. Safroneeva E, Pan Z, King E, et al, Consortium of Eosinophilic Gastrointestinal Disease Researchers. Long-lasting dissociation of esophageal eosinophilia and symptoms after dilation in adults with eosinophilic esophagitis. Clin Gastroenterol Hepatol 2022;20(4):766–75.e4.

45. Straumann A, Blanchard C, Radonjic-Hoesli S, et al. A new eosinophilic esophagitis (EoE)-like disease without tissue eosinophilia found in EoE families. Allergy 2016;71(6):889–900.

46. Greuter T, Straumann A, Fernandez-Marrero Y, et al. Characterization of eosinophilic esophagitis variants by clinical, histological, and molecular analyses: A cross-sectional multi-center study. Allergy 2022;77(8):2520–33.

47. Sonnenberg A, Turner KO, Genta RM. Associations of microscopic colitis with other lymphocytic disorders of the gastrointestinal tract. Clin Gastroenterol Hepatol 2018;16(11):1762–7.

48. Straumann A, Conus S, Grzonka P, et al. Anti-interleukin-5 antibody treatment (mepolizumab) in active eosinophilic oesophagitis: a randomised, placebo-controlled, double-blind trial. Gut 2010;59(1):21–30.

49. Assa'ad AH, Gupta SK, Collins MH, et al. An antibody against IL-5 reduces numbers of esophageal intraepithelial eosinophils in children with eosinophilic esophagitis. Gastroenterology 2011;141(5):1593–604.

50. Spergel JM, Rothenberg ME, Collins MH, et al. Reslizumab in children and adolescents with eosinophilic esophagitis: results of a double-blind, randomized, placebo-controlled trial. J Allergy Clin Immunol 2012;129(2):456–63.

51. Safroneeva E, Straumann A, Coslovsky M, et al, International Eosinophilic Esophagitis Activity Index Study Group. Symptoms have modest accuracy in detecting endoscopic and histologic remission in adults with eosinophilic esophagitis. Gastroenterology 2016;150(3):581–90.e4.

52. Heil A, Kühlewindt T, Godat A, et al. Histological phenotyping in eosinophilic esophagitis: Localized proximal disease is infrequent, but associated with less severe disease and better disease outcome. Int Arch Allergy Immunol 2024; 185(1):63–72 (Accepted for publication).

Histopathology of Eosinophilic Gastrointestinal Diseases Beyond Eosinophilic Esophagitis

Nicoleta C. Arva, MD, PhD[a],*, Anas Bernieh, MD[b],
Oscar Lopez-Nunez, MD[b], Maria Pletneva, MD, PhD[c],
Guang-Yu Yang, MD, PhD[d], Margaret H. Collins, MD[e]

KEYWORDS

- Eosinophilia • Immune therapy • Genotype–phenotype correlations

KEY POINTS

- Eosinophils are normal cellular constituents of the gastric, small, and large bowel lamina propria with a crescendo-decrescendo distribution. Cutoff values for peak eosinophil count were established for each segment to aid in the diagnosis of eosinophilic gastrointestinal diseases (EGID).
- The histopathologic diagnosis of EGID is a diagnosis of exclusion, after other conditions that can present with lamina propria eosinophilia have been excluded.
- In addition to evaluating eosinophil inflammation to generate a peak eosinophil count, assessing additional histopathologic abnormalities is important because those abnormalities may contribute to persistent symptoms in patients whose biopsies are devoid of eosinophils.
- The molecular signature of eosinophilic gastritis and eosinophilic duodenitis is similar to that of eosinophilic enteritis, whereas eosinophilic colitis shows minimal evidence of a strong allergic T_H2 immune response.

[a] Department of Pathology, Nationwide Children's Hospital, 700 Childrens Drive, Columbus, OH 43205, USA; [b] Division of Pathology and Laboratory Medicine, Cincinnati Children's Hospital Medical Center, 3333 Burnet Avenue, Cincinnati, OH 45229, USA; [c] Department of Pathology, University of Utah, 2000 Circle of Hope, Room 3100, Salt Lake City, UT 84112, USA; [d] Department of Pathology, Northwestern University Feinberg School of Medicine, 303 East Chicago Avenue, Chicago, IL 60611, USA; [e] Division of Pathology and Laboratory Medicine, ML1035, Cincinnati Children's Hospital Medical Center, 3333 Burnet Avenue, Cincinnati, OH 45229, USA
* Corresponding author.
E-mail address: nicoleta.arva@nationwidechildrens.org

Immunol Allergy Clin N Am 44 (2024) 369–381
https://doi.org/10.1016/j.iac.2024.01.008
0889-8561/24/© 2024 Elsevier Inc. All rights reserved.
immunology.theclinics.com

BACKGROUND

Eosinophilic gastrointestinal diseases (EGID) are chronic inflammatory conditions characterized by persistent gastrointestinal (GI) symptoms and elevated levels of activated eosinophils in the GI tract tissue. Recently, updated consensus recommendations for EGID nomenclature for both clinical and research use have been achieved: EGID remains the umbrella term replacing "eosinophilic gastroenteritis," and specific naming conventions by location of GI tract involvement are recommended, such as eosinophilic gastritis (EoG), eosinophilic enteritis (EoN; including eosinophilic duodenitis [EoD], eosinophilic jejunitis, or ileitis), and eosinophilic colitis (EoC).[1] The diagnosis of these conditions is challenging: symptoms are generally nonspecific (early satiety, nausea and vomiting, abdominal pain and cramping, bloating, and diarrhea) and overlap with other common GI conditions.[2] In addition, considering the rarity of the disease, pathologists tend to overlook mild or moderate increases in the density of eosinophils in GI biopsy specimens.[3] As opposed to eosinophilic esophagitis (EoE), where the presence of any intraepithelial eosinophil is considered abnormal, eosinophils are normal constituents of the lamina propria in other locations of the GI tract. Surprisingly, the normal numbers of lamina propria eosinophils along the GI tract have rarely been investigated, and most studies focused on pediatric patients.[4–7] The results demonstrated similar findings, showing a crescendo-decrescendo distribution of eosinophils, with the highest density in the cecum, and lowest in the stomach and rectum. Therefore, cutoff values have been suggested to help pathologists with the diagnosis of EGID.[8] However, establishing the exact cutoff value for peak eosinophil counts is further complicated by population-related geographic differences in the normal distribution of eosinophils along the GI tract.[9] Previous literature suggested that the histologic diagnosis of EoG is established when the peak eosinophil count is 30/high power field (HPF) or greater in 5 HPF or greater or 70/HPF or greater in 3 HPF or greater; excess eosinophils in the small intestine could be considered a multiple of the maximum count found in normal biopsies, such as 2 × 26/HPF or 52/HPF in duodenal mucosa and 2 × 28/HPF or 56/HPF in ileum for a diagnosis of EoN; EoC is diagnosed histologically if peak eosinophil count is a multiple of the peak count per HPF in normal biopsies, including 2 × 50/HPF or 100/HPF in cecum and ascending colon, 2 × 42/HPF or 84/HPF in transverse and descending colon, and 2 × 32/HPF or 64/HPF in rectosigmoid mucosa.[8] As per the Food and Drug Administration, 30 or greater eosinophils per HPF in 3 or greater HPFs is an accepted definition for EoD for certain clinical trials purposes.[3] Very recently, the joint European and North American Society For Pediatric Gastroenterology, Hepatology and Nutrition guidelines on childhood EGID have been published and suggested threshold peak eosinophil counts for the diagnosis of these disorders: 30 or greater eosinophils/HPF for EoG, 50/HPF or greater for EoD, 60/HPF or greater in the terminal ileum, 100/HPF or greater in the cecum/ascending colon, 80/HPF or greater in the transverse and descending colon, and 60/HPF or greater in the sigmoid colon and rectum.[10] EGID can frequently coexist with one another: about 43% of children with EoG have concurrent EoE and 21% have EoN.[11]

PATHOGENESIS OF EOSINOPHILIC GASTROINTESTINAL DISEASES

The pathogenesis of EoG is related to a T_H2 immune response. When compared with gastric samples from control patients, subjects diagnosed with EoG contain CD3+ T cells that are mainly CD8+; the CD8/CD4 ratio is comparable in EoG and control biopsy samples. However, gastric regulatory T (CD3+CD4+FOXP3+) and T_H2 (CD3+CD4+GATA3+) cell levels are increased in EoG versus controls and correlate with gastric eosinophil level. In addition, CD3+CD8+ cells and CD3+CD4+FOXP3+ cells are interferon-γ and interleukin (IL)-10 producers, whereas CD3+CD4+GATA3+ T cells produce IL-4, IL-5, and IL-13. Gastric IL4, IL5, and IL13 mRNA levels correlate with histologic features of EoG.[12] Tissue mast cells counts have also been shown to be increased in patients with EoG. Moreover, mast cell–specific transcripts and transcripts for other cytokines such as IL17, CCL26 were upregulated, whereas decreased IL33 transcripts were observed.[13,14] Although the mechanisms of disease in EoG seem similar to those of EoE and transcript profiling revealed changes in 8% of the genome in gastric tissue from patients with EoG, only 7% of this EoG transcriptome overlap with that of EoE.[13]

Many patients with EoG have coexisting eosinophilic inflammation in multiple GI segments; the esophagus represents the most common secondary site. Increased peripheral blood eosinophil counts are also observed in subjects with EoG and positively correlate with peak gastric eosinophil counts.[13] These findings suggest that EoG is a systemic disorder associated with blood and extragastric eosinophilia.

Transcriptome analysis of EoD revealed 382 differentially expressed genes between EoD and normal controls with enrichment in genes involved in IL-4/IL-13 signaling, mast cells, and myeloid progenitor cells, establishing EoD as part of a spectrum of EGID associated with type T_H2 immunity.[15]

EoC seems to have a different pathogenesis. Transcriptome analysis from patients diagnosed with histologic EoC demonstrated 987 differentially expressed genes between EoC and healthy subjects.[16] However, there was minimal transcriptomic overlap and minimal evidence of a strong allergic type T_H2 immune response in EoC compared with other EGID such as EoE and EoG. Comparing type 2–related gene expression showed that the main chemotactic factor for EoC was likely CCL11, whereas it was CCL26 for both EoE and EoG. Expression of type 2 cytokines (IL13, IL4, and IL5) was not increased in patients with EoC. Instead, decreased cell cycle and increased apoptosis were found in EoC compared with control samples.[16] EoC transcriptome–based scores were reversible with disease remission and also differentiated EoC from inflammatory bowel disease (IBD).

HISTOPATHOLOGIC EVALUATION OF MUCOSAL BIOPSIES FOR THE DIAGNOSIS OF EOSINOPHILIC GASTROINTESTINAL DISEASE

"Eosinophilic gastroenteritis" (the original term used to describe what is currently known as non-EoE EGID) was initially subclassified as mucosal type presenting with protein loss, a mural form affecting motility and a serosal group leading to ascites rich in eosinophils.[17] However, those previous studies were performed on resected specimens; currently, large surgical excisions are not performed as part of EGID treatment and the diagnosis is usually established by evaluating endoscopic biopsy material, which analyzes only the mucosal layer.

Eosinophil counts and other features of the EoE histologic scoring system (EoEHSS)[18] may be subjected to interobserver variability in EoE, particularly in the eyes of inexperienced pathologists.[19,20] Although similar studies related to other EGID are lacking, there is variability in pathology practice when it comes to counting and reporting eosinophils in other segments of the GI tract. This is due to frequent absence of significant endoscopic findings,[21] lack of specific patients' symptoms in a high number of subjects[7] and low disease awareness, which might result in pathologists not fully appreciating the value of enumerating eosinophils in the GI tract beyond esophagus. Pathologists should be alert to these entities, aware of the new nomenclature[1] and should realize that a diagnosis of EGID is one of exclusion. Low and medium power examination of the tissue should help in identifying the number of tissue pieces present in the sample, their appropriate orientation, as well as determining the area with the highest eosinophil density to perform the count.

Guidelines defining a countable eosinophil in the GI tract have been established,[3] and 3 different appearances have been recognized: (1) intact cell with eosinophilic granules and intact bilobed nucleus; (2) well-defined cell with eosinophilic granules and a partial nucleus; or (3) a discrete cluster of eosinophil granules at least in part limited by a membrane, even if there is no clearly discernible nucleus. Granules haphazardly scattered in the lamina propria should not be counted. Moreover, eosinophils in areas below the muscularis mucosae should not be counted, even if intact. Some cases may exhibit dense eosinophilic infiltration, in which eosinophils seem to coalesce in indistinct sheets of granules. An accurate count is difficult to achieve in these instances; estimating a bilobed nucleus as one eosinophil as a means of approximating the number of eosinophils in an area of apparently coalesced cells might facilitate the count. Descriptive pathology reports, emphasizing the presence of multiple aggregates of eosinophils, would also be appropriate. Regardless of the GI segment involved (stomach, small bowel, or large bowel), an increased number of eosinophils in the lamina propria is frequently associated with increased interglandular/cryptal spaces (**Fig. 1**) and formation and periglandular/cryptal collars (circumferential rings of 1–2 layers of eosinophils around glands/crypts; **Fig. 2**). Intraepithelial eosinophils (either within surface epithelium or as eosinophilic glandulitis/cryptitis) may be observed (see **Fig. 2**), and more severe cases will have eosinophilic abscesses. The number of intraepithelial eosinophils must be significant, as occasional ones might be seen, particularly in pediatric patients unrelated to EGID.[6] Extracellular granules can be prominent.

In addition, EGID can also exhibit specific histopathologic changes based on the location along the GI tract. In cases of EoG involving the body/fundus (oxyntic mucosa), eosinophils tend to be located mainly between the oxyntic glands and seem squeezed (**Fig. 3**). In the antrum, their common location is usually basal/subepithelial (**Fig. 4**). Changes that are not related to the eosinophilic infiltrate may be seen in EoG, such as epithelial damage with mucin depletion (**Fig. 5**) and foveolar hyperplasia, lamina propria fibroplasia, smooth muscle hyperplasia (**Fig. 6**), and presence of other inflammatory infiltrates, notably neutrophils. Similar to EoEHSS, a scoring system was

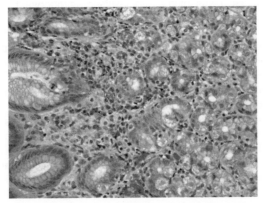

Fig. 1. EoG: Eosinophil sheets with increased interglandular spaces (hematoxylin-eosin stain, 200×).

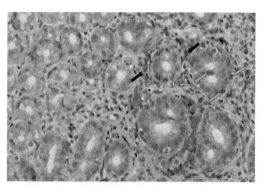

Fig. 2. EoG: Eosinophils collars with few layers of eosinophils arranged circumferentially around glands, black arrows. Adjacent glands have few intraepithelial eosinophils, gray arrows (hematoxylin-eosin stain, 200×).

designed for EoG[14] based on the evaluation of 11 histologic features: lamina propria eosinophil sheets, periglandular circumferential collars, eosinophils in surface epithelium, eosinophil glandulitis, eosinophil gland abscesses, eosinophils in muscularis mucosa, lamina propria fibroplasia, lamina propria smooth muscle hyperplasia, reactive epithelial changes, acute inflammatory cells, and surface erosion/ulceration. Each feature is scored by using a 3-point scale (0: absent; 1: mild/moderate; and 2: marked), with a maximum score for each biopsy specimen of 22. Three histologic features (lamina propria eosinophil sheets, periglandular circumferential collars, and eosinophil glandulitis) correlate strongly with EoG gene expression profile being the most effective histopathologic features at capturing biological processes underlying the molecular signature of EoG.[14]

In the small bowel, the subcryptal areas tend to be the first to be populated by eosinophils in cases with mild to moderate increases (**Fig. 7**). Increased density of lamina propria eosinophils will induce crypts to become distanced from each other (**Fig. 8**). When infiltrates are more marked, the eosinophils aggregate also toward the tip of the villi, which may become wider and shorter (**Fig. 9**). Villous blunting with crypt hyperplasia and reactive epithelial changes may be present in more severe cases but

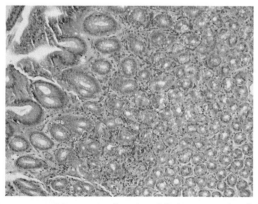

Fig. 3. EoG: Oxyntic mucosa with squeezed eosinophils between glands (hematoxylin-eosin stain, 200×).

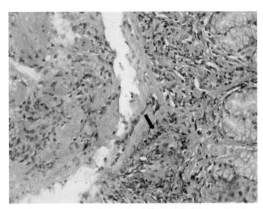

Fig. 4. EoG involving the antrum, with an eosinophilic infiltrate located at the base, between the glands and muscularis mucosa, arrow (hematoxylin-eosin stain, 200×).

mild-to-moderate eosinophilia seems to have little influence on the duodenal morphology. Among histologic features seen in EoD, lamina propria eosinophil sheets seem to be the most associated with transcriptomic changes.[15]

In EoC, crypt architectural distortion and crypt loss may be present (**Figs. 10** and **11**). A histologic score was also designed in EoC based on the severity (0: absent, 1: mild/moderate, and 2: marked) of the following pathologic features: acute crypt abscess, acute cryptitis, acute inflammation, crypt architectural abnormalities, crypt dropout/loss, crypt epithelial injury, crypts partly destroyed by eosinophilic inflammation, eosinophil crypt abscess, eosinophil cryptitis, eosinophils in muscularis mucosa/submucosa, eosinophils in surface epithelium, granulomas, lamina propria eosinophil sheets, lymphocytes in surface epithelium, overall eosinophilic inflammation, pericryptal circumferential eosinophil collars, subcryptal eosinophil aggregates, subcryptal lymphoplasmacytosis, and surface epithelial injury.[16] Histologic findings commonly observed in EoC biopsies, such as overall eosinophilic inflammation, pericryptal circumferential eosinophil collars, and lamina propria eosinophil sheets have been shown to highly correlate with the EoC transcriptome.[16]

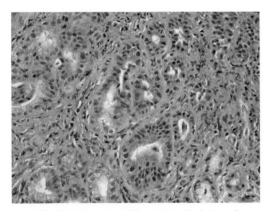

Fig. 5. EoG: Reactive epithelial changes with mucin depletion (hematoxylin-eosin stain, 400×).

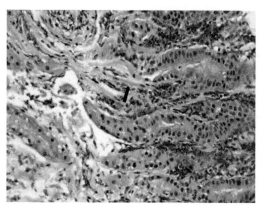

Fig. 6. EoG: Smooth muscle hyperplasia, arrow (hematoxylin-eosin stain, 200×).

Immunohistochemistry (IHC) is rarely used for the diagnosis of EGID. Newer studies have demonstrated that eosinophil peroxidase IHC in conjunction with automated image analysis can facilitate the histologic diagnosis of eosinophilic duodenitis.[22]

INFLUENCE OF EOSINOPHIL-DEPLETING BIOLOGIC AGENTS ON HISTOPATHOLOGY IN EOSINOPHILIC GASTROINTESTINAL DISEASE

Considering the T_H2 immune response in the pathogenesis of EoG, and the presence of high levels of IL-5 mRNA in the gastric mucosa of patients with EoG,[12] clinical trials analyzing the efficacy of benralizumab have been conducted.[23,24] Benralizumab is a humanized monoclonal antibody against the α chain of the IL-5 receptor, which is expressed by mature eosinophils, eosinophil progenitor cells, and basophils. It has been shown to deplete eosinophils in the blood, bone marrow, and airway mucosal and submucosal tissues by antibody-dependent cell-mediated cytotoxicity.[25] It has been approved for the treatment of severe eosinophilic asthma and possible other eosinophil-associated diseases.[26,27] Patients with EoG treated with benralizumab demonstrated significant reduction in peak gastric eosinophil counts, EoG histology total score, and histology inflammatory score compared with placebo group.[24]

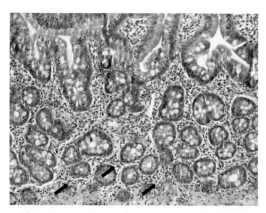

Fig. 7. EoN: Subcryptal/basal eosinophilic infiltrate, arrows (hematoxylin-eosin stain, 200×).

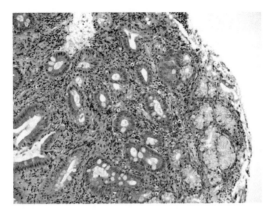

Fig. 8. EoN: Lamina propria eosinophils with increased intercryptal distance (hematoxylin-eosin, 400×).

However, no significant changes were noted in the EoG histology structural score between the cohorts. Gastric epithelial changes persisted despite treatment. Moreover, GI mast cells were generally unchanged.[23] These results suggest that the pathogenesis of EGID also involves mechanisms that are independent of eosinophilia.

Differential Diagnosis

Histopathologic diagnosis of EGID is frequently one of exclusion because other entities characterized by mucosal GI eosinophilia must be ruled out. Parasitic disease can present with blood eosinophilia, GI symptoms or both, depending on the infectious agent. Increased eosinophil count in the blood is a common finding in tropical developing countries and is strongly associated with the presence of parasitic disease, particularly intestinal helminth infestation,[28] whereas *Giardia intestinalis* and *Cryptosporidium* species induce GI symptoms (mainly diarrhea) but without blood eosinophilia.[29] In contrast, hookworm (*Ancylostoma duodenale* and *Necator americanus*) and Strongyloidiasis (*Strongyloides stercoralis*) can present with both blood and tissue eosinophilia.[30] In these situations, a stool sample for ova and parasites

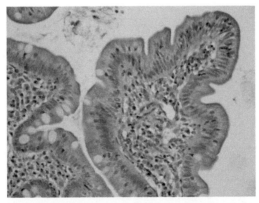

Fig. 9. EoN: Eosinophilic infiltrate toward the tip of the villi with associated villous blunting and intraepithelial eosinophils within surface epithelium (hematoxylin-eosin, 400×).

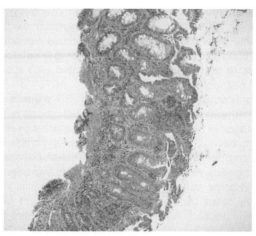

Fig. 10. EoC: Mild crypt architectural distortion (hematoxylin-eosin, 100×).

and appropriate serology can elucidate the diagnosis. *Helicobacter pylori* infection has also been linked to increased eosinophilic infiltrates in the gastric mucosa, with persistence of high numbers of lamina propria eosinophils particularly after eradication therapy.[31]

When accompanied by blood hypereosinophilia (absolute eosinophil count ≥1500/ mm[3]), EGID may be related to hypereosinophilic syndrome (HES), occurring as an isolated GI disorder (HES/EGID overlap) or as part of a multisystem HES. The clinical presentation and management of both groups are remarkably similar. When associated with HES, GI tissue eosinophilia seems to involve multiple gut segments in the vast majority (67%) of the patients, with 17% of the subjects having all 4 areas (esophagus, stomach, small bowel, and large bowel) affected.[32]

Vasculitis and connective tissue disorders may present with GI tissue eosinophilia. Eosinophilic granulomatosis with polyangiitis, formerly known as Churg-Strauss syndrome, a multisystemic disorder belonging to the small and medium vessel antineutrophil cytoplasmic antibody–associated vasculitis presents with eosinophilic organ infiltrations, especially in lungs, heart, and GI system. When affecting the GI tract,

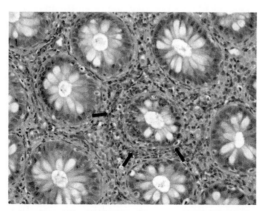

Fig. 11. EoC: Sheets of eosinophils separating the crypts and formation of eosinophilic collars, arrows (hematoxylin-eosin, 200×).

patients may develop intestinal obstruction or perforation[33,34] suggesting mural involvement, which might be difficult to detect on histopathologic analysis of only mucosal biopsies. Interstitial and angiocentric granulomas composed of eosinophilic necrotic matrix surrounded by giant cells and palisading lymphocytes accompanied by fibrinoid necrosis of the vessel wall and associated with eosinophilic infiltrates are the prototypical histopathologic findings.[35]

Early studies describing mucosal biopsies from IBD patients revealed mucosal eosinophilia compared with healthy controls. An IBD diagnosis is associated with an older age at presentation, a significant inflammatory picture with elevated sedimentation rate and hematochezia.[36] On histopathology, signs of chronic inflammation such as more prominent crypt distortion, crypt loss, and Paneth cell metaplasia raise suspicion for IBD. The significance of eosinophils in IBD has also been investigated, with conflicting results. In some studies, the severity of eosinophilic inflammation in patients with ulcerative colitis seems to be the most significant predictor of lack of response to therapy in adults.[37] Another study revealed also that increased mucosal eosinophilia and IL-5 levels in resected colon of patients with Crohn disease were associated with endoscopic recurrence.[38] Reducing ileal eosinophils in Crohn-like murine model reversed the histologic and molecular signatures of remodeling (goblet cell hyperplasia, muscularis propria hypertrophy, villus blunting, and expression of inflammatory and remodeling genes), suggesting that eosinophils participate in intestinal architectural changes in Crohn disease.[39] However, the PROTECT study[40] examined rectal biopsies from children with ulcerative colitis who were not previously treated and found that low peak eosinophil counts (32/HPF) correlated with more severe activity scores at diagnosis, and the need to escalate therapy to tumor necrosis factor-α at weeks 12 and 52.[40,41] Interestingly, in the study by Mark and colleagues,[36] of the 19 non-IBD, non-EoC subjects with colonic eosinophilia, 2 were diagnosed with microscopic (1 collagenous and 1 lymphocytic) colitis.

Similarly, collagenous gastritis enters the differential diagnosis of EoG. There seems to be a histologic evolution of the disease: the first stage is characterized by inactive gastritis, then eosinophilia develops, and finally marked collagen deposition occurs.[42] Performing Gomori trichrome stain when there is persistent gastric eosinophilia to highlight the patchy thickening of the subepithelial collagen bands (>10 μm) may lead to the correct diagnosis. Tenascin IHC also highlights the subepithelial collagen and seems to be a more sensitive method of collagen detection in biopsies from patients with subtle subepithelial collagen.[43]

Some cases of active celiac disease may demonstrate an eosinophilic infiltration in the duodenal mucosa[44] and must be differentiated from EoN. Mucosal eosinophilia is more obvious in advanced histologic stages of celiac disease, suggesting that eosinophils may play a role in mucosal damage.[45] In fact, a correlation between EoE and celiac disease was suggested by occasional case reports[46] but studies with larger cohorts found this association to be likely incidental and not causal.[47]

Functional dyspepsia, a common condition defined by unexplained pain or discomfort centered in the upper abdomen, has demonstrated duodenal eosinophilia.[48] Increased eosinophilic density was significantly associated with early satiety, postprandial fullness, and abdominal pain in subjects with functional dyspepsia.

GI tract eosinophilia is also a known posttransplant complication and its etiology in this setting has been related to antirejection medication. It seems to affect patients who are transplanted earlier in life and who have pretransplant atopy.[49] Interestingly, transplanted patients that develop EGID seem to have a denser eosinophilic infiltrate in the graft biopsies when they develop rejection episodes.[50] Other morphologic features can point toward drug-induced eosinophilia and include endocrine cell aggregates, presence of multiple confluent apoptotic bodies and hypereosinophilic (degenerated) crypts with crypt distortion.[51]

DISCLOSURES

M. Pletneva is a consultant for Allakos. M.H. Collins is a consultant for Allakos, Arena/Pfizer, AstraZeneca, Calypso Biotech, EsoCap Biotech, GlaxoSmithKline, Receptos/Celgene/BMS, Regeneron Pharmaceuticals, Robarts Clinical Trials Inc./Alimentiv, Inc. and Shire, a Takeda company. N.C. Arva, A. Bernieh, O. Lopez-Nunez, and G-Y. Yang do not have conflicts of interest.

REFERENCES

1. Dellon ES, Gonsalves N, Abonia JP, et al. International Consensus Recommendations for Eosinophilic Gastrointestinal Disease Nomenclature. Clin Gastroenterol Hepatol 2022;20(11):2474–84.e3.
2. Gonsalves N. Eosinophilic gastrointestinal disorders. Clin Rev Allergy Immunol 2019;57(2):272–85.
3. Turner KO, Collins MH, Walker MM, et al. Quantification of Mucosal Eosinophils for the Histopathologic Diagnosis of Eosinophilic Gastritis and Duodenitis: A Primer for Practicing Pathologists. Am J Surg Pathol 2022;46(4):557–66.
4. Lowichik A, Weinberg AG. A quantitative evaluation of mucosal eosinophils in the pediatric gastrointestinal tract. Mod Pathol 1996;9(2):110–4.
5. Talley NJ, Walker MM, Aro P, et al. Non-ulcer dyspepsia and duodenal eosinophilia: an adult endoscopic population-based case-control study. Clin Gastroenterol Hepatol 2007;5(10):1175–83.
6. DeBrosse CW, Case JW, Putnam PE, et al. Quantity and distribution of eosinophils in the gastrointestinal tract of children. Pediatr Dev Pathol 2006;9(3):210–8.
7. Turner KO, Sinkre RA, Neumann WL, et al. Primary Colonic Eosinophilia and Eosinophilic Colitis in Adults. Am J Surg Pathol 2017;41(2):225–33.
8. Collins MH, Capocelli K, Yang GY. Eosinophilic Gastrointestinal Disorders Pathology. Front Med 2018;4:261.
9. Koutri E, Patereli A, Noni M, et al. Distribution of eosinophils in the gastrointestinal tract of children with no organic disease. Ann Gastroenterol 2020;33(5):508–15.
10. Papadopoulou A, Amil-Dias J, Auth MK, et al. Joint ESPGHAN/NASPGHAN Guidelines on Childhood Eosinophilic Gastrointestinal Disorders beyond Eosinophilic Esophagitis. J Pediatr Gastroenterol Nutr 2023. https://doi.org/10.1097/MPG.0000000000003877.
11. Ko HM, Morotti RA, Yershov O, et al. Eosinophilic gastritis in children: clinicopathological correlation, disease course, and response to therapy. Am J Gastroenterol 2014;109(8):1277–85.
12. Ben-Baruch Morgenstern N, Shoda T, Rochman Y, et al. Local type 2 immunity in eosinophilic gastritis. J Allergy Clin Immunol 2023;152(1):136–44.
13. Caldwell JM, Collins MH, Stucke EM, et al. Histologic eosinophilic gastritis is a systemic disorder associated with blood and extragastric eosinophilia, T H2 immunity, and a unique gastric transcriptome. J Allergy Clin Immunol 2014;134(5):1114–24.
14. Shoda T, Wen T, Caldwell JM, et al. Molecular, endoscopic, histologic, and circulating biomarker-based diagnosis of eosinophilic gastritis: multi-site study. J Allergy Clin Immunol 2020;145(1):255–69.
15. Shoda T, Rochman M, Collins MH, et al. Molecular analysis of duodenal eosinophilia. J Allergy Clin Immunol 2023;151(4):1027–39.

16. Shoda T, Collins MH, Rochman M, et al. Consortium of Eosinophilic Gastrointestinal Diseases Researchers (CEGIR). Evaluating Eosinophilic Colitis as a Unique Disease Using Colonic Molecular Profiles: A Multi-Site Study. Gastroenterology 2022;162(6):1635–49.

17. Klein NC, Hargrove RL, Sleisenger MH, et al. Eosinophilic gastroenteritis. Medicine (Baltimore) 1970;49(4):299–319.

18. Collins MH, Martin LJ, Alexander ES, et al. Newly developed and validated eosinophilic esophagitis histology scoring system and evidence that it outperforms peak eosinophil count for disease diagnosis and monitoring. Dis Esophagus 2017;30(3):1–8.

19. Stucke EM, Clarridge KE, Collins MH, et al. Value of an additional review for eosinophil quantification in esophageal biopsies. J Pediatr Gastroenterol Nutr 2015;61(1):65–8.

20. Vieira MC, Gugelmin E3, Percicote AP, et al. Intra and interobserver agreement of histopathological findings in pediatric patients with eosinophilic esophagitis. J Pediatr 2022;98(1):26–32.

21. Pesek RD, Reed CC, Collins MH, et al. Association between endoscopic and histologic findings in a multicenter retrospective cohort of patients with non-esophageal eosinophilic gastrointestinal disorders. Dig Dis Sci 2020;65(7): 2024–35.

22. Hasan SH, Taylor S, Garg S, et al. Diagnosis of Pediatric Non-Esophageal Eosinophilic Gastrointestinal Disorders by Eosinophil Peroxidase Immunohistochemistry. Pediatr Dev Pathol 2021;24(6):513–22.

23. Kuang FL, De Melo MS, Makiya M, et al. Benralizumab Completely Depletes Gastrointestinal Tissue Eosinophils and Improves Symptoms in Eosinophilic Gastrointestinal Disease. J Allergy Clin Immunol Pract 2022;10(6):1598–605.e2.

24. Kliewer KL, Murray-Petzold C, Collins MH, et al. Benralizumab for eosinophilic gastritis: a single-site, randomised, double-blind, placebo-controlled, phase 2 trial. Lancet Gastroenterol Hepatol 2023. S2468-S1253(23)00145-0.

25. Kolbeck R, Kozhich A, Koike M, et al. MEDI-563, a humanized anti-IL-5 receptor alpha mAb with enhanced antibody-dependent cell-mediated cytotoxicity function. J Allergy Clin Immunol 2010;125(6):1344–53.

26. Laviolette M, Gossage DL, Gauvreau G, et al. Effects of benralizumab on airway eosinophils in asthmatic patients with sputum eosinophilia. J Allergy Clin Immunol 2013;132(5):1086–96.

27. Kuang FL, Legrand F, Makiya M, et al. Benralizumab for PDGFRA-negative hypereosinophilic syndrome. N Engl J Med 2019;380(14):1336–46.

28. Lee D, Albenberg L, Compher C, et al. Diet in the Pathogenesis and Treatment of Inflammatory Bowel Diseases. Gastroenterology 2015;148(6):1087–106.

29. Fletcher S, Van Hal S, Andresen D, et al. Gastrointestinal pathogen distribution in symptomatic children in Sydney, Australia. Journal of epidemiology and global health 2013;3(1):11–21.

30. Mehta P, Furuta GT. Eosinophils in Gastrointestinal Disorders: Eosinophilic Gastrointestinal Diseases, Celiac Disease, Inflammatory Bowel Diseases, and Parasitic Infections. Immunol Allergy Clin 2015;35(3):413–37.

31. Genta RM, Lew GM, Graham DY. Changes in the gastric mucosa following eradication of Helicobacter pylori. Mod Pathol 1993;6(3):281–9.

32. Kuang FL, Curtin BF, Alao H, et al. Single-Organ and Multisystem Hypereosinophilic Syndrome Patients with Gastrointestinal Manifestations Share Common Characteristics. J Allergy Clin Immunol Pract 2020;8(8):2718–26.

33. Vaglio A, Corradi D, Ronda N, et al. Large bowel obstruction heralding Churg-Strauss syndrome. Am J Gastroenterol 2004;99(3):562–3.

34. Ikoma N, Fischer UM, Covinsky M, et al. Ileal perforation in a young female with Churg-Strauss syndrome. Am Surg 2014;80(1):94–6.

35. Lie JT. Illustrated histopathologic classification criteria for selected vasculitis syndromes. American College of Rheumatology Subcommittee on Classification of Vasculitis. Arthritis Rheum 1990;33(8):1074–87.

36. Mark J, Fernando SD, Masterson JC, et al. Clinical Implications of Pediatric Colonic Eosinophilia. J Pediatr Gastroenterol Nutr 2018;66(5):760–6.

37. Zezos P, Patsiaoura K, Nakos A, et al. Severe eosinophilic infiltration in colonic biopsies predicts patients with ulcerative colitis not responding to medical therapy. Colorectal Dis 2014;16(12):O420–30.

38. Dubucquoi S, Janin A, Klein O, et al. Activated eosinophils and interleukin 5 expression in early recurrence of Crohn's disease. Gut 1995;37(2):242–6.

39. Masterson JC, McNamee EN, Jedlicka P, et al. CCR3 Blockade Attenuates Eosinophilic Ileitis and Associated Remodeling. Am J Pathol 2011;179(5):2302–14.

40. Hyams JS, Davis S, Mack DR, et al. Factors associated with early outcomes following standardised therapy in children with ulcerative colitis (PROTECT): a multicentre inception cohort study. Lancet Gastroenterol Hepatol 2017;2(12): 855–68.

41. Hyams JS, Davis Thomas S, Gotman N, et al. Clinical and biological predictors of response to standardised paediatric colitis therapy (PROTECT): a multicentre inception cohort study. Lancet 2019;393(10182):1708–20.

42. Klein J, Wilkins BJ, Verma R, et al. Collagenous Gastritis Masquerading as Eosinophilic Gastritis. ACG Case Rep J 2021;8(2):e00527.

43. Arnason T, Brown IS, Goldsmith JD, et al. Collagenous gastritis: a morphologic and immunohistochemical study of 40 patients. Mod Pathol 2015;28(4):533–44.

44. Colombel JF, Torpier G, Janin A, et al. Activated eosinophils in adult coeliac disease: evidence for a local release of major basic protein. Gut 1992;33(9):1190–4.

45. Brown IS, Smith J, Rosty C. Gastrointestinal pathology in celiac disease: a case series of 150 consecutive newly diagnosed patients. Am J Clin Pathol 2012; 138(1):42–9.

46. Kagalwalla AF, Shah A, Ritz S, et al. Cow's milk protein-induced eosinophilic esophagitis in a child with gluten-sensitive enteropathy. J Pediatr Gastroenterol Nutr 2007;44(3):386–8.

47. Ahmed OI, Qasem SA, Abdulsattar JA, et al. Esophageal eosinophilia in pediatric patients with celiac disease: is it a causal or an incidental association? J Pediatr Gastroenterol Nutr 2015;60(4):493–7.

48. Walker MM, Aggarwal KR, Shim LS, et al. Duodenal eosinophilia and early satiety in functional dyspepsia: confirmation of a positive association in an Australian cohort. J Gastroenterol Hepatol 2014;29(3):474–9.

49. Ozdogan E, Doganay L, Can D, et al. Disease Course and Treatment Response of Eosinophilic Gastrointestinal Diseases in Children With Liver Transplantation: Long-Term Follow-Up. Am J Gastroenterol 2021;116(1):188–97.

50. Bush JW, Mohammad S, Melin-Aldana H, et al. Eosinophilic density in graft biopsies positive for rejection and blood eosinophil count can predict development of post-transplant digestive tract eosinophilia. Pediatr Transplant 2016;20(4): 540–51.

51. Star KV, Ho VT, Wang HH, et al. Histologic features in colon biopsies can discriminate mycophenolate from GVHD-induced colitis. Am J Surg Pathol 2013;37(9): 1319–28.

Dietary Management of Non-EoE Eosinophilic Gastrointestinal Diseases

Mirna Chehade, MD, MPH[a],*, Bethany Doerfler, MS, RDN[b],
Dan Atkins, MD[c]

KEYWORDS

- Eosinophilic gastrointestinal disease • Eosinophilic gastritis • Eosinophilic enteritis
- Malnutrition • Elimination diet • Feeding difficulties • Food triggers

KEY POINTS

- Some patients with non–eosinophilic esophagitis eosinophilic gastrointestinal diseases (non-EoE EGIDs) respond to elimination diets, but more prospective studies are needed to determine the optimal approach to dietary restriction that provides the best therapeutic outcomes while having the least negative impact on quality of life.
- Patients with non-EoE EGIDs often present with a compromised nutritional status at baseline due to disease-specific inflammation and complications, and they require remediation of nutritional status prior to the initiation of therapeutic diets.
- Although most patients with non-EoE EGIDs are atopic, elimination diets informed by immunoglobulin (Ig) E–mediated sensitization to foods identified through skin testing or measurement of food-specific IgE levels have not outperformed empiric elimination diets.

BACKGROUND

Nature of the Problem: Clinical Presentation and Complications of Non–Eosinophilic Esophagitis Eosinophilic Gastrointestinal Diseases

Eosinophilic gastrointestinal diseases (EGIDs) are chronic, immune-mediated diseases of various segments of the gastrointestinal (GI) tract characterized by GI symptoms and eosinophil-predominant inflammation in the absence of other potential causes of GI tissue eosinophilia.[1] EGIDs encompass eosinophilic esophagitis (EoE)

[a] Mount Sinai Center for Eosinophilic Disorders, Icahn School of Medicine at Mount Sinai, One Gustave L. Levy Place, Box 1198, New York, NY 10029, USA; [b] Department of Gastroenterology & Hepatology, Northwestern Feinberg School of Medicine, Digestive Health Center, 259 East Erie, Suite 1600, Chicago, IL 60611, USA; [c] Department of Pediatrics, Allergy and Immunology, Gastrointestinal Eosinophilic Diseases Program, University of Colorado School of Medicine, Children's Hospital Colorado, 13123 E. 16th Avenue, Aurora, CO 80045, USA
* Corresponding author. Icahn School of Medicine at Mount Sinai, One Gustave L. Levy Place, Box 1198, New York, NY 10029.
E-mail address: mirna.chehade@mssm.edu

Immunol Allergy Clin N Am 44 (2024) 383–396
https://doi.org/10.1016/j.iac.2024.01.009
0889-8561/24/© 2024 Elsevier Inc. All rights reserved.

immunology.theclinics.com

and non-EoE EGIDs, which are named based upon the affected GI segment. Non-EoE EGIDs include eosinophilic gastritis (EoG), enteritis (EoN), and colitis. When the specific location affected by eosinophilic inflammation in the small intestine is known, EoN can be further specified as eosinophilic duodenitis (EoD), jejunitis, or ileitis.[1] Non-EoE EGIDs are patchy diseases involving 1 or multiple segments of the GI tract. Furthermore, the eosinophil-predominant inflammation can involve 1 or more of the mucosal, muscular, or serosal layers of a specific segment.[2]

Patients with non-EoE EGIDs have various clinical and endoscopic manifestations based on disease location, depth, and extent of involvement. Nutritional deficiencies commonly result from either food avoidance or the inability to absorb required nutrients. Patients with the mucosal variant, which is the most common, present with 1 or more symptoms, which include abdominal pain, nausea, vomiting, diarrhea, and gas/bloating.[3] Patients with severe mucosal disease can experience significant weight loss, or lack of weight gain, and growth failure in the case of children.[4,5] Other complications include anemia due to bleeding ulcers, malabsorption, malnutrition, and/or blood loss due to associated protein-losing enteropathy (PLE).[4–7] Patients with PLE develop edema in dependent areas due to protein and albumin losses and can leak immunoglobulin (Ig) G into the gut lumen, including specific antibodies made in response to vaccinations, potentially rendering them vulnerable to preventable infections.[8]

Patients with the muscular variant present clinically with obstructive symptoms, including gastric outlet obstruction when the eosinophilic inflammation is in the stomach or bowel obstruction when the small intestine is involved. This often results in abdominal distention and repeated vomiting.[2,9] The least common serosal variant of non-EoE EGIDs typically presents with ascites, either alone or in combination with various other GI symptoms related to involvement of other layers of the GI tract, such as nausea and vomiting.[2,9]

Symptoms related to non-EoE EGIDs and their complications result in a variety of nutritional deficiencies that require timely diagnosis and proper management in order to optimize nutritional intake for the promotion of adequate and timely recovery in response to treatment, while also supporting catch-up weight gain and growth.

Evaluation: Importance of Reviewing the Diet

The diet of patients with non-EoE EGIDs must be thoroughly assessed by taking a detailed dietary history so that nutritional deficiencies and/or malnutrition secondary to non-EoE EGIDs complications can be promptly identified and corrected. Nutritional outcome goals in children include appropriate weight gain, including catch-up growth, dietary expansion when appropriate, and reaching feeding milestones, whereas nutritional goals in adults include correction of nutritional deficiencies and returning to or maintaining an appropriate weight. Dietary assessment, including food preferences, is also required to aid in determining whether dietary elimination therapy is a viable option for a given non-EoE EGIDs patient.

Approach: Nutritional Assessment

Non-EoE EGIDs can negatively impact the nutritional status of patients directly due to both the pathophysiology of the disease and its complications and through dietary restrictions when foods thought to exacerbate GI symptoms are removed by the patient or the treating provider. Failure to thrive has been reported in children with non-EoE EGIDs.[10,11] Various symptoms in patients with non-EoE EGIDs can have a negative impact on their nutritional status, resulting in specific deficiencies that require precise nutritional interventions (**Table 1**).

Table 1

Gastrointestinal and nutrition impact symptoms common in non–eosinophilic esophagitis eosinophilic gastrointestinal diseases

GI and nutrition Impact Symptoms	Clinical Presentation	Possible Causes	Medical Evaluation	Nutritional Intervention
Abdominal pain and early satiety	Food avoidance Reduced oral intake Weight loss Malnutrition	Active EGIDs Delayed gastric emptying	CBC with differential, CMP Gastric emptying scan	Frequent small meals Energy-dense foods Oral enteral nutritional supplementation with safe ingredients
Nausea, vomiting, and diarrhea	Food avoidance Reduced oral intake Dehydration	Active EGIDs Delayed gastric emptying	Gastric emptying scan[a] CMP, CBC with differential Urine-specific gravity Fecal elastase	Oral rehydration solutions Removal of suspected food triggers Supplemental oral nutrition
Weight loss	Failure to thrive	Sub-optimal calorie intake	Nutrition assessment and calorie counts	Nutrition assessment
	Muscle loss Fatigue	Malabsorption ARFID	CBC with differential, CMP Rule out other causes (stool for calprotectin, stool culture)	Scheduled meals Supplemental oral nutrition Possible nutritional support with enteral access
Edema	Hypoalbuminemia Hypoproteinemia Loss of muscle mass Fatigue Hair loss	Active EGIDs Poor protein intake Rapid weight loss	CMP Iron panel with ferritin Stool alpha-1-trypsin IgG level Rule out other causes (TSH, T3/T4)	Adequate calorie intake Increase total protein Amino acid–based formula supplementation
Anemia	Fatigue	Malnutrition	CBC with differential	Nutrition assessment to evaluate dietary adequacy
	Exercise intolerance	Intestinal malabsorption	Iron panel with ferritin	Provide supplementation to correct serum abnormalities
		Bleeding ulcer	Vitamin B12 level and folate	Include fortified gluten-free grains

Abbreviations: ARFID, Avoidant/restrictive food intake disease; CBC, complete blood count; CMP, comprehensive metabolic profile; EGIDs, eosinophilic gastrointestinal diseases; GI, gastrointestinal; IgG, immunoglobulin G; TSH, .thyroid-stimulating hormone.

[a] To be considered in patients with dyspepsia despite histologic remission.

Approach: Tools to Assess Nutritional Status

For both children and adults, anthropometric assessment and physical nutrition assessment comprise the nutrition-focused physical examination. Among adults, malnutrition risk should be considered in the context of chronic illness and social circumstances. Several factors including the percentage of weight loss, diminished calorie intake, and loss of both muscle and fat stores factor into a diagnosis of malnutrition.[12] Among children, anthropometry includes weight, length (recumbent length for children<24 months of age and standing 2–20 years), and head circumference (for children<36 months). Growth parameters should be plotted on pediatric growth charts (World Health Organization charts for infants and children from birth to 24 months).[13] Proper growth assessment is used to calculate growth patterns (Z-scores). In children, this assessment should include attainment of feeding milestones, oral motor development, and food aversions that increase nutrition risk. Children on elimination diets may exhibit signs of height stunting even before weight loss. A loss of growth velocity should trigger a referral to a registered dietitian.[13]

In adults, additional assessment tools which determine nutritional status by also accounting for nutrition impact symptoms is the patient-generated subjective global assessment (PGSGA) and its abridged version (abPGSGA). These are practical, valid tools that can be used clinically to quickly classify nutrition status in the outpatient setting. Previously used in oncology populations, the abPGSGA includes subjective and objective data regarding changes in weight, dietary intake, nutrition symptoms, and physical functioning and allows for nutrition status rankings (mild–severely malnourished).[14,15]

Fig. 1 provides a clinician's pocket guide to quickly assess nutrition risk in both children and adults with non-EoE EGIDs.

Approach: Additional Nutritional Challenges to Consider

There are several nutritional considerations unique to patients with non-EoE EGIDs that may stem from GI nutrition impact symptoms (such as dysphagia, pain, malabsorption, and food refusal) as well as from elimination diets used to treat non-EoE EGIDs. In addition, developmental milestones related to feeding need to be considered in young children. Oral motor and oral sensory development occur predominantly within the first 3 years of life and require careful monitoring if dietary intake is modified for treatment.[16,17]

Social determinants of health including family food budget and access to low-allergen foods are important to consider when developing a nutrition care plan. Shopping for specialized foods commonly recommended while on an empiric elimination diet can increase the cost of food.[18] In addition, amino acid–based formulas can be expensive and are not universally covered by medical insurance.[19]

The goal of dietary restriction therapy is not only to improve nutritional status and treat disease but also to provide protection of bone health, maintenance of muscle mass, and promotion of a diverse microbiome. There are many functional aspects of foods to consider. **Table 2** and **Fig. 2** integrate the interplay of the food matrix on health outcomes.

CURRENT EVIDENCE: ALLERGY EVALUATION OF PATIENTS WITH NON–EOSINOPHILIC ESOPHAGITIS EOSINOPHILIC GASTROINTESTINAL DISEASES
Evidence Pointing Toward an Allergic Etiology for Non–Eosinophilic Esophagitis Eosinophilic Gastrointestinal Diseases

Emerging research studies point toward a type 2 allergic etiology in non-EoE EGIDs, especially in children.[20] The allergy cytokines interleukin (IL) 4, IL-5, and IL-13 were

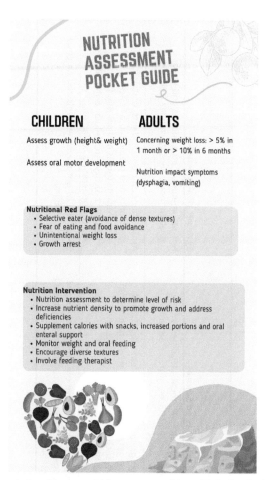

Fig. 1. Clinician's pocket guide to quickly assess nutrition risk in both children and adults with non–eosinophilic esophagitis eosinophilic gastrointestinal diseases.

shown to be upregulated in gastric tissue of children with EoG.[20] In addition, mast cell transcripts and mast cell numbers were shown to be increased in gastric/duodenal tissue of patients with EoG/EoD.[20,21]

The connection of an allergic response to foods in particular was demonstrated by Prussin and colleagues[22] who found abundant IL-5(+) peanut-specific Th2 cells in patients with EoG and peanut allergy, as opposed to IL-5(−) peanut-specific Th2 cells in patients with peanut allergy without EoG, indicating a link between food allergy and eosinophil-dominant immunopathology in patients with non-EoE EGIDs.

Additional Testing: Allergy Evaluation

As noted in EoE, a significant portion of non-EoE EGIDs patients have comorbid atopic disease.[3] Thus, a fundamental aspect of the initial evaluation of non-EoE EGIDs patients is to identify the triggers and severity of coexisting allergic diseases such as food allergy, atopic dermatitis, allergic rhinitis, or asthma. Optimal control of comorbid allergic diseases is an important aspect of holistic non-EoE EGIDs management. The recognition of seasonal worsening of non-EoE EGIDs correlating with an increase in

Table 2
Metabolic benefits of a diverse dietary pattern beyond the gut

Nutrients	Hypoallergenic Food Sources	Systemic Health Benefits
Protein, calories, calcium, vitamin D, vitamin A, vitamin B12, phosphorus	Fortified vegan milk, meats, legumes, whole grains, fortified juices, gluten-free whole grains, seeds	Normal immune status, muscle and linear growth, bone density, cellular function
Folate, B vitamins, fiber, iron, trace minerals, essential fatty acids	Fortified grains, dark green leafy vegetables, root vegetables, legumes, whole gluten-free grains such as millet, oats, quinoa, and buckwheat	Anticarcinogenic antioxidants, dietary probiotics and prebiotics, bile acid sequestrants (gums and soluble fibers), transport of oxygen, cellular antioxidants, energy generating co-factors
Phenolic compounds and antioxidants	Berries, extra-virgin olive oil, green tea, yellow/orange root vegetables and fruits, green leafy vegetables	Reduction of gut methane levels and mucosal permeability

Body System Impacted by EGID: Implications for Health

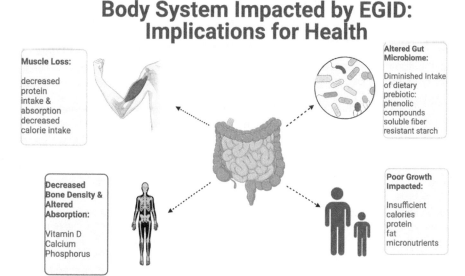

Muscle Loss:

decreased protein intake & absorption decreased calorie intake

Altered Gut Microbiome:

Diminished Intake of dietary prebiotic: phenolic compounds soluble fiber resistant starch

Decreased Bone Density & Altered Absorption:

Vitamin D Calcium Phosphorus

Poor Growth Impacted:

Insufficient calories protein fat micronutrients

Fig. 2. Nutrients and body systems impacted by altered nutritional intake and absorption in non–eosinophilic esophagitis eosinophilic gastrointestinal. (Created with BioRender.com.)

symptoms of other allergic disease may aid in identifying non-EoE EGIDs triggers or suggest the need to proactively increase non-EoE EGIDs treatment or avoid foods with pollen cross-reactive allergens at specific times of the year. Identifying and documenting patient-perceived food allergies and intolerances are key due to their impact on diet and nutrition, as they often complicate attempts at dietary management of non-EoE EGIDs by further limiting dietary choices. IgE-mediated sensitization to a potential allergen is documented by prick skin testing and/or the measurement of serum allergen–specific IgE levels. However, IgE-mediated sensitization is not a reliable predictor of whether a specific allergen is a non-EoE EGIDs trigger.[5] IgE-mediated allergy is defined not by sensitization alone but by sensitization combined with reproducible symptoms upon exposure. Thus, using sensitization alone to diagnose allergy leads to overdiagnosis. As a result, skin testing and/or the measurement serum food allergen–specific IgE levels should be limited to allergens suggested by the history. The use of large panels of skin tests or serum allergen–specific IgE levels is not recommended. Although uncommon, some patients are sensitized to a food before removal or become sensitized to an eliminated food allergen while on an elimination diet.[23] As a result, skin testing prior to the reintroduction of a major food allergen can help determine whether a food is best reintroduced at home or under medical supervision. Patients with non-EoE EGIDs on elimination diets should be informed that developing IgE-mediated allergy to an eliminated food, although rare, can occur and not to ignore symptoms with accidental exposures or attempted reintroduction of the avoided food.

THERAPEUTIC OPTIONS: DIET AS A TREATMENT MODALITY

While non-EoE EGIDs are a group of heterogeneous diseases, an allergic etiology has been suspected for at least a subset of patients with the disease. This has led to several historical attempts at treating non-EoE EGIDs with a dietary elimination approach resembling that used in patients with EoE, with success achieved using more restrictive diets.

Dietary Elimination Therapies

Clinical evidence for the efficacy of dietary restriction in patients with non-EoE EGIDs stems from early studies of children with non-EoE EGIDs treated with elemental diet with good clinical response. In 2006, Chehade and colleagues[8] published data on the therapeutic response to elimination diets in a retrospective study of children with EoG and/or EoD with associated PLE. The study included 6 children, with age at symptom onset ranging from 2 to 31 months and age at diagnosis ranging from 16 to 42 months. They had significant gastric and/or duodenal eosinophilia (peak gastric antral eosinophils 43–300/ high-power microscopy field [HPF] and peak duodenal eosinophils 30–88/HPF). While the clinical response was variable to food elimination diets, response to an elemental diet consisting of exclusive feeding with a non-allergenic amino acid–based formula was excellent. A limited number of solid foods of low allergenic potential were continued in the diet of 3 children. All patients experienced rapid resolution of symptoms and their anemia and hypoalbuminemia in less than 4 weeks. No histologic follow-up was obtained. In discussions 2.5 to 5.5 years later, parents of these children indicated that some food-responsive symptoms persisted, but all patients had tolerated gradual addition of various foods to their diet. The number of foods tolerated over time did not correlate with food-specific IgE levels, again highlighting the cell-mediated rather than IgE-mediated response to food in non-EoE EGIDs.

Ko and colleagues[5] later reported on results of empiric dietary interventions in another retrospective study of children with EoG. In that study of 30 children, median age at diagnosis was 7.5 years (range 0.2–15.2 years), and 17 received dietary restriction therapy. Diets included either an elemental diet, consisting of feeding with a nonallergenic amino acid–based formula while allowing concurrent consumption of 1 to 12 foods (6 patients), an empiric 6-food elimination diet in addition to removal of red meat (avoidance of milk, wheat, egg, soy, nuts, seafood, red meats; 6 patients), and empiric avoidance of 1 to 3 common food allergens (milk, egg, soy, and/or wheat; 5 patients). Of the 17 children treated with dietary restriction therapy, 14 (82%) had clinical response, defined by resolution of symptoms. Fourteen patients had repeat upper endoscopy with biopsies following dietary intervention, 11 of whom (78%) had histologic response (peak gastric eosinophils <10/HPF). All histologic responders to the dietary restriction therapy also had clinical response to that therapy. Response to diet did not correlate with skin prick test results to foods or serum food-specific IgE levels, again emphasizing the non-IgE-mediated nature of the food response in non-EoE EGID.

Confirmation of the efficacy of the empiric elimination diet for children with EoG was recently demonstrated by Ng and colleagues[24], in a retrospective study of 20 patients entirely comprised of children of Asian ancestry and median age of 15 months (range 3–192 months), who were started on a proton pump inhibitor (PPI) concurrently with an empiric elimination diet as a first-line therapy, consisting of avoidance of 1 to 6 of the common food allergens. The diet was individualized based on dietary history, symptoms related to food ingestion, and co-existence of IgE-mediated food allergies. As in other pediatric EoG studies[5], some of these patients had concurrent EoD or esophageal eosinophilia. Nine (45%) had 4 or more foods eliminated from their diet. The top foods eliminated were milk (90%) and soy (85%), followed by egg, wheat, nuts, and seafood (30%–45%). Clinical, endoscopic, and histologic remissions were achieved in 94.7%, 81.3%, and 68.8%, respectively, following this combination therapy. Although concurrent PPI therapy may have at least partially contributed to some of the responses seen, the data still provide insight as to the potential utility of this combination therapy with PPI and empiric elimination diets in children with non-EoE EGIDs.

More recently, a new type of empiric elimination diet, which is less restrictive than an elemental diet, but more restrictive than the 6-food elimination diet, was tested in children with non-EoE EGIDs by Nagashima and colleagues in Japan[25], and the results were retrospectively reported. The diet consisted of exclusive feeding with an amino acid–based formula in addition to fruits, vegetables, tubers, and roots. Seven children, aged 2 to 17 years, with refractory disease to less restrictive empiric elimination diets and/or pharmacologic therapies, 4 of whom with associated PLE, were transitioned to this dietary therapy regimen for at least 2 weeks. Five children were symptomatic before starting the diet and showed clinical improvement. No histologic follow-up was available. A decrease in the peripheral eosinophil count was seen in 6 patients, and serum albumin improved in those with PLE, with resolution of their secondary edema.

It appears that age plays a factor in the success rate of food restriction therapy in children. In a study of 12 children with EoG/EoD with associated anemia and hypoproteinemia secondary to PLE, Katz and colleagues[26] identified 2 subsets, those that responded to milk elimination, with amelioration of signs and symptoms, and those that were nonresponsive to this diet and often required pharmacologic therapy for clinical relief. Milk-responsive patients had earlier disease onset, namely in infancy (presenting age 5.2 ± 3.9 months vs 4.0 ± 3.3 years in nonresponsive patients). Milk reintroduction was clinically tolerated when added at 30 to 36 months of age, while earlier reintroduction was associated with clinical and histologic disease relapse. Note that before receiving pharmacologic therapy, the refractory subset of patients underwent subsequent elimination of multiple foods from their diet based on results of standard allergy tests including skin prick tests and serum food-specific IgE levels without success, pointing again toward the non-IgE–mediated mechanism of food responsiveness in patients with EoG/EoD.

This observation of age-related response to diet was also observed by Ng and colleagues[24] several years later in their cohort described earlier. EoG patients with symptom onset in childhood (>12 months) were generally more severe than those with infantile-onset EoG patients (age at presentation ≤12 months); they were more likely to have anemia and more likely to suffer from PLE. In addition, a greater proportion of patients from the childhood-onset group required more extensive food eliminations, with more than half having ≥4 foods eliminated from their diet. Despite this, the childhood-onset EoG group had poorer endoscopic and histologic remission rates, with half of the patients exhibiting a refractory disease course.

The response to dietary restriction therapy does not appear to be limited to children, as an elemental diet was recently demonstrated to be effective in adults with non-EoE EGIDs. Gonsalves and colleagues[27] recently published results of a prospective single-center clinical trial using elemental diet therapy for adult patients with EoG and/or EoD that is refractory to standard of care therapies, including an empiric 6-food elimination diet for a subset of patients. They were exclusively fed a non-allergenic amino acid–based formula orally under close supervision by a dietitian for a total of 6 weeks, with clinical, endoscopic, and histologic follow-up. Fifteen out of 19 patients, mean age 37.7 years, completed the study. All patients achieved histologic disease remission at 6 weeks as defined by peak gastric/duodenal eosinophils less than 30/HPF. On average, eosinophil levels significantly decreased (from 50 to 11 eos/HPF in the stomach, $P < .001$, and from 49 to 16 in the duodenum, $P = .001$). Additionally, clinical and endoscopic improvements were observed. Thirteen out of 15 patients elected to reintroduce foods afterward, 1 food at a time, with clinical and histologic follow-ups.

Nearly all patients had disease recurrence with specific food introductions, suggesting a dominant role for food allergens in adults with EoG and EoD. Multiple foods were suspected/identified as triggers in these patients based on symptoms and/or histology. Specifically, 11/13 reacted to grains and proteins such as oats, legumes, and poultry. All participants had symptoms with the top 8 allergens such as wheat, dairy, eggs, soy, nuts, and seafood.

Furthermore, successful empiric dietary elimination therapy was also recently described by Okimoto and colleagues[28] in a retrospective study of their patients with non-EoE EGIDs in Japan. Of 34 adults with non-EoE EGIDs, mean age 41.6 years, 13 patients were treated with an empiric 6-food elimination diet, consisting of avoidance of milk, wheat, egg, soy, peanut/tree nuts, and seafood. Eleven of those patients had experienced disease relapse with reduced corticosteroids, and the remaining 2 patients did not receive prior therapy. All 13 patients had symptom improvement on the diet. Food triggers were identified in 9 patients, and 7 were reported to be maintained in remission without corticosteroids, though the investigators did not specify how remission was defined. Milk and soy were the most commonly identified food triggers in these patients.

In summary, data from children and adults, both from the US and from Asia, though mostly limited to retrospective studies, point toward the presence of food triggers in the pathogenesis of non-EoE EGIDs. As a result, dietary elimination therapy is a viable treatment option for patients with these diseases. Prospective studies using various empiric elimination diets for children and adults with non-EoE EGIDs are needed to determine their optimal efficacy while minimizing nutritional and social complications.

Which Patients to Select for Dietary Elimination Therapy

The choice to use elimination diet therapy is best reached through shared decision-making after a thorough presentation and discussion of the pros and cons of each available therapy. In addition, individual aspects of the patient's situation such as age, feeding skills, baseline nutritional status, baseline food avoidance, food preferences, food availability, disease severity, motivation, social support, and socioeconomic factors must be considered. Children old enough to participate should be included in the decision to optimize adherence and avoid significant preventable negative impact on their quality of life.

Dietary Elimination Therapy Implementation: Nutritional Tips

The ultimate goal of diet therapy is to provide the least restrictive pattern of eating that offers nutrient density and enhances therapeutic outcomes. Effective nutrition interventions integrate nutrition assessment, education of safer food substitutes which are equally nutrient dense, and nutritional monitoring. **Table 3** illustrates common nutrition problems in patients with non-EoE EGIDs that need to be addressed, especially when a dietary elimination therapy is initiated.

DISCUSSION
Future Directions: Diet in Non–Eosinophilic Esophagitis Eosinophilic Gastrointestinal Diseases

Numerous questions surround the role of diet in the pathophysiology and management of non-EoE EGIDs. For example, are food antigens truly the only or even the most common drivers of non-EoE EGIDs? Can the specific allergens driving disease be identified and used to develop testing to accurately predict food provocateurs in an individual patient? Rather than specific food antigens driving disease, could dietary differences or other environmental influences on the microbiome in different segments

Table 3 Troubleshooting common nutritional complications	
Texture-selective eater	Develop ladder of textures within food groups to try (ie, apple juice, applesauce, cooked chunky apples, freeze dried and fresh) Involve both a dietitian and feeding therapist to offer acceptable substitutes while increasing textures Limit excessive snacking to optimize mealtimes
Excessive food group restriction	Shared decision-making with the patient and family to begin with the least restrictive food group removal Emphasis on food substitution vs avoidance Supplement diet with allergy-free enteral option
Diminished social eating	Strategize safe places for dining Encourage friends and family to bring low-allergen dishes for communal eating. Bring restaurant card with avoided foods when dining out. Choose social events that do not revolve around mealtimes only.
Reduced calorie and protein intake	Offer allergy-appropriate low-volume, energy-dense foods Create structured meals and snacks Integrate hypoallergenic oral enteral nutrition Increase liquid calories meals with addition of 100% juices and non-dairy milks with safe ingredients

of the gut drive disease in some patients? Will biologics be able to control disease while allowing continued ingestion or dietary reintroduction of food triggers? Unfortunately, research of this population is even more difficult than studying patients with EoE given there are significantly fewer patients with non-EoE EGIDs, making it more difficult to accumulate large cohorts for study. In addition, less invasive methods, such as transnasal endoscopy, the esophageal string test or the cytosponge, currently being studied in the evaluation of response to dietary therapies in patients with EoE, are currently lacking for non-EoE EGIDs. Therefore, endoscopies with biopsies requiring sedation or anesthesia are currently required for disease monitoring or assessment of response to therapies. In a sense, the issues involving non-EoE EGIDs echo those encountered with EoE years ago. Thus, the significant progress made in the awareness, recognition, definition, diagnosis, and management of EoE over the past decades supports an optimistic view that similar advances in the field of non-EoE EGIDs are on the horizon.

SUMMARY

Dietary restriction therapy has a role in treating children and adults with non-EoE EGIDs. Nutrition assessment and addressing nutritional concerns are a key component of management for all non-EoE EGIDs patients, even when dietary restriction is not used for treatment as these patients are at risk of nutritional deficiencies due to food avoidant behaviors and the pathophysiology of the disease process leading to poor nutrient absorption depending on the section, layer and extent of the GI tract involved. Although the majority of patients with non-EoE EGIDs are atopic and benefit from assessment and control of co-existing food and environmental allergies, IgE-mediated sensitization is not a reliable predictor of whether a specific food is an non-EoE EGIDs trigger. This is supported by studies revealing that test-directed elimination diets do not outperform empiric elimination diets. Deciding on how extensive empiric dietary elimination should be is a process best approached by shared decision-making with patients and their families considering nutritional, cultural, and lifestyle factors.

CLINICS CARE POINTS

- The majority of patients with non-EoE EGIDs have comorbid allergic disease. Accurate diagnosis and optimal management of these allergic conditions is an essential aspect of non-EoE EGIDs care.

- Some patients with non-EoE EGIDs respond to dietary avoidance of specific food allergens. Therefore, dietary elimination therapy should be considered in patients with non-EoE EGIDs.

- Involvement of a registered dietitian to provide an initial nutrition assessment of children and adults with non-EoE EGIDs and to oversee the proper execution and management of elimination diets is key.

- The initial elimination diet is implemented for a predetermined relatively brief period of time, to aid in identifying food triggers. A plan for food reintroduction accompanied by monitoring for GI inflammation by endoscopies with GI biopsies is an essential aspect of dietary elimination therapy. Symptoms alone are not a reliable indicator of disease status.

- Patients with non-EoE EGIDs often suffer from micronutrient abnormalities. A detailed clinical review and serum assessment of visceral proteins, electrolytes, micronutrients and blood counts are warranted. A plan for remediation of biochemical and nutritional abnormalities should be in place before beginning elimination diet therapy.

DISCLOSURE

M. Chehade is currently serving or has served as consultant for Regeneron, Adare/Ellodi, AstraZeneca, Sanofi, Bristol Myers Squibb, Recludix Pharma, Nexstone Immunology, Allakos, Shire/Takeda, and Phathom, and is currently receiving or has received research funding from Regeneron, United States, Allakos, Shire/Takeda, AstraZeneca, United Kingdom, Adare/Ellodi, Bristol-Myers Squibb, United States, Danone, v. B. Doerfler has served on speakers bureaus for Nutricia North America, on advisory boards for Trellus Health LLC, and received honoraria from PRIMED CME and ACHL Healthcare. D. Atkins has nothing to disclose.

REFERENCES

1. Dellon ES, Gonsalves N, Abonia JP, et al. International consensus recommendations for eosinophilic gastrointestinal disease nomenclature. Clin Gastroenterol Hepatol 2022;20(11):2474–2484 e2473.
2. Klein NC, Hargrove RL, Sleisenger MH, et al. Eosinophilic gastroenteritis. Medicine (Baltim) 1970;49(4):299–319.
3. Chehade M, Kamboj AP, Atkins D, et al. Diagnostic delay in patients with eosinophilic gastritis and/or duodenitis: a population-based study. J Allergy Clin Immunol Pract 2021;9(5):2050–2059 e2020.
4. Papadopoulou A, Amil-Dias J, Auth MK, et al. Joint ESPGHAN/NASPGHAN Guidelines on Childhood Eosinophilic Gastrointestinal Disorders Beyond Eosinophilic Esophagitis. J Pediatr Gastroenterol Nutr 2024;78(1):122–52.
5. Ko HM, Morotti RA, Yershov O, et al. Eosinophilic gastritis in children: clinicopathological correlation, disease course, and response to therapy. Am J Gastroenterol 2014;109(8):1277–85.

6. Lam AY, Gonsalves N. "Tickle me pink": update in eosinophilic gastrointestinal disorders. Curr Opin Gastroenterol 2023;39(1):36–42.

7. Prussin C. Eosinophilic gastroenteritis and related eosinophilic disorders. Gastroentorol Clin North Am 2014;43(2):3 17–27.

8. Chehade M, Magid MS, Mofidi S, et al. Allergic eosinophilic gastroenteritis with protein-losing enteropathy: intestinal pathology, clinical course, and long-term follow-up. J Pediatr Gastroenterol Nutr 2006;42(5):516–21.

9. Talley NJ, Shorter RG, Phillips SF, et al. Eosinophilic gastroenteritis: a clinicopathological study of patients with disease of the mucosa, muscle layer, and subserosal tissues. Gut 1990;31(1):54–8.

10. Chehade M, Jones SM, Pesek RD, et al. Phenotypic characterization of eosinophilic esophagitis in a large multicenter patient population from the consortium for food allergy research. J Allergy Clin Immunol Pract 2018;6(5):1534–1544 e1535.

11. Alhmoud T, Hanson JA, Parasher G. Eosinophilic gastroenteritis: an underdiagnosed condition. Dig Dis Sci 2016;61(9):2585–92.

12. White JV, Guenter P, Jensen G, et al. Consensus statement: academy of nutrition and dietetics and american society for parenteral and enteral nutrition: characteristics recommended for the identification and documentation of adult malnutrition (undernutrition). JPEN - J Parenter Enter Nutr 2012;36(3):275–83.

13. Groetch M, Venter C, Skypala I, et al. Dietary therapy and nutrition management of eosinophilic esophagitis: a work group report of the american academy of allergy, asthma, and immunology. J Allergy Clin Immunol Pract 2017;5(2):312–324 e329.

14. Doerfler B, Allen TS, Southwood C, et al. Medical nutrition therapy for patients with advanced systemic sclerosis (MNT PASS): a pilot intervention study. JPEN - J Parenter Enter Nutr 2017;41(4):678–84.

15. Gabrielson DK, Scaffidi D, Leung E, et al. Use of an abridged scored Patient-Generated Subjective Global Assessment (abPG-SGA) as a nutritional screening tool for cancer patients in an outpatient setting. Nutr Cancer 2013;65(2):234–9.

16. Delaney AL, Arvedson JC. Development of swallowing and feeding: prenatal through first year of life. Dev Disabil Res Rev 2008;14(2):105–17.

17. Chehade M, Meyer R, Beauregard A. Feeding difficulties in children with non-IgE-mediated food allergic gastrointestinal disorders. Ann Allergy Asthma Immunol 2019;122(6):603–9.

18. Asher Wolf W, Huang KZ, Durban R, et al. The six-food elimination diet for eosinophilic esophagitis increases grocery shopping cost and complexity. Dysphagia 2016;31(6):765–70.

19. Schultz F, Warren CM, Chehade M, et al. When supplemental formula is essential: overcoming barriers to hypoallergenic formula access for patients with food allergies. J Allergy Clin Immunol Pract 2023;11(9):2686–92.

20. Caldwell JM, Collins MH, Stucke EM, et al. Histologic eosinophilic gastritis is a systemic disorder associated with blood and extragastric eosinophilia, TH2 immunity, and a unique gastric transcriptome. J Allergy Clin Immunol 2014;134(5):1114–24.

21. Reed CC, Genta RM, Youngblood BA, et al. Mast cell and eosinophil counts in gastric and duodenal biopsy specimens from patients with and without eosinophilic gastroenteritis. Clin Gastroenterol Hepatol 2021;19(10):2102–11.

22. Prussin C, Lee J, Foster B. Eosinophilic gastrointestinal disease and peanut allergy are alternatively associated with IL-5+ and IL-5(-) T(H)2 responses. J Allergy Clin Immunol 2009;124(6):1326–1332 e1326.

23. Ho HE, Chehade M. Development of IgE-mediated immediate hypersensitivity to a previously tolerated food following its avoidance for eosinophilic gastrointestinal diseases. J Allergy Clin Immunol Pract 2018;6(2):649–50.

24. Ng LQ, Loh W, Ong JX, et al. Clinical, histopathological features and efficacy of elimination diet and proton-pump inhibitor therapy in achieving histological remission in Asian children with eosinophilic gastritis. J Paediatr Child Health 2022; 58(7):1244–50.

25. Nagashima S, Yamamoto M, Inuzuka Y, et al. Tolerability and safety of a new elimination diet for pediatric eosinophilic gastritis and duodenitis. Allergol Int 2023; 72(2):306–15.

26. Katz AJ, Twarog FJ, Zeiger RS, et al. Milk-sensitive and eosinophilic gastroenteropathy: similar clinical features with contrasting mechanisms and clinical course. J Allergy Clin Immunol 1984;74(1):72–8.

27. Gonsalvos N, Doerfler B, Zalewski A, et al. Prospective study of an amino acid-based elemental diet in an eosinophilic gastritis and gastroenteritis nutrition trial. J Allergy Clin Immunol 2023;152(3):676–88.

28. Okimoto E, Ishimura N, Ishihara S. Clinical Characteristics and Treatment Outcomes of Patients with Eosinophilic Esophagitis and Eosinophilic Gastroenteritis. Digestion 2021;102(1):33–40.

Pharmacologic Management of Non–Eosinophilic Esophagitis Eosinophilic Gastrointestinal Diseases

Evan S. Dellon, MD, MPH[a],*, Sandeep K. Gupta, MD[b]

KEYWORDS

- Non–eosinophilic esophagitis eosinophilic gastrointestinal diseases
- Pharmacologic therapy • Trials • Outcomes

KEY POINTS

- Medical treatment of non–eosinophilic esophagitis (EoE) eosinophilic gastrointestinal diseases (EGIDs) is challenging.
- Because of the rarity of these conditions, data on specific treatments, outcomes, predictors of response, recurrence rates, and management algorithms are limited, and recent pediatric guidelines had universal agreement on the statement that "there is a lack of randomized controlled trials assessing the efficacy of the available treatment options for non-EoE EGIDs."
- Nevertheless, pharmacologic options exist and are used, though all are off-label for conditions like eosinophilic gastritis, eosinophilic enteritis, and eosinophilic colitis.

INTRODUCTION

Medical treatment of non–eosinophilic esophagitis (EoE) eosinophilic gastrointestinal diseases (EGIDs) is challenging. Because of the rarity of these conditions,[1] data on specific treatments, outcomes, predictors of response, recurrence rates, and management algorithms are limited, and recent pediatric guidelines had universal agreement on the statement that "there is a lack of randomized controlled trials assessing the efficacy of the available treatment options for non-EoE EGIDs."[2] Nevertheless, pharmacologic options exist and are used, though all are off-label for conditions like eosinophilic gastritis (EoG), eosinophilic enteritis (EoN), and eosinophilic colitis (EoC). While

[a] Division of Gastroenterology and Hepatology, Department of Medicine, Center for Esophageal Diseases and Swallowing, University of North Carolina School of Medicine, 130 Mason Farm Road, Chapel Hill, NC 27599-7080, USA; [b] Division of Pediatric Gastroenterology, Hepatology and Nutrition, University of Alabama at Birmingham/Children's of Alabama, 1600 7th Avenue South, Birmingham, AL 35233-1785, USA
* Corresponding author.
E-mail address: edellon@med.unc.edu

Immunol Allergy Clin N Am 44 (2024) 397–406
https://doi.org/10.1016/j.iac.2024.01.010
0889-8561/24/© 2024 Elsevier Inc. All rights reserved.

the mainstays of treatment are corticosteroids, with "topical" delivery preferred over systemic, a number of other non-biologic treatments have been reported, including proton-pump inhibitors (PPIs), mast-cell stabilizers like cromolyn and ketotifen, and immunomodulators.[2–5] With the increasing understanding of non-EoE EGID pathogenesis, including the presumed allergic basis of EoG and EoN with T2-predominant inflammation,[6–8] targeted treatments can now be studied, including those in the biologic and small-molecule classes. In this article, the authors will review data related to corticosteroids, non-biologic treatments such as small molecules, and biologic treatments for non-EoE EGIDs. The authors will also discuss medications that are under development and potential therapeutic targets, highlighting an expanding pipeline for drug development for this complex set of conditions.

CORTICOSTEROID TREATMENTS

Both topical and systemic corticosteroids have been used in the treatment of non-EoE EGIDs,[9–12] with reported response rates of 90% in some instances.[13] Systemic prednisone use is reported at doses of 5 to 60 mg/d followed by a taper over 4 to 6 weeks.[11,13,14] Due to a sub-segment of patients who may relapse or experience continuous disease, intermittent or chronic low-dose corticosteroid use may be needed.[13,14]

Topical budesonide has fewer systemic side effects due to first-pass hepatic metabolism, and its enteric-coated formulations can be adapted for more distal non-EoE EGIDs. Doses of 0.25 to 9 mg of viscous slurry or enteric-coated budesonide have been used for eosinophilic gastroenteritis.[11,15] A retrospective study of 44 patients with eosinophilic gastroenteritis compared 6-food elimination diet (SFED) plus montelukast to SFED plus prednisone or SFED plus budesonide.[16] Here, SFED-prednisone and SFED-budesonide were superior to SFED with montelukast. Two different formulations of budesonide were used in this study—Entocort was used for patients with inflammation in the stomach and duodenum and Budenofalk was used for inflammation in the ileum and colon; budesonide doses ranged from 1 mg twice daily to 3 mg 3 times daily, depending on age. In a study of 8 children with non-EoE EGIDs, targeted combinations of crushed, opened, and intact budesonide capsules were associated with significant improvement in gastric eosinophil counts.[17] In another study, a significant decrease in gastric eosinophils was observed in a subset of pediatric EoE patients treated with fluticasone who also had elevated gastric eosinophils.[18] This suggests that fluticasone may be helpful, particularly in patients with predominant gastric involvement.[2] In a retrospective multicenter study from the US of 108 patients with EoC, 19% of children were treated with enteric-coated budesonide capsules.[19] After 6 months of treatment, those who underwent repeat colonoscopy showed a decrease in mucosal eosinophilia with crushed corticosteroids, but the changes did not reach statistical significance.

Based on these data, the joint European Society for Pediatric Gastroenterology Hepatology and Nutrition (ESPGHAN)/North American Society for Pediatric Gastroenterology, Hepatology, and Nutrition (NASPGHAN) guidelines on childhood EGIDs have a number of statements related to steroid treatment, including 2 recommendations per expert opinion.[2] Oral systemic steroids should be "considered to induce remission in individual patients with non-EoE EGIDs and that their use should be undertaken after thorough discussion with the patient and parents about their benefits and risks" (strong strength of recommendation with 100% agreement); and topical steroids are conditionally recommended to be considered in "selected patients with non-EoE EGIDs" (weak strength of recommendation with 96% agreement).[2]

OTHER NON-BIOLOGIC TREATMENTS
Proton-Pump Inhibitors

The data on PPIs in non-EoE EGIDs are surprisingly limited. Lansoprazole improved mucosal eosinophilia in a toddler with eosinophilic gastroenteritis.[20] The mechanism of the effect of PPIs in EoE has been hypothesized to involve the blockade of inter-leukin (IL)-4 and IL-13 activity as well as acid suppression.[21] Unlike for EoE, there is a conspicuous dearth of data on the use of PPI and dosing of PPI in non-EoE EGIDs. Another confounder is that PPI therapy might be used due to the presence of mucosal erosions and ulcerations especially if noted in the upper gastrointestinal (GI) tract.

Mast-Cell Stabilizers

There have been sporadic case reports on the use of mast-cell stabilizers like sodium cromoglycate (cromolyn) and ketotifen in non-EoE EGIDs. Two adults, in a report from 1990, responded to cromolyn 300 mg 4 times daily after failing exclusion diets.[22] Addi-tional reports of adult patients with small intestine and/or colonic eosinophilic GI dis-ease report symptomatic improvement with cromolyn of 100 mg daily to 200 mg 4 times daily.[23,24] Ketotifen, which is both a mast-cell stabilizer and antihistamine, at doses 2to 4 mg/d induced symptomatic improvement within 1 to 4 months in 6 pa-tients with gastric, duodenal, and/or colonic EGID.[25] Four of these 6 patients under-went repeat endoscopy and all 4 patients had endoscopic and histologic remission.

Leukotriene Inhibitors

Leukotrienes are chemoattractants for eosinophils and there are case reports of mon-telukast used in cases of non-EoE EGIDs; in fact, esophageal leukotriene levels were elevated in a subset of patients with EoE and gastroduodenitis.[26] A teenager with eosinophilic infiltrations in the esophagus, stomach, ileum, and colon, who initially responded to prednisone 40 mg daily, was able to wean off prednisone after starting montelukast 10 mg daily and remained symptom-free at the 24-month follow-up.[27] A 27-year-old male with serosal eosinophilic duodenitis (EoD) was weaned off predni-sone within 4 weeks after starting montelukast 10 mg daily, and remained symptom-free at the 20-month follow-up.[28] A 13-year-old female with mucosal eosinophilia of her esophagus, stomach, and duodenum experienced symptom resolution with mon-telukast 10 mg daily after previously failing cromolyn, ranitidine, and hydroxyzine.[29] While these reports provide alternate non-corticosteroid options for some patients, the ESPGHAN/NASPGHAN guidelines found insufficient data to make recommenda-tions for or against the use of mast-cell stabilizers or leukotriene antagonists for non-EoE EGIDs.[2]

Other Therapies and Combination Therapy

Some case reports include immunosuppressants, such as azathioprine or 6-mercap-topurine, in steroid-dependent refractory non-EoE EGIDs as well as Th2 inhibitors (eg, suplatast tosilate).[30] Azathioprine induces apoptosis of T and B cells and the usual dose for patients with eosinophilic gastroenteritis is similar to that used in patients with inflammatory bowel diseases (2–2.5 mg/kg) and lower doses may not be effec-tive.[30] It should be noted that other patient series have not demonstrated significant beneficial use of immunomodulators in eosinophilic gastroenteritis, and more detailed studies are needed to evaluate any potential benefit.[2]

Apart from case reports, no studies have systematically investigated the role of combination therapy in non-EoE EGIDs.[2]

BIOLOGIC TREATMENTS

While a number of biologics could have a potential role in the non-EoE EGIDs,[31] only 2 have been tested in clinical trials to date, and other data are from case reports or series. Because of this, recent pediatric EGID guidelines had a 90% agreement with the statement that "there is insufficient data to make a recommendation for or against the use of biological drugs in treating childhood non-EoE EGIDs."[2] However, the field is rapidly evolving and biologics may become an important treatment modality for these diseases, particularly in order to spare systemic steroids.

Lirentelimab

Lirentelimab is an antibody against the sialic acid–binding immunoglobulin-like lectin 8 (Siglec-8) receptor which is largely localized to eosinophils and mast cells.[32] This medication depletes eosinophils through antibody-dependent cell-mediated cytotoxicity and apoptosis and inhibits mast cells, and thus has a strong rationale for use in EGIDs. In a phase 2 randomized, double-blind, placebo-controlled, clinical trial, 65 patients with EoG or EoD were randomized to receive either placebo or 2 doses of lirentelimab, which was given as 4 doses of a monthly intravenous infusion.[33] In the combined lirentelimab group, the primary endpoint was achieved as the mean GI eosinophil count decreased by 86% versus an increase of 9% in the placebo group ($P<.001$). In addition, a composite symptom score (accounting for 8 GI symptoms: abdominal pain, nausea, vomiting, early satiety, loss of appetite, abdominal cramping, bloating, diarrhea) decreased by 48% with active medication compared to a 22% decrease with placebo ($P = .004$). Based on these promising results, a phase 3 study was conducted (NCT04322604). While this has not been published, results were released.[34] Of 180 patients randomized, 85% treated with lirentelimab achieved histologic response, defined as ≤ 4 eosinophils per high-power field (eos/hpf) in the stomach or ≤ 15 eos/hpf in the duodenum, compared to just 5% in placebo ($P<.001$). However, the change in symptoms were similar between the active and placebo groups ($P = .343$). Because the study did not achieve both co-endpoints, lirentelimab is not currently being pursued for non-EoE EGIDs, and work remains ongoing to understand the discrepancy between the phase 2 and phase 3 results.

Benralizumab

Benralizumab is an antibody against the IL-5 receptor alpha. When this receptor is activated, eosinophils are depleted from the body though an antibody-dependent cell-mediated cytotoxicity mechanism. This medication is Food and Drug Administration (FDA) approved for the treatment of eosinophilic asthma and demonstrated proof of concept for treating pathologic GI tract eosinophilic infiltration in a clinical trial for hypereosinophilic syndrome.[35] In that study, Kuang and colleagues[36] studied a subset of 7 of the 20 patients treated who had GI tract involvement from the hypereosinophilic syndrome and showed that there was a marked reduction (to counts of zero eos/hpf) in multiple segments of the GI tract where eosinophilis were previously elevated. In additional analyses, however, they showed a heterogenous clinical response with some persistent symptoms and non-eosinophil–related epithelial changes.[36] Based on these proof-of-concept data, an investigator-initiated, phase 2, randomized, double-blind, placebo-controlled trial was conducted where 13 patients received monthly benralizumab for 12 weeks and 13 received placebo.[37] In the benralizumab arm, 77% of patients achieved the primary endpoint, defined as the proportion in histologic remission (>30 eos/hpf), compared to 8% in the placebo group ($P = .001$), and similar significant decreases compared to placebo were seen for the peak eosinophil counts

Table 1 Pharmacologic treatments for non–eosinophilic esophagitis eosinophilic gastrointestinal diseases	
Corticosteroids	• Systemic: prednisone • Topical: budesonide (various formulations targeted to the area of involvement)
Acid suppressors	• Proton-pump inhibitors • Histamine H-2 receptor antagonists
Mast-cell stabilizers	• Cromolyn • Ketotifen
Leukotriene inhibitors	• Montelukast
Other small-molecules	• 6-mercaptopurine • Azathioprine • Methotrexate
Biologic medications	• Lirentelimab (anti–Siglec 8) • Dupilumab (anti–IL-4RA) • Cendakimab (anti–IL-13) • Benralizumab (anti–IL-5RA) • Reslizumab (anti–IL-5) • Mepolizumab (anti–IL-5) • Vedolizumab (anti-integrin) • Omalizumab (anti-IgE)
Combination therapies	• Combination of above and/or diet
Emerging agents and potential targets	• Sphingosine-1-phosphate receptor modulators • Janus kinase inhibitors • Antibodies against other cytokines like IL-15 or alarmins like TSLP • Antibodies against KIT that deplete mast cells • Calcineurin inhibitors

Abbreviations: IgE, immunoglobulin E; IL, interleukin; IL-4RA, interleukin-4 receptor alpha; IL-5RA, interleukin-5 receptor alpha; Siglec-8, sialic acid–binding immunoglobulin-like lectin 8; TSLP, thymic stromal lymphopoietin.

and an EoG histology total score. However, there were no significant differences between the active and placebo groups for endoscopic severity (as measured by the EoG Endoscopic Reference Score[38]) and patient-reported outcomes (as measured by the Severity of Dyspepsia Assessment and the Patient-Reported Outcome Measurement Information System short-form questionnaire), although the study was not powered for these symptom outcomes. A phase 3 study of benralizumab for EoG was started (NCT5251909) but is no longer recruiting as per clinicaltrials.gov.

Dupilumab, Mepolizumab, Vedolizumab, and Cendakimab

Based on pathogenic parallels with EoE, as well as emerging mechanisms of disease in EoG and EoN, additional biologics are either under study or are being tested in non-EoE EGIDs.[31] Dupilumab, a monoclonal antibody against the IL-4 receptor alpha and the first FDA-approved medication for EoE,[39,40] has been reported in a few case series to be effective for EoG and/or EoN and might lead to some tolerance of causative foods in selected patients.[41–44] Though these data are limited, the strong proof of concept has led to an investigator-initiated phase 2, randomized, double-blind, placebo-controlled trial of dupilumab for EoG with or without EoD (NCT03678545), and a phase 3 study of dupilumab for a similar patient population has been announced (NCT05831176).

Mepolizumab is an antibody against soluble IL-5 and is approved for eosinophilic asthma, hypereosinophilic syndrome, and eosinophilic granulomatosis with polyangiitis. It has previously been tested in EoE with a good effect on histology response but without consistent symptom benefit.[45–48] Limited case report and anecdotal data suggest that it may have benefit for EoG and EoN,[49,50] but further study is required.

Vedolizumab, an antibody against the α7β4 integrin, prevents lymphocyte egress from the blood into the bowel and is approved for inflammatory bowel disease. It has not been studied in a clinical trial setting for EoE or non-EoE EGIDs, but there are case reports of some patients having clinical and histologic benefit with this medication.[51,52]

Cendakimab is an antibody against soluble IL-13 that has shown benefit in a phase 2 study of EoE[53] with a phase 3 study in EoE ongoing (NCT04753697). As it is an experimental agent, there are no case reports of its use in non-EoE EGIDs, but a clinical trial is ongoing in Japanese patients with EoG/EoN (NCT05214768).

SUMMARY AND FUTURE DIRECTIONS

The pharmacologic treatment of non-EoE EGIDs remains challenging because of a lack of approved treatments and a scarcity of clinical trial–level data. However, the field is evolving rapidly, based in part on lessons learned from EoE and in part on advances in the knowledge of pathogenic mechanisms of the disease (**Table 1**). If a patient opts for pharmacologic treatment, the approach should generally be individualized based on patient preference, shared decision-making, and also an understanding of the extent and severity of the underlying disease and comorbidities.[5] If the EGID is mild, then a PPI or a topical steroid targeted to the area(s) of involvement would make sense; erosions and ulcerations could also merit addition of treatment with a PPI. However, with more severe disease or complications (large ulceration, stenoses, anemia, ascites, malnutrition, and so forth), systemic steroids may be required, with plans to taper and transition to topical steroids or possibly an immunomodulator.[4] If there are overlapping comorbidities that merit treatment with an approved medication for that other condition, but that might also benefit the EGID (though off-label for this disease class), this strategy could be considered. Examples could include a patient with translocation-negative hypereosinophilic syndrome and with multiple organ systems involved (including the GI tract) being treated with mepolizumab, a patient with severe eosinophilic asthma and EoG/EoN being treated with benralizumab, or a patient with severe atopic dermatitis and EoG/EoN being treated with dupilumab. However, given there are no approved medications, it is also important to remember to offer these patients the option to be enrolled in a clinical trial. Patient recruitment is critical to ongoing efforts to develop new treatments.

To that end, there are a number of therapeutic targets in addition to the ones discussed earlier that could be investigated in the near future, some of which are already being assessed in EoE. These include sphingosine-1-phosphate receptor modulators, Janus kinase inhibitors, antibodies against other cytokines like IL-15 or alarmins like thymic stromal lymphopoietin, antibodies against KIT that deplete mast cells, calcineurin inhibitors, or agents that might help to induce immune tolerance. With this, an evolving understanding of treatment outcomes, clinical trial endpoints, and ongoing dialog with regulatory agencies are also critical to ultimately achieve drug approval in this field to benefit patients with non-EoE EGIDs.[54] With the rapidly increasing knowledge and treatment options, the future appears to be bright for the development of new, safe, and effective pharmacologic options for these patients with non-EoE EGIDs.

CLINICS CARE POINTS

- Clinical care of patients with non-EoE EGIDs should take the following into consideration:
  - Recent societal guidelines establish normal and abnormal mucosal eosinophil counts in various segments of the GI tract in pediatric patients[2]
  - Currently accepted treatments are primarily based on case reports and small-scale studies. Shared decision-making and individualization of care are of importance.
  - Treatment decisions should consider the segment and layer of GI tract involved and to be targeted, the severity of disease, and the age of the patient.
  - Disease extent may vary over time as may disease behavior.
- Oral corticosteroids may be considered to induce remission followed by dose reduction over a period of weeks.
- Topical corticosteroids such as budesonide may be swallowed as intact capsules with intent to treat inflammation of the distal small bowel or colon. Crushed enteric-coated granules of opened capsules may be swallowed to treat more proximal disease in the stomach, while opened capsule with the granules intact can target the duodenum and jejunum.
- Other reported pharmacologic treatments such as PPI, mast-cell stabilizers, leukotriene receptor antagonists, and immunomodulators have variable responses with limited published literature.
- While biologics are being actively studied in patients with non-EoE EGIDs, their off-label use might warrant consideration in some situations.
- Given the scarcity of rigorous treatment data for non-EoE EGIDs, providers should consider enrolling appropriate non-EoE EGID patients in clinical trials to help advance the field.

DISCLOSURE

E.S. Dellon: Research funding: Adare/Ellodi, Allakos, ARENA, United States/Pfizer, AstraZeneca, United Kingdom, Eupraxia, Canada, GSK, Meritage, Miraca, Nutricia, United States, Celgene, United States/Receptos/BMS, Regeneron, United States, Revolo, Shire/Takeda. Consultant: Abbott, Abbvie, Adare/Ellodi, Aimmune, Akesobio, Alfasigma, ALK, Allakos, Amgen, Aqilion, Arena/Pfizer, Aslan, AstraZeneca, Avir, Biorasi, Calypso, Celgene/Receptos/BMS, Celldex, Eli Lilly, EsoCap, Eupraxia, Ferring, GSK, Gossamer Bio, Holoclara, Invea, Knightpoint, Landos, LucidDx, Morphic, Nexstone Immunology/Uniquity, Nutricia, Parexel/Calyx, Phathom, Regeneron, Revolo, Robarts/Alimentiv, Salix, Sanofi, Shire/Takeda, Target RWE, Upstream Bio; Educational grant: Allakos, Aqilion, Holoclara, Invea.

S.K. Gupta: Research funding: Adare/Ellodi, Allakos, Regeneron, Shire/Takeda. Consultant: Adare/Ellodi, Allakos, Celgene/Receptos/BMS, PeerViewRegeneron, Shire/Takeda.

REFERENCES

1. Jensen ET, Martin CF, Kappelman MD, et al. Prevalence of Eosinophilic Gastritis, Gastroenteritis, and Colitis: Estimates From a National Administrative Database. J Pediatr Gastroenterol Nutr 2016;62:36–42.
2. Papadopoulou A, Amil-Dias J, Auth MK, et al. Joint ESPGHAN/NASPGHAN Guidelines on Childhood Eosinophilic Gastrointestinal Disorders beyond Eosinophilic Esophagitis. J Pediatr Gastroenterol Nutr 2023. https://doi.org/10.1097/MPG.0000000000003877.

3. Walker MM, Potter M, Talley NJ. Eosinophilic gastroenteritis and other eosinophilic gut diseases distal to the oesophagus. Lancet Gastroenterol Hepatol 2018;3(4):271–80.

4. Gonsalves N. Eosinophilic Gastrointestinal Disorders. Clin Rev Allergy Immunol 2019;57(2):272–85.

5. Dellon ES. Eosinophilic Gastrointestinal Diseases Beyond Eosinophilic Esophagitis. Am J Gastroenterol 2022;117(5):697–700.

6. Caldwell JM, Collins MH, Stucke EM, et al. Histologic eosinophilic gastritis is a systemic disorder associated with blood and extragastric eosinophilia, TH2 immunity, and a unique gastric transcriptome. J Allergy Clin Immunol 2014; 134(5):1114–24.

7. Shoda T, Wen T, Caldwell JM, et al. Molecular, endoscopic, histologic, and circulating biomarker-based diagnosis of eosinophilic gastritis: Multi-site study. J Allergy Clin Immunol 2020;145(1):255–69.

8. Shoda T, Hochman M, Collins MH, et al. Molecular Analysis of Duodenal Eosinophilia. J Allergy Clin Immunol 2023;151:1027–39.

9. Chang JY, Choung RS, Lee RM, et al. A shift in the clinical spectrum of eosinophilic gastroenteritis toward the mucosal disease type. Clin Gastroenterol Hepatol 2010;8(8):669–75 [quiz: e88].

10. Talley NJ, Shorter RG, Phillips SF, et al. Eosinophilic gastroenteritis: a clinicopathological study of patients with disease of the mucosa, muscle layer, and subserosal tissues. Gut 1990;31(1):54–8.

11. Reed C, Woosley JT, Dellon ES. Clinical characteristics, treatment outcomes, and resource utilization in children and adults with eosinophilic gastroenteritis. Dig Liver Dis 2015;47(3):197–201.

12. Alfadda AA, Storr MA, Shaffer EA. Eosinophilic colitis: epidemiology, clinical features, and current management. Therap Adv Gastroenterol 2011;4(5):301–9.

13. Pineton de Chambrun G, Gonzalez F, Canva JY, et al. Natural history of eosinophilic gastroenteritis. Clin Gastroenterol Hepatol 2011;9(11):950–956 e1.

14. Chen MJ, Chu CH, Lin SC, et al. Eosinophilic gastroenteritis: clinical experience with 15 patients. World J Gastroenterol 2003;9(12):2813–6.

15. Tan AC, Kruimel JW, Naber TH. Eosinophilic gastroenteritis treated with non-enteric-coated budesonide tablets. Eur J Gastroenterol Hepatol 2001;13(4):425–7.

16. Fang S, Song Y, Zhang S, et al. Retrospective study of budesonide in children with eosinophilic gastroenteritis. Pediatr Res 2019;86(4):505–9.

17. Kennedy K, Muir AB, Grossman A, et al. Modified oral enteric-coated budesonide regimens to treat pediatric eosinophilic gastroenteritis, a single center experience. J Allergy Clin Immunol Pract 2019;7(6):2059–61.

18. Ammoury RF, Rosenman MB, Roettcher D, et al. Incidental Gastric Eosinophils in Patients With Eosinophilic Esophagitis: Do They Matter? J Pediatr Gastroenterol Nutr 2010;51(6):723–6.

19. Pesek RD, Reed CC, Muir AB, et al. Increasing Rates of Diagnosis, Substantial Co-Occurrence, and Variable Treatment Patterns of Eosinophilic Gastritis, Gastroenteritis, and Colitis Based on 10-Year Data Across a Multicenter Consortium. Am J Gastroenterol 2019;114(6):984–94.

20. Yamada Y, Toki F, Yamamoto H, et al. Proton pump inhibitor treatment decreased duodenal and esophageal eosinophilia in a case of eosinophilic gastroenteritis. Allergol Int 2015;64(Suppl):S83–5.

21. Cheng E, Zhang X, Huo X, et al. Omeprazole blocks eotaxin-3 expression by oesophageal squamous cells from patients with eosinophilic oesophagitis and GORD. Gut 2013;62:824–32.

22. Di Gioacchino M, Pizzicannella G, Fini N, et al. Sodium cromoglycate in the treatment of eosinophilic gastroenteritis. Allergy 1990;45(3):161–6.

23. Moots RJ, Prouse P, Gumpel JM. Near fatal eosinophilic gastroenteritis responding to oral sodium chromoglycate. Gut 1988;29(9):1282–5.

24. Pérez-Millán A, Martín-Lorente JL, López-Morante A, et al. Subserosal eosinophilic gastroenteritis treated efficaciously with sodium cromoglycate. Dig Dis Sci 1997;42(2):342–4.

25. Melamed I, Feanny SJ, Sherman PM, et al. Benefit of ketotifen in patients with eosinophilic gastroenteritis. Am J Med 1991;90(3):310–4.

26. Gupta SK, Peters-Golden M, Fitzgerald JF, et al. Cysteinyl leukotriene levels in esophageal mucosal biopsies of children with eosinophilic inflammation: are they all the same? Am J Gastroenterol 2006;101(5):1125–8.

27. Quack I, Sellin L, Buchner NJ, et al. Eosinophilic gastroenteritis in a young girl–long term remission under Montelukast. BMC Gastroenterol 2005;5:24.

28. Schwartz DA, Pardi DS, Murray JA. Use of montelukast as steroid-sparing agent for recurrent eosinophilic gastroenteritis. Dig Dis Sci 2001;46(8):1787–90.

29. Neustrom MR, Friesen C. Treatment of eosinophilic gastroenteritis with montelukast. J Allergy Clin Immunol 1999;104(2 Pt 1):506.

30. Abou Rached A, El Hajj W. Eosinophilic gastroenteritis: Approach to diagnosis and management. World J Gastrointest Pharmacol Ther 2016;7(4):513–23.

31. Dellon ES, Spergel JM. Biologics in eosinophilic gastrointestinal diseases. Ann Allergy Asthma Immunol 2023;130(1):21–7.

32. Legrand F, Cao Y, Wechsler JB, et al. Sialic acid-binding immunoglobulin-like lectin (Siglec) 8 in patients with eosinophilic disorders: Receptor expression and targeting using chimeric antibodies. J Allergy Clin Immunol 2019;143(6):2227–37.e10.

33. Dellon ES, Peterson KA, Murray JA, et al. Anti-Siglec-8 Antibody for Eosinophilic Gastritis and Duodenitis. N Engl J Med 2020;383(17):1624–34.

34. Available at: https://investor.allakos.com/news-releases/news-release-details/allakos-announces-topline-phase-3-data-enigma-2-study-and-phase. Accessed September 2, 2023.

35. Kuang FL, Legrand F, Makiya M, et al. Benralizumab for PDGFRA-Negative Hypereosinophilic Syndrome. N Engl J Med 2019;380(14):1336–46.

36. Kuang FL, De Melo MS, Makiya M, et al. Benralizumab Completely Depletes Gastrointestinal Tissue Eosinophils and Improves Symptoms in Eosinophilic Gastrointestinal Disease. J Allergy Clin Immunol Pract 2022;10(6):1598–605.e2.

37. Kliewer KL, Murray-Petzold C, Collins MH, et al. Benralizumab for eosinophilic gastritis: a single-site, randomised, double-blind, placebo-controlled, phase 2 trial. Lancet Gastroenterol Hepatol 2023;8(9):803–15.

38. Hirano I, Collins MH, King E, et al. Prospective Endoscopic Activity Assessment for Eosinophilic Gastritis in a Multisite Cohort. Am J Gastroenterol 2022;117(3):413–23.

39. Dellon ES, Rothenberg ME, Collins MH, et al. Dupilumab in Adults and Adolescents with Eosinophilic Esophagitis. N Engl J Med 2022;387(25):2317–30.

40. Hirano I, Dellon ES, Hamilton JD, et al. Dupilumab Efficacy and Safety in Adult Patients With Active Eosinophilic Esophagitis: A Randomized Double-Blind Placebo-Controlled Phase 2 Trial. Am J Gastroenterol 2017;112(Suppl 1). AB 20 (ACG 2017).

41. Arakawa N, Yagi H, Shimizu M, et al. Dupilumab Leads to Clinical Improvements including the Acquisition of Tolerance to Causative Foods in Non-Eosinophilic Esophagitis Eosinophilic Gastrointestinal Disorders. Biomolecules 2023;13(1).

42. Mori F, Renzo S, Barni S, et al. Dupilumab treatment of eosinophilic gastrointestinal disease in an adolescent. Pediatr Allergy Immunol 2023;34(6):e13973.

43. Patel N, Goyal A, Thaker A, et al. A Case Series on the Use of Dupilumab for Treatment of Refractory Eosinophilic Gastrointestinal Disorders. J Pediatr Gastroenterol Nutr 2022;75(2):192–5.

44. Watanabe S, Uchida H, Fujii R, et al. The efficacy of dupilumab in induction and maintenance of remission in an adult patient with steroid-dependent eosinophilic enteritis (EoN). Clin J Gastroenterol 2023;16(4):527–31.

45. Stein ML, Collins MH, Villanueva JM, et al. Anti-IL-5 (mepolizumab) therapy for eosinophilic esophagitis. J Allergy Clin Immunol 2006;118(6):1312–9.

46. Straumann A, Conus S, Grzonka P, et al. Anti-interleukin-5 antibody treatment (mepolizumab) in active eosinophilic oesophagitis: a randomised, placebo-controlled, double-blind trial. Gut 2010;59(1):21–30.

47. Assa'ad AH, Gupta SK, Collins MH, et al. An antibody against IL-5 reduces numbers of esophageal intraepithelial eosinophils in children with eosinophilic esophagitis. Gastroenterology 2011;141(5):1593–604.

48. Dellon ES, Peterson KA, Mitlyng BL, et al. Mepolizumab for treatment of adolescents and adults with eosinophilic oesophagitis: a multicentre, randomised, double-blind, placebo-controlled clinical trial. Gut 2023;72:1828–37.

49. Han D, Lee JK. Severe asthma with eosinophilic gastroenteritis effectively managed by mepolizumab and omalizumab. Ann Allergy Asthma Immunol 2018; 121(6):742–3.

50. Caruso C, Colantuono S, Pugliese D, et al. Severe eosinophilic asthma and aspirin-exacerbated respiratory disease associated to eosinophilic gastroenteritis treated with mepolizumab: a case report. Allergy Asthma Clin Immunol 2020;16:27.

51. Kim HP, Reed CC, Herfarth HH, et al. Vedolizumab Treatment May Reduce Steroid Burden and Improve Histology in Patients With Eosinophilic Gastroenteritis. Clin Gastroenterol Hepatol 2018;16(12):1992–4.

52. Grandinetti T, Biedermann L, Bussmann C, et al. Eosinophilic Gastroenteritis: Clinical Manifestation, Natural Course, and Evaluation of Treatment with Corticosteroids and Vedolizumab. Dig Dis Sci 2019;64(8):2231–41.

53. Hirano I, Collins MH, Assouline-Dayan Y, et al. RPC4046, a Monoclonal Antibody Against IL13, Reduces Histologic and Endoscopic Activity in Patients With Eosinophilic Esophagitis. Gastroenterology 2019;156:592–603.e10.

54. Rothenberg ME, Hottinger SKB, Gonsalves N, et al. Impressions and aspirations from the FDA GREAT VI Workshop on Eosinophilic Gastrointestinal Disorders Beyond Eosinophilic Esophagitis and Perspectives for Progress in the Field. J Allergy Clin Immunol 2022;149:844–53.

Moving?

Make sure your subscription moves with you!

To notify us of your new address, find your **Clinics Account Number** (located on your mailing label above your name), and contact customer service at:

Email: **journalscustomerservice-usa@elsevier.com**

800-654-2452 (subscribers in the U.S. & Canada)
314-447-8871 (subscribers outside of the U.S. & Canada)

Fax number: 314-447-8029

Elsevier Health Sciences Division
Subscription Customer Service
3251 Riverport Lane
Maryland Heights, MO 63043

*To ensure uninterrupted delivery of your subscription, please notify us at least 4 weeks in advance of move.

Printed and bound by CPI Group (UK) Ltd, Croydon, CR0 4YY

03/10/2024

01040471-0009